Expert Consultations in Gynecological Cancers

BASIC AND CLINICAL ONCOLOGY

Editor

Bruce D. Cheson, M.D.

National Cancer Institute
National Institutes of Health
Bethesda, Maryland

ADDITIONAL VOLUMES IN PREPARATION

Expert
Consultations
in
Gynecological
Cancers

edited by

Maurie Markman
Cleveland Clinic Cancer Center and
Cleveland Clinic Foundation, Cleveland,
and The Ohio State University School of Medicine,
Columbus, Ohio

Jerome L. Belinson
Cleveland Clinic Foundation, Cleveland,
and The Ohio State University, Columbus, Ohio

Marcel Dekker, Inc.   New York•Basel•Hong Kong

ISBN: 0-8247-9768-X

The publisher offers discounts on this book when ordered in bulk quantities. For more information, write to Special Sales/Professional Marketing at the address below.

This book is printed on acid-free paper.

Marcel Dekker, Inc.
270 Madison Avenue, New York, New York 10016

Current printing (last digit):
10 9 8 7 6 5 4 3 2 1

Printed in the United States of America

Preface

This book was conceived from the numerous informal discussions we all have had after reviewing cases daily with our colleagues. At national meetings, when panels of experts are assembled, formally or informally, we've frequently been fascinated with the diversity of opinions that exist based on a known body of information applied to relatively straightforward cases. When the cases become more unusual, the variations increase and many surprising management schemes ensue. If the classic textbooks and medical literature are the suppliers of the raw materials, the consultants' interpretation of these resources and their experience create the final product that, with hope, will lead to the best results for our patients.

We have assembled a variety of cases for our consultants. These cases vary from routine events we all see in our practices to extremely rare occurrences possibly never encountered by the consultants. It turns out to be quite easy to write cases with no good answers and interesting to see how "experts" handle such cases. There were many times we could have supplied much more information. This likely would have resulted in greater similarity as well as less information in the consultation. However, it is important to recognize that while a lack of details allows more variability it also does not allow experts to get answers to questions they think are important. Case 13 is a good example of this, since the actual histological diagnosis was not supplied. Even when all key information is supplied it is evident there can be several acceptable, quite different approaches to a problem. The reader should appreciate that a formal medical consultation is a very complex event that is extremely difficult to duplicate in print. There is no way to account for the interactions between the doctor and the patient and the variations in our individual abilities in taking a history, reviewing x-rays and pathology, and doing a physical exam.

The authors were asked to provide a formal consultation as they would in the hospital chart. They received the cases (without the titles of the cases we have included for the reader), and it was recommended that the responses be under two pages in length. We asked the consultants to provide just a few references they believed to be the "best" references on the topic of the case. As a result, we believe the reader is presented with, collectively, a great set of references and, by consensus, within each case the "best of the best."

However, the reader should recognize the inevitable delay between writing the consultations and their publication. For example, BRCA1 and BRCA 2 have been identified and sequenced since the submission of Cases 1 through 4. Now genetic testing, with all its complexities, is a reality. Therefore, the discussions of Cases 1 through 4 would likely include dialogue on whom to test, informed consent, and pre- and post-test counseling, as well as the risks and benefits of testing.

There is one overriding theme that needs special emphasis: Over the years, as clever as we might have been as diagnosticians or surgeons, it is frequently our access to good pathology that has allowed us as consultants to make a major contribution to the evaluation and management of our patients. The importance of pathology review, along with all prior records and radiographic examinations, cannot be overemphasized. We are indebted to our many expert consultants who were willing to publish examples of how they think, not just how they report the literature.

We dedicate this book to our wives, Tomes and Maureen, and our children, Meg, Jon, Tim, Betsey, Suzanne, Raman, Tyler and Patrick.

Maurie Markman
Jerome L. Belinson

Contents

Contents

Contributors

Mark David Adelson, M.D. Comprehensive Gynecology, P.C., Crouse Business Center, Syracuse, New York

David S. Alberts, M.D. Professor of Medicine and Pharmacology, and Deputy Director, University of Arizona Cancer Center, Tucson, Arizona

Ronald D. Alvarez, M.D. Department of Obstetrics and Gynecology, Division of Gynecologic Oncology, University of Alabama, Birmingham, Alabama

Ann Anderson, M.D. Assistant Professor of Pathology, Albert Einstein College of Medicine, Long Island Jewish Medical Center, New Hyde Park, New York

Barrie Anderson, M.D. Professor, Division of Gynecologic Oncology, University of Iowa Hospital and Clinics, John and Mary Pappajohn Clinic Cancer Center, Iowa City, Iowa

Patrick S. Anderson, M.D. Assistant Professor, Department of Obstetrics and Gynecology, Division of Gynecologic Oncology, Albert Einstein College of Medicine of Yeshiva University, Montefiore Medical Center, Bronx, New York

Harrison George Ball, III, M.D. Associate Professor and Director, Division of Gynecologic Oncology, Department of Obstetrics and Gynecology, Tufts University School of Medicine, New England Medical Center, Boston, Massachusetts

Richard R. Barakat, M.D. Clinical Assistant Surgeon, Gynecology Service,

Department of Surgery, Memorial Sloan-Kettering Cancer Center, New York, New York

Hugh R. K. Barber, M.D.   Director, Department of Obstetrics and Gynecology, Lenox Hill Hospital, New York, New York

Scott I. Bearman, M.D.   Bone Marrow Transplant Program, University of Colorado Health Sciences Center, Denver, Colorado

Jonathan S. Berek, M.D.   Director, Gynecologic Oncology Service, Department of Obstetrics and Gynecology, UCLA School of Medicine and Jonsson Comprehensive Cancer Center, UCLA Medical Center, Los Angeles, California

Ross Stuart Berkowitz, M.D.   Director of Gynecology and Gynecologic Oncology, Brigham and Women's Hospital and Dana-Farber Cancer Institute, Boston, Massachusetts

Michael L. Berman, M.D.   Professor, Division of Gynecologic Oncology, University of California, Irvine, Irvine Medical Center, Department of Obstetrics and Gynecology, Orange, California

Luca Bocciolone, M.D.   European Institute of Oncology, Division of Gynecology, Milan, Italy

Robert A. Burger, M.D.   Clinical Instructor, Division of Gynecologic Oncology, Department of Obstetrics and Gynecology, University of California, Irvine, Orange, California

Pablo J. Cagnoni, M.D.   Bone Marrow Transplant Program, University of Colorado Health Sciences Center, Denver, Colorado

Joanna M. Cain, M.D.   Associate Professor, Division of Gynecologic Oncology, Department of Obstetrics and Gynecology, University of Washington Medical Center, Seattle, Washington

Stephen A. Cannistra, M.D.   Dana-Farber Cancer Institute, Boston, Massachusetts

John A. Carlson, Jr., M.D.   Associate Professor, Director, Division of Gynecologic Oncology, Department of Obstetrics and Gynecology, Thomas Jefferson University, Philadelphia, Pennsylvania

Pamela J. Carney, M.D. Medical Fellow Specialist and Instructor, University of Minnesota, Minneapolis, Minnesota

Linda F. Carson, M.D. Director, Gynecology/Oncology, Department of Obstetrics and Gynecology, University of Minnesota, Minneapolis, Minnesota

Murray Joseph Casey, M.D. Professor and Chairman, Department of Obstetrics and Gynecology, Creighton University School of Medicine, Omaha, Nebraska

Weldon E. Chafe, M.D. Associate Professor and Co-Director, Division of Gynecologic Oncology, Department of Obstetrics and Gynecology, Eastern Virginia Medical School, Norfolk, Virginia

Joseph T. Chambers, Ph.D., M.D. Associate Professor, Department of Obstetrics and Gynecology, Yale University School of Medicine, New Haven, Connecticut

Setsuko K. Chambers, M.D. Associate Professor, Gynecologic Oncology, Department of Obstetrics and Gynecology, Yale University School of Medicine, New Haven, Connecticut

M. Dwight Chen, M.D. Fellow, Department of Obstetrics and Gynecology, Medical School, University of Minnesota, Minneapolis, Minnesota

Judy Cheng, M.D. Gynecologic Oncology, Department of Obstetrics and Gynecology, Riverside Regional Medical Center, Newport News, Virginia

Max A. Clark, D.O. Assistant Professor, Division of Gynecology, Department of Obstetrics and Gynecology, Wright State University, Dayton, Ohio

William A. Cliby, M.D. Assistant Professor of Obstetrics and Gynecology, Department of Obstetrics and Gynecology, Mayo Clinic, Rochester, Minnesota

Nicoletta Colombo, M.D. European Institute of Oncology, Division of Gynecology, Milan, Italy

John T. Comerci, M.D. Fellow, Department of Obstetrics and Gynecology, Division of Gynecologic Oncology, Albert Einstein College of Medicine of Yeshiva University, Montefiore Medical Center, Bronx, New York

Larry J. Copeland, M.D. Director, Gynecologic Oncology, Division of Gynecologic Oncology, Ohio State University College of Medicine, Columbus, Ohio

William T. Creasman, M.D. Sims Hester Professor and Chairman, Department of Obstetrics and Gynecology, Medical University of South Carolina, Charleston, South Carolina

John L. Currie, M.D. Professor and Chairman, Department of Obstetrics and Gynecology, Dartmouth–Hitchcock Medical Center, Lebanon, New Hampshire

John P. Curtin, M.D. Gynecology Service, Department of Surgery, Memorial Sloan-Kettering Cancer Center, New York, New York

Gunter Deppe, M.D. Professor of Medicine, Division of Gynecologic Oncology, Department of Obstetrics and Gynecology, Wayne State University, Hutzel Hospital, Detroit, Michigan

Charles J. Dunton, M.D. Associate Professor, Division of Gynecologic Oncology, Department of Obstetrics and Gynecology, Thomas Jefferson University, Philadelphia, Pennsylvania

John H. Edmonson, M.D. Consultant in Medical Oncology, Professor of Oncology, Mayo Clinic, Rochester, Minnesota

Babak Edraki, M.D. Instructor, Gynecologic Oncology, Department of Obstetrics and Gynecology, Yale University School of Medicine, New Haven, Connecticut

Stephen S. Falkenberry, M.D. Department of Obstetrics and Gynecology, Women and Infants Hospital and Brown University, Providence, Rhode Island

Gini F. Fleming, M.D. Assistant Professor of Medicine, Section of Hematology/Oncology, University of Chicago Medical Center, Chicago, Illinois

Peter Fleming, M.D. Department of Radiation Oncology, Cleveland Clinic Foundation, Cleveland, Ohio

Ernest W. Franklin, III, M.D. Clinical Professor of Gynecology, Mercer University School of Medicine, Atlanta, Georgia

Michael L. Friedlander, M.D. Department of Clinical Oncology, Prince of Wales Hospital, Randwick, New South Wales, Australia

Walter H. Gajewski, M.D. Gynecologic Oncologist, Department of Obstetrics and Gynecology, Women and Infants Hospital and Brown University, Providence, Rhode Island

David Gal, M.D. Professor of Clinical Obstetrics and Gynecology, New York University School of Medicine, and Associate Director, Gynecologic Oncology, North Shore University Hospital, Manhasset, New York

Holly H. Gallion, M.D. Associate Professor, Department of Obstetrics and Gynecology, University of Kentucky Medical Center, Lexington, Kentucky

Mary M. Gallenberg, M.D. Assistant Professor of Obstetrics and Gynecology, Mayo Clinic, Rochester, Minnesota

David M. Gershenson, M.D. Professor and Deputy Chairman, Department of Gynecology, University of Texas M.D. Anderson Cancer Center, Houston, Texas

Susan K. Gibbons, M.D. Regional Radiation Oncology Program, Albany Medical Center, Albany, New York

Robert E. Girtanner, Jr., M.D. Associate Professor of Gynecology, Division of Gynecologic Oncology, Department of Obstetrics and Gynecology, Baylor College of Medicine, Houston, Texas

Jeffrey M. Goldberg, M.D. Senior Fellow, Department of Gynecologic Oncology, Roswell Park Cancer Institute, Buffalo, New York

Michael I. Goldberg, M.D. Clinical Professor and Chief, Division of Gynecologic Oncology, UMD-Robert Wood Johnson Medical School, New Brunswick, New Jersey

Donald P. Goldstein, M.D. Assistant Clinical Professor of Obstetrics and Gynecology and Reproductive Biology, Division of Gynecologic Oncology, Brigham and Women's Hospital, Boston, Massachusetts

Cornelius O. Granai, M.D. Division Director, Department of Obstetrics and Gynecology, Women and Infants Hospital and Brown University, Providence, Rhode Island

Jianan Graybill, M.D. Radiation Oncologist, Department of Radiation Oncology, St. John's Health System, Anderson, Indiana

Neville F. Hacker, M.D. Associate Professor of Obstetrics and Gynecology, University of New South Wales, and Director of Gynecologic Oncology, Royal Hospital for Women, Paddington, Australia

Charles R. Harrison, M.D. Director, Gynecologic Oncology, National Naval Medical Center, Uniformed Services University of the Health Sciences, Gynecologic Oncology, Department of Obstetrics and Gynecology, National Naval Medical Center, Bethesda, Maryland

Ellen M. Hartenbach, M.D. Assistant Professor, University of Wisconsin, Madison, Madison, Wisconsin

Philip C. Hoffman, M.D. University of Chicago Medical Center, Chicago, Illinois

Howard D. Homesley, M.D. Professor and Head, Section of Gynecologic Oncology, Comprehensive Cancer Center of the Bowman Gray School of Medicine, Wake Forest University, Winston-Salem, North Carolina

Michael P. Hopkins, M.D. Chairman and Professor, Department of Obstetrics and Gynecology, Northeastern Ohio University College of Medicine, Akron General Medical Center, Akron, Ohio

William J. Hoskins, M.D. Attending Surgeon and Chief, Gynecology Service, Department of Surgery, Memorial Sloan-Kettering Cancer Center, New York, New York

Malcolm G. Idelson, M.D. Gynecologic Oncologist, Vassar Brothers Hospital and St. Francis Hospital, Poughkeepsie, New York

Mike F. Janicek, M.D. Clinical Assistant Professor, Division of Gynecologic Oncology, Sylvester Comprehensive Cancer Center, University of Miami Hospital and Clinics, Miami, Florida

Maureen A. Jarrell, M.D. Gynecologic Oncologist, Greensboro, North Carolina

Scott Jennings, M.D. Assistant Professor and Director, Division of Gynecologic Oncology, Department of Obstetrics and Gynecology, Medical University of South Carolina, Charleston, South Carolina

Roy B. Jones, Ph.D., M.D. Bone Marrow Transplant Program, University of Colorado Health Sciences Center, Denver, Colorado

Howard W. Jones, III, M.D. Professor of Obstetrics and Gynecology, and Director of Gynecologic Oncology, Vanderbilt University, Nashville, Tennessee

A. Robert Kagan, M.D., F.A.C.R. Chief, Department of Radiation Oncology, Kaiser Permanente Medical Center, Los Angeles, California

Alan L. Kaplan, M.D. Professor and Chief, Division of Gynecologic Oncology, Baylor College of Medicine, Houston, Texas

Edward J. Kaplan, M.D. Assistant Professor, Department of Radiation Oncology, New York Hospital–Cornell Medical Center, New York, New York

John J. Kavanagh, M.D. Chief, Section of Gynecologic Medical Oncology, University of Texas, M.D. Anderson Cancer Center, Houston, Texas

Alexander W. Kennedy, M.D. Head, Gynecologic Oncology, Cleveland Clinic Foundation, Cleveland, Ohio

Henry M. Keys, M.D. Professor and Chairman, Radiation Oncology, Albany Medical College, Albany, New York

Maureen A. Killackey, M.D. Director, Gynecologic Oncology, St. Luke's–Roosevelt Hospital Center, New York, New York

Ernest I. Kohorn, M.D. Professor of Gynecology, Department of Obstetrics and Gynecology, Yale University School of Medicine, New Haven, Connecticut

Hans-B. Krebs, M.D. Clinical Associate Professor, Fairfax Hospital, Annandale, Virginia

Gunnar B. Kristensen, M.D. Assistant Chairman, Gynecologic Oncology, Norwegian Radium Hospital, Montebello, Oslo, Norway

Leo D. Lagasse, M.D. Professor, Obstetrics and Gynecology, UCLA, and Director, Gynecologic Oncology, Department of Obstetrics and Gynecology, Cedars Sinai Medical Center, Los Angeles, California

Tally Levy, M.D. Fellow, Department of Gynecologic Oncology, Baylor College of Medicine, Houston, Texas

Lois Loescher, R.N., M.S. Arizona Cancer Center, Tucson, Arizona

Harry J. Long, M.D. Consultant in Medical Oncology, Mayo Clinic, Rochester, Minnesota

John L. Lovecchio, M.D. Professor of Clinical Obstetrics and Gynecology, Cornell University Medical College, and Director, Gynecologic Oncology, Northshore University Hospital, Manhasset, New York

Henry T. Lynch, M.D. Creighton University School of Medicine, Omaha, Nebraska

Cynthia T. Macri, M.C., F.A.C.O.G., F.A.C.S. Assistant Head, Gynecologic Oncology, Department of Obstetrics and Gynecology, National Naval Medical Center, Bethesda, Maryland

Angelo Maggioni, M.D. European Institute of Oncology, Division of Gynecology, Milan, Italy

Javier F. Magrina, M.D. Associate Professor, Mayo Graduate School of Medicine, and Chair, Gynecologic Surgery and Oncology, Scottsdale, Arizona

Francis J. Major, M.D. Director, Gynecologic Oncology, Presbyterian/St. Lukes Hospital, Denver, Colorado

John H. Malfetano, M.D. Director, Gynecologic Oncology, Albany Medical College, Albany, New York

Vinay K. Malviya, M.D. Associate Professor, Division of Gynecologic Oncology, Wayne State University School of Medicine, Detroit, Michigan

Alberto Manetta, M.D. Associate Professor, Department of Obstetrics and Gynecology, Division of Gynecologic Oncology, University of California Irvine Medical Center, Orange, California

William J. Mann, M.D. Gynecologic Oncologist, Obstetrics and Gynecology Residency Program Director, Riverside Regional Medical Center, Newport News, Virginia

William P. McGuire, III, M.D. Emory Clinic, Department of Medical Oncology, Atlanta, Georgia

Andrew W. Menzin, M.D. Fellow, Division of Gynecologic Oncology, Department of Obstetrics and Gynecology, Hospital of the University of Pennsylvania, University of Pennsylvania Medical Center, Philadelphia, Pennsylvania

Michael Method, M.D., M.P.H. Assistant Clinical Professor, Division of Gynecologic Oncology, Department of Obstetrics and Gynecology, Sylvester Comprehensive Cancer Center, University of Miami School of Medicine, Miami, Florida

John J. Mikuta, M.D. Franklin Payne Professor, Division of Gynecologic Oncology, Department of Obstetrics and Gynecology, University of Pennsylvania Medical Center, Philadelphia, Pennsylvania

Bradley J. Monk, M.D. Assistant Professor and Director of Gynecologic Oncology, Department of Obstetrics and Gynecology, Texas Tech University Health Sciences Center, Lubbock, Texas

Thomas W. Montag, M.D. HOPE—A Women's Cancer Center, Asheville, North Carolina

Fredrick J. Montz, M.D. Associate Professor, Gynecologic Oncology Service, Center for Health Sciences, Department of Obstetrics and Gynecology, UCLA School of Medicine, Los Angeles, California

David H. Moore, M.D. Associate Professor, Gynecologic Oncology, Department of Obstetrics and Gynecology, Indiana University Medical Center, University Hospital, Indianapolis, Indiana

George W. Morley, M.D. Associate Chair, Department of Obstetrics and Gynecology, University of Michigan Medical Center, Ann Arbor, Michigan

Rodrigue Mortel, M.D. Professor and Chairman, Department of Obstetrics and Gynecology, The Milton S. Hershey Medical Center, Pennsylvania State University, Hershey, Pennsylvania

Franco Muggia, M.D. Kenneth Norris Jr. (USC) Cancer Center, Los Angeles, California

James H. Nelson, Jr., M.D. Obstetrician and Gynecologist-In-Chief, Stamford Hospital, Stamford, Connecticut

James L. Nicklin, M.D. Wesley Medical Center, Auchenflower, Australia

Najmosama Nikrui, M.D. Assistant Professor, Department of Obstetrics and Gynecology, Harvard Medical School, and Assistant Gynecologist, Department of Gynecology, Ambulatory Care Center, Massachusetts General Hospital, Boston, Massachusetts

Jonathan M. Niloff, M.D. Director, Division of Gynecologic Oncology, Beth Israel Hospital, Boston, Massachusetts

Datta Nori, M.D. Director of Oncology, and Professor and Chairman, Department of Radiation Oncology, The New York Hospital-Cornell Medical Center, New York, New York

Franco Odicino, M.D. Universitá di Brescia, European Institute of Oncology, Milan, Italy

Olufunmilayo I. Olopade, M.D. Assistant Professor, Department of Medicine, Section of Hematology/Oncology, University of Chicago Medical Center, Chicago, Illinois

George A. Omura, M.D. University of Alabama at Birmingham, Birmingham, Alabama

Robert F. Ozols, M.D. Senior Vice President, Medical Science, Fox Chase Cancer Center, Philadelphia, Pennsylvania

Robert C. Park, M.D. Distinguished Professor, Uniformed Services University of the Health Sciences, Walter Reed Army Medical Center, Department of Obstetrics and Gynecology, Washington, D. C.

Edward E. Partridge, M.D. Associate Professor and Division Director, Department of Obstetrics and Gynecology, Division of Gynecologic Oncology, University of Alabama at Birmingham, Birmingham, Alabama

Sergio Pecorelli, M.D. Professor and Chairman, Gynecologic Oncology, Universitá de Brescia, European Institute of Oncology, Milan, Italy

Manuel A. Penalver, M.D. Professor of Obstetrics and Gynecology, Department of Obstetrics/Gynecology, Division of Gynecology, University of Miami School of Medicine, Sylvester Comprehensive Cancer Center, Miami, Florida

Ivy A. Petersen, M.D. Department of Radiation Oncology, Mayo Clinic, Rochester, Minnesota

Garth D. Phibbs, M.D. Clinical Associate Professor of Obstetrics and Gynecology, Medical College of Ohio, Toledo, Ohio

M. Steven Piver, M.D. Chief, Department of Gynecologic Oncology, and Clinical Professor of Gynecology, Roswell Park Memorial Institute, Buffalo, New York

Edward S. Podczaski, M.D. Associate Professor, Department of Obstetrics and Gynecology, Division of Gynecologic Oncology, Pennsylvania State University, Hershey, Pennsylvania

Karl C. Podratz, M.D., Ph.D. Professor and Chairman, Department of Obstetrics and Gynecology, Mayo Clinic, Rochester, Minnesota

R. Gerald Pretorius, M.D. Director, Gynecology, Robert C. Byrd Health Sciences Center of West Virginia University, Morgantown, West Virginia

Marcus E. Randall, M.D. Professor and Chairman, Department of Radiation Oncology, Indiana University School of Medicine, Indianapolis, Indiana

Eddie Reed, M.D. Chief, Clinical Pharmacology Branch, National Cancer Institute, Bethesda, Maryland

Bonnie S. Reichman, M.D. Director of Medical Oncology, Strang–Cornell Breast Cancer Center, New York, New York

Richard Reid, M.D. Assistant Professor, Obstretics and Gynecology, Wayne State University School of Medicine, and Director, Gynecologic Laser Service, Sinai Hospital of Detroit, The Carson Centre, Southfield, Michigan

James A. Roberts, M.D., M.S. Director, Division of Gynecologic Oncology, University of Michigan Hospital, Ann Arbor, Michigan

Thomas F. Rocereto, M.D. Professor of Clinical Obstetrics and Gynecology, Division of Gynecologic Oncology, Cancer Center of Southern New Jersey, University Medical Center/Cooper Hospital, Camden, New Jersey

Michael Rodriguez, M.D. Assistant Professor, Division of Gynecologic Oncology, University Hospitals, Cleveland, Ohio

Lynda D. Roman, M.D. Assistant Professor of Obstetrics and Gynecology,

Division of Gynecologic Oncology, Women's and Children's Hospital, Los Angeles, California

Peter G. Rose, M.D. Associate Professor, Department of Obstetrics and Gynecology, University MacDonald Women's Hospital, and University Ireland Cancer Center, Cleveland, Ohio

Stephen C. Rubin, M.D. Professor and Director, University of Pennsylvania Medical Center, Division of Gynecologic Oncology, Department of Obstetrics and Gynecology, Philadelphia, Pennsylvania

Carolyn D. Runowicz, M.D. Director, Department of Obstetrics and Gynecology, Division of Gynecologic Oncology, Albert Einstein College of Medicine of Yeshiva University, Montefiore Medical Center, Bronx, New York

Thomas J. Rutherford, M.D. Assistant Professor, Gynecologic Oncology, Department of Obstetrics and Gynecology, Yale University School of Medicine, New Haven, Connecticut

Richardo Sainz de la Cuesta, M.D. Fellow, Department of Gynecology, Massachusetts General Hospital, Boston, Massachusetts

Andrew K. Saltzman, M.D. Division of Gynecologic Oncology, Naval Medical Center, San Diego, San Diego, California

Duncan Savage, M.D. Regional Radiation Oncology Program, Albany Medical Center, Albany, New York

Jerrold P. Saxton, M.D. Department of Radiation Oncology, Cleveland Clinic Foundation, Cleveland, Ohio

Mary Jo Schmitz, M.D., Capt., M.C., U.S.A.F. Fellow, Gynecologic Oncology, Department of Obstetrics and Gynecology, National Naval Medical Center, Bethesda, Maryland

Peter E. Schwartz, M.D. Professor, Department of Obstetrics and Gynecology, Yale University School of Medicine, New Haven, Connecticut

Thomas V. Sedlacek, M.D. Chairman, Department of Gynecology, The Graduate Hospital, Philadelphia, Pennsylvania

Vicki L. Seltzer, M.D. Chairman, Obstetrics and Gynecology, Long Island

Jewish Medical Center, and Professor, Gynecology and Obstetrics, Albert Einstein College of Medicine, New Hyde Park, New York

Neal Semrad, M.D. Assistant Regional Director Gynecologic Oncology, Kaiser Permanente, Southern California Permanente Medical Group, Los Angeles, California

Bernd-Uwe Sevin, M.D., Ph.D. Professor, Division of Gynecologic Oncology, University of Miami Medical School, Sylvester Comprehensive Cancer Center, Miami, Florida

Sharon Sheffield, M.D. Jones Institute of Reproductive Medicine, Norfolk, Virginia

Hugh M. Shingleton, M.D. J. Marion Sims Professor and Chairman, Department of Obstetrics and Gynecology, University of Alabama at Birmingham, Birmingham, Alabama

Elizabeth J. Shpall, M.D. University of Colorado Health Sciences Center, Denver, Colorado

Mario Sideri, M.D. Universitá di Brescia, European Institute of Oncology, Milan, Italy

Loren Simovitch, M.D. University of Miami School of Medicine, Sylvester Comprehensive Cancer Center, Miami, Florida

Daniel H. Smith, M.D. Director, Gynecologic Oncology, Columbia-Presbyterian Medical Center, New York, New York

James L. Speyer, M.D. Professor of Clinical Medicine, Division of Medical Oncology, New York University Medical Center, New York, New York

Darcy V. Spicer, M.D. Kenneth Norris Jr. (USC) Cancer Center, Los Angeles, California

Adriana Suarez, M.D. University of Miami School of Medicine, Sylvester Comprehensive Cancer Center, Miami, Florida

Gregory P. Sutton, M.D. Mary Fendrich Hulman Professor and Chief, Section of Gynecologic Oncology, Division of Gynecologic Oncology, Department of

Obstetrics and Gynecology, Indiana University School of Medicine, and University Hospital, Indianapolis, Indiana

Robert F. Taylor, M.D.   Milwaukee, Wisconsin

Peyton T. Taylor, Jr., M.D.   Richard N. and Louise R. Crockett Professor, and Director, Division of Gynecologic Oncology, University of Virginia Health Sciences Center, Charlottesville, Virginia

Wim Ten Bokkel Huinink, M.D.   Medical Oncologist, The Netherlands Cancer Institute, Amsterdam, The Netherlands

Antonella Tessadelli, M.D.   Universitá di Brescia, European Institute of Oncology, Milan, Italy

James T. Thigpen, M.D.   Professor of Medicine and Director, Division of Oncology, Department of Medicine, University of Mississippi Medical Center, Jackson, Mississippi

Gillian M. Thomas, BSc., M.D., F.R.C.P.   Associate Professor, Department of Obstetrics and Gynecology, University of Toronto, Toronto-Bayview Regional Cancer Centre, North York, Ontario, Canada

Daniel H. Tobias, M.D.   Department of Obstetrics and Gynecology, Division of Gynecologic Oncology, Albert Einstein College of Medicine of Yeshiva University, Montefiore Medical Center, Bronx, New York

Edward L. Trimble, M.D.   National Cancer Institute, Bethesda, Maryland

Claus Tropé, M.D.   Chairman, Department of Gynecologic Oncology, Gynecologic Section, Norwegian Radium Hospital, Oslo, Norway

Leo B. Twiggs, M.D.   Professor and Head, Department of Obstetrics and Gynecology, and Director, Woman's Cancer Center, University of Minnesota, Minneapolis, Minnesota

Lucien Vanuystel, M.D.   Universitá di Brescia, European Institute of Oncology, Milan, Italy

Polly Vaughan, M.D.   Jones Institute of Reproductive Medicine, Norfolk, Virginia

Steven E. Waggoner, M.D. Section of Gynecologic Oncology, University of Chicago Medical Center, Chicago, Illinois

Robert C. Wallach, M.D. Professor, Clinical Obstetrics and Gynecology, Beth Israel Medical Center, New York, New York

Watson G. Watring, M.D. Regional Director, Gynecologic Oncology and Pelvic Surgery, Kaiser Permanente, Southern California Permanente Medical Group, Los Angeles, California

Maurice J. Webb, M.D. Professor in Obstetrics and Gynecology, Mayo Clinic, Rochester, Minnesota

Kenneth D. Webster, M.D. Department of Gynecology, Cleveland Clinic Foundation, Cleveland, Ohio

John C. Weed, Jr., M.D. Professor and Director, Division of Gynecologic Oncology, University of Kansas School of Medicine, Kansas University Hospital, Kansas City, Kansas

Stephen D. Williams, M.D. Director, Indiana University Cancer Center, Indianapolis, Indiana

Timothy O. Wilson, M.D. Division of Gynecologic Surgery, Mayo Clinic, Rochester, Minnesota

Joseph L. Yon, M.D. Head, Section of Gynecologic Oncology, Virginia Mason Clinic, Seattle, Washington

Expert
Consultations
in
Gynecological
Cancers

1

Prevention of Ovarian Cancer in Young Women with a Strong Family History of Ovarian Cancer

CASE

Your patient, a 37-year-old woman, is found to have developed stage III ovarian cancer. She asks your advice on how to reduce the risk of ovarian cancer in her 14- and 12-year-old daughters. Your patient has one sister who developed ovarian cancer at age 48 and her mother died of breast cancer at age 62.

PHYSICIAN'S RESPONSE

JAMES SPEYER

The advice to the patient must be expressed in terms of what we think the risk of her daughters developing ovarian cancer is, what (if anything) we might do about it, and how they can be followed over time. As her daughters are young, we are likely to learn more about this before they are at full risk for developing a cancer. In addition, we need to balance our concerns and interest in surveillance with a concern that we not make these young women cancer-phobic out of proportion to their risk of developing a cancer.

The patient has one first-degree relative with ovarian cancer, her sister. The typical high-risk kindreds have been defined as having two first-degree relatives. The daughters therefore have significantly increased risk (possibly as high as 40%) of developing an ovarian cancer in their lifetimes. Ovarian cancers can

1

occur at earlier ages in these families. The lifetime risk of a patient with one first-degree relative is less (approximately 2.5%).

There is no history of colon cancer or endometrial cancer. It is unlikely, then, that the patient is part of a Lynch type II kindred, a more common kind of ovarian cancer family. This syndrome appears to be associated with a defect in DNA repair enzymes on chromosome 2 and 3.

Finally, the patient does have a mother with breast cancer. Families with linked ovarian and breast cancer are described. It must be emphasized that these represent only a small percent of all patients with these cancers. Most families with hereditary breast and ovarian cancer have linkage to the recently described BRCA1 gene on chromosome 17q. Testing for the presence of this gene may be available in the near future. This would permit more accurate assessment as to whether the daughters carry this increased risk.

Assuming the daughters either carry the BRCA1 gene or that they may be part of an increased-risk ovarian kindred, the options for remedy are limited. Prophylactic oophorectomy has been advocated by some for many years, particularly after such patients pass their reproductive phase. This is not a guaranteed solution, though. In one series of patients at high risk for developing ovarian cancer who were treated with prophylactic oophorectomy, 3 of 28 women developed a disseminated carcinoma histopathologically similar to ovarian cancer, suggesting that this disease can also arise from the peritoneal lining. The recommendation of the National Institutes of Health (NIH) consensus panel for patients at high risk is to have prophylactic oophorectomy after childbearing or by age 35.

There are also provocative new data from Hartge et al. suggesting that the risk of developing ovarian cancer is related to the total number of ovulations that a woman has had. Ovarian cancer risk declines with the number of pregnancies, extended use of oral contraceptives, and increased duration of breast feeding. These observations need to be confirmed and the relative health risks of multiple pregnancies, oral contraceptive use, or early induced menopause need to be considered. Prospective clinical trials to confirm these observations should certainly be considered. Patients at increased risk will also be candidates for chemoprevention strategies as they become available.

Finally, because of increased risk in the patient's daughters, they are candidates for careful screening. Starting at age 20, they should have annual bimanual examinations, CA-125 (tumor marker) determinations, and transvaginal ultrasound. They will certainly be candidates for better screening tests as they become available.

One might argue that the daughters should get pregnant early and often (this would also reduce the risk of breast cancer), followed by oral contraceptives and or oophorectomy. These are pretty strong remedies when we are not completely certain of our data or these patients' actual risk. We place a heavy burden on patients with this kind of information. Continued studies of family pedigrees and search for biomolecular markers are mandatory.

References

Jacobs N. Genetic, biochemical, and multimodal approaches to screening for ovarian cancer. Gynecol. Oncol. 1994; 55:S22–S27.

Hartge P, Whittemore AS, Itnyre J, et al. Rates and risks of ovarian cancer in subgroups of US white women. Obstet Gynecol 1995 in press.

National Institutes of Health. Consensus Development Conference Statement Ovarian Cancer: Screening, treatment, and follow-up. Gynecol Oncol 1994; 55:S4–S14.

Whittemore AS. Characteristics relating to ovarian cancer risk: Implications for prevention and detection. Gynecol Oncol 1994; 55:S15–S19.

PHYSICIAN'S RESPONSE

SCOTT JENNINGS

Approximately 7% of women with epithelial ovarian cancer are noted to have one or more family members diagnosed with ovarian cancer, but the diagnosis of a true hereditary ovarian cancer syndrome is rare. In order to characterize this patient's hereditary syndrome, and, even more importantly, to estimate the risks carried by other members of her family, it is critical that she have a family pedigree constructed after confirmation of the diagnoses of the other afflicted family members. Recall bias has unfortunately overestimated the incidence of familial ovarian cancer in many studies, and it is extremely important that valid hospital records, pathology reports, and/or death certificates be utilized for the individual estimation of risk for specific patients. Importantly, it is also vital that both cases of ovarian cancer in this family be confirmed as being epithelial. If true, this patient's family appears to fulfill many of our clinical expectations of the most common of the hereditary ovarian cancer syndromes, that of the breast-ovary syndrome. Specifically, this family exhibits two first-degree relatives with ovarian cancer and one with breast cancer; the two family members found to have ovarian cancer were diagnosed well before the median age of 59 described for sporadic ovarian cancer. Patients with suspected hereditary ovarian cancer syndromes, be they breast-ovary cancer, Lynch type II, or site-specific ovarian cancer, should be targeted for education and intensive surveillance.

Breast cancer is considerably more common than ovarian cancer, and a great deal of interest has focused on familial clustering of this disease. King described a gene in 1990 that may be responsible for as many as 2% of cases of breast cancer and an uncertain fraction of ovarian cancer. Although positional cloning isolated the sequence in question that appears to confer this risk of both breast and ovarian cancer (the so-called BRCA1 gene), this work to patients has not yet been applied to patients prospectively and many controversial subtleties are sure to arise as "screening" with BRCA1 begins.

The BRCA1 gene is sure to play an extraordinarily important role in defining which female family members of affected pedigrees have an elevated risk of ovarian and breast cancer and which probably do not. Until the BRCA1 tests are widely available (anticipated 2 to 5 years hence), however, we will have to rely upon clinical information to supply us with most of the information we can offer our patients. Fortunately, the two daughters of the patient in question are both young enough to anticipate some benefit from the maturation of the BRCA1 marker.

Early Detection

In the meantime, we must continue the process of education and careful risk assessment for our patients at risk for hereditary ovarian cancer. At the present time, there is insufficient information to demonstrate the utility of screening studies for the early detection of ovarian cancer, as mammography putatively offers for breast cancer. There is early evidence from many centers in the United States and Britain that noninvasive imaging studies, possibly coupled with serum tumor markers, may be useful in certain populations at risk for the development of ovarian cancer. These studies will remain unqualified, however, until randomized studies are available to demonstrate their real application in the detection of early-stage ovarian cancer. Until randomized studies are completed, it seems prudent to encourage all women at risk for hereditary ovarian cancer to enroll in one of the many clinical trials in progress at this time (local chapters of the American Cancer Society can provide lists of such studies). Serial transvaginal sonography and selected tumor markers (probably CA-125, OVX1, and possibly others) appear to be the best available methods for early detection of ovarian malignancy, but once again, we will not gain the knowledge we need to further our understanding of the early detection for these uniquely important patients unless they are referred to these important clinical trials.

Prevention

The concept of prevention of ovarian cancer is a particularly thorny issue due to the low incidence of the disease and lack of a true premalignant phase. Prophylactic oophorectomy at the completion of childbearing has relatively strong backing in the United States and Britain. However, it is unknown by how much this realistically lowers the risk of cancer, given the finding of peritoneal carcinomatosis indistinguishable from serous ovarian cancer in women following prior oophorectomy. In a National Cancer Institute registry study, 11% of 28 women who underwent recommended prophylactic oophorectomy because of the presence of two or more first-degree family members with ovarian cancer were found to subsequently develop peritoneal carcinomatosis. To keep these preliminary data in context, retrospective studies suggest that bilateral oophorectomy in women in their forties may diminish the risk of ovarian cancer by as much as 12% in nonhereditary ovarian cancer. Despite a lack of hard evidence either way, it seems reasonable to continue to recommend prophylactic oophorectomy at age 35 or at the completion of childbearing in carefully selected women with strong evidence of the presence of the breast-ovary cancer syndrome. Although some investigators have recommended delaying oophorectomy in women with a family history of ovarian cancer until they reach their later forties, one should understand that the incident age of ovarian cancer in the breast-ovary cancer syndrome is indeed earlier than that of those patients with simply a strong family history of ovarian cancer alone. Careful discussions of the surgical risks, the possibility of subsequent peritoneal carcinomatosis (possibly as high as 11%), and the pros and cons of hormone replacement therapy following surgical castration at an early age are mandatory for physicians who care for these women.

Besides surgical intervention, it is known that oral contraceptives reduce the risk of ovarian cancer in women with no hereditary risk for the disease. Analyses from the University of California/San Francisco demonstrate that even in women with a 5% lifetime risk of ovarian cancer due to the presence of a single first-degree relative with ovarian cancer, the lifetime risk of ovarian cancer may be reduced by 50% with the use of oral contraceptives for 10 years or more. Although this finding has not been replicated in the breast-ovary cancer syndrome in question here, it seems reasonable to anticipate these same reductions in risk (if not more).

The other side of the coin for this patient's daughters is the issue of what measures may impact on their risk of breast cancer. As opposed to the uncertainty in the early detection of ovary cancer, it seems apparent that annual mammography, probably beginning at age 30 years, is useful in the early detection of breast cancer in patients with familial breast cancer. Prophylactic mastectomy for the prevention of breast cancer is even more circumspect than prophylactic oophorectomy. Many investigators no longer recommend prophylactic mastectomy given the lack of epidemiologic data supporting this approach, the difference of opinion regarding what comprises adequate breast removal, and the lack of simple reconstructive implants that were available until recently. It is uncertain if the use of oral contraceptives are an important factor in the development of breast cancer, but rare studies have suggested a marginal effect on the incidence of breast cancer in early, long-term users of oral contraceptives.

References

Kerlkoske K, Brown JS, Grady DG. Should women with familial ovarian cancer undergo prophylactic oophorectomy? Obstet Gynecol 1992; 80:700–707.

Schwartz PE. The role of prophylactic oophorectomy in the avoidance of ovarian cancer. Int J Gynecol Obstet 1992; 39:175–184.

PHYSICIAN'S RESPONSE

VICKI SELTZER

It is important to begin with a very thorough family history and pedigree analysis. In addition to asking about all other family members who have had breast and ovarian cancer, it is essential to know about other malignancies in both male and female relatives.

Factors that have been demonstrated to reduce the risk of ovarian cancer are increasing length of oral contraceptive use, increasing number of pregnancies, and increasing duration of lactation. Hartge has estimated that more than half of all ovarian cancers in women in the United States might have been prevented if all had used oral contraceptives for at least 4 years. Although the use of oral contraceptives is likely of great benefit in primary prevention, Hartge's estimate is based on the assumptions that the currently used low-dose oral contraceptives exert the same protective effect as the older higher-dose formulations and that the protective effects last throughout life; neither of these assumptions has yet been proven to be true.

Tubal ligation and hysterectomy have both been associated with reduction in ovarian cancer risk, although further confirmatory data are needed. There are some possible risk factors for which evidence is inconclusive but which are modifiable. These include consumption of dietary fat and of milk products and also coffee consumption. There are data implicating infertility in increased ovarian cancer risk, as well as data suggesting that the use of fertility drugs increases risk.

Of all of the aforementioned factors that may reduce risk, which ones make sense for the patient's daughters? If they have no contraindications to oral contraceptive use, this may be an appropriate method for reducing risk. If they have children, they should be encouraged to breast-feed. Although data regarding dietary modification are inconclusive, it is reasonable to encourage a low-fat diet and to avoid excessive consumption of coffee.

Although screening for ovarian cancer in the low-risk population is considered by most to be inappropriate, there is greater potential utility for screening higher-risk individuals. At present, endovaginal ultrasound plus serum CA-125 evaluation are the modalities utilized. For individuals at risk for a hereditary ovarian cancer, the age of occurrence is usually earlier than that of the typical patient. In addition, since this patient was found to have ovarian cancer at age 37, I would begin to screen her daughters approximately a decade earlier.

Depending upon the entire family pedigree, these girls may be at increased risk for a variety of other malignancies, and obviously they would need screening for these as well.

The BRCA1 gene has been sequenced, and it is expected many other genes that which confer increased risk for a variety of malignancies will be sequenced by the time these young girls reach the age at which they will be at increased risk to develop malignancies. There are specific recommendations that exist today for prophylactic oophorectomy at age 35 or when childbearing is completed for women believed to be at *very high risk* for ovarian cancer. However, by the time these girls reach an age at which they will be at increased risk, it is likely that they will be able to be tested to determine whether they carry alleles conferring such risk.

References

Hartge P, Whittemore AS, Itnyre J, et al. Rates and risks of ovarian cancer in subgroups of U.S. white women. Obstet Gynecol 1995. In press.

Whittemore AS. Characteristics relating to ovarian cancer risk: Implications for prevention and detection. Gynecol Oncol 1994; 55:S15–S19.

PHYSICIAN'S RESPONSE

JONATHAN S. BEREK

This patient, like her sister, was unfortunately found to have advanced ovarian cancer when she was still premenopausal. Based on this fact, her sister's diagnosis of ovarian cancer at age 48, and her mother's death due to cancer at age 62, the patient is probably a member of a pedigree with breast/ovarian familial cancer syndrome or with the site-specific ovarian familial cancer syndrome. With either pedigree, there is a clear concern that her daughters are at risk for the development of premenopausal epithelial ovarian cancer and/or breast cancer. While the precise pattern of heritability is unclear, the patient could be at increased risk because she is a member of an adverse pedigree. In both of these pedigrees, the age of onset of the disease can be as much as a decade earlier than the usual age of diagnosis, i.e., around the average age of menopause at 51 years of age, versus the average age of diagnosis of ovarian cancer in general, i.e., at 61 years of age.

At this time, there is no way to determine with certainty the absolute risk for her daughters. A proper and thorough pedigree analysis should be performed. In women with a pedigree like that of this patient, if there is a mutation in the BRCA1 gene, the risk of developing ovarian cancer may be as high as 50%, because of the autosomal dominant inheritance pattern of this syndrome. If the patient has inherited the defective gene, then her lifetime risk of the development of breast cancer may be even higher, i.e., 85% (1).

Screening for ovarian cancer in the offspring of women who have had ovarian cancer apparently as part of a familial or hereditary pattern has been performed using transvaginal ultrasound and CA-125 (2). However, it is uncertain that this approach is, in fact, sensitive enough to detect early ovarian cancer in these high-risk patients. Furthermore, it is unclear if screening with these modalities in the general population is warranted, because only about one-half of stage I tumors can be ascertained before they have metastasized. The concern would be that this approach might be falsely reassuring and that an ovarian cancer could be missed.

In general, in women who may be at this very high risk for the development of premenopausal ovarian cancer should undergo prophylactic oophorectomy at the age of 35 or as soon as possible after the completion of their families. Hopefully, over the next decade the development of tests for mutations in the BRCA1 and other genetic loci will be able to determine which offspring of women from high-risk pedigrees in fact carry these mutations and require oophorectomy. Conversely, absence of such identifiable mutations might permit the preservation of ovaries in some women. We must await the development of such specific tests for those areas of the genome that are responsible for these hereditary ovarian cancer syndromes.

References

1. Hall JM, Lee MK, Newman B, et al: Linkage of early-onset familial breast cancer to chromosome 17q21 Science 1990; 250:1684.
2. Bourne T, Whitehead MI, Campbell S, et al. Ultrasound screening for familial ovarian cancer. Gynecol Oncol 1991; 43:92.

2

Family History of Ovarian and Breast Cancer

CASE

You are asked to see a 25-year-old woman in consultation. Her mother has just been diagnosed as having ovarian cancer and she asks your opinion as to how she should be followed in the future.

Review of the patient's family history reveals that her mother developed ovarian cancer (stage IIIC) at age 44, two maternal aunts were found to have breast cancer at ages 42 and 53, and her grandmother died of "some type of cancer which filled her abdomen with fluid" at age 49. Your patient has two brothers but no sisters. She has been married 2 years and is now considering starting a family.

Physical examination is unremarkable.

PHYSICIAN'S RESPONSE

GREG SUTTON

Although it is difficult to be certain about the diagnosis of ovarian cancer in this patient's grandmother, the clinical picture is highly suggestive of an epithelial ovarian malignancy. Before firm recommendations are offered, therefore, an attempt should be made to retrieve hospital summaries or pathology reports regarding this relative.

Perhaps the strongest risk factor for epithelial ovarian cancer is a family history of this disease. Although the overwhelming majority of women with ovarian cancer have sporadic or nonhereditary disease, approximately 3% come from families in which one of three hereditary ovarian cancer syndromes exist. The first is the Lynch type II syndrome, which may include endometrial cancer, colon cancer not associated with polyposis (and generally occurring in the right colon), prostate cancer, and epithelial cancer of the ovary. The second is the "site-specific" ovarian cancer syndrome, and the third is the breast/ovarian cancer syndrome.

The patient presented above is likely to come from a family in which the breast/ovarian cancer syndrome is present. This syndrome is associated with germ-line mutations localized to a gene on chromosome 17q and known as BRCA1. BRCA1 is a tumor-suppressor gene much like p53; an inherited mutation in one allele predisposes the carrier to breast or ovarian cancer. Approximately 87% of breast/ovarian cancer families are felt to be linked to BRCA1; the median age of onset of breast cancer for BRCA1 carriers is less than 45 years. The presence of a mutation in BRCA1 may confer a breast cancer risk of 54% and an ovarian cancer risk of 30% by age 60. Although the patient presented above is only 25 years of age, BRCA1 testing as part of a research protocol at one of a number of centers should be considered; the results of such testing would allow her to make an informed decision regarding the initiation of a family and to allow counseling regarding prophylactic mastectomy and/or oophorectomy, since the risks of developing breast or ovarian cancer in a woman *not* carrying a BRCA1 mutation fall to around 10 and 2%, respectively—similar to those of the general population.

Since DNA-based testing for breast cancer susceptibility is not commercially available, it is important that the patient under consideration be referred to the medical genetics department of a regional referral hospital participating in the identification and cataloging of BRCA1 mutations. Since such operations are technically challenging and the understanding of mutations is in an early stage, it is important that the patient be properly informed about the difficulty of providing a yes-no answer, particularly when innocuous sequence changes that may not affect the function of a given gene are identified (neutral polymorphisms). If, after testing, this patient is considered at risk for ovarian/breast cancer, surveillance breast and pelvic examinations as well as mammography, vaginal ultrasound, and CA-125 screening should be considered annually until surgery can be completed after childbearing.

References

Easton DF, Ford D, Bishop DT, and the Breast Cancer Linkage Consortium. Breast and ovarian cancer incidence in BRCA1-mutation carriers. Am J Hum Genet 1995; 56:265–271.

Hoskins KF, Stopfer JE, Calzone KA, et al. Assessment and counseling for women with a family history of breast cancer: A guide for clinicians. JAMA 1995; 273:577–585.

PHYSICIANS' RESPONSE

M. PIVER
J. GOLDBERG

This young woman certainly has a very disconcerting family history. There are a number of reasons why she is at very high risk for the development of a malignancy. First, she has one first-degree relative (her mother) who has confirmed ovarian cancer. Most cases of ovarian cancer are sporadic; thus the majority of people with just one first-degree relative with ovarian cancer are not at risk for hereditary ovarian cancer. However, approximately 5 to 10% of ovarian cancer cases may be hereditary, and relatives of these patients have a significantly increased risk of ovarian cancer. Therefore, as a group, women with one first-degree relative with ovarian cancer have a relative risk of 4.5 compared to the general population, equivalent to a lifetime risk of approximately 8.0% (compared to 1.8% for the general population).

Second, the patient's grandmother very likely had ovarian cancer as well. While it is possible for both the patient's mother and grandmother to have been afflicted due to random chance, the likelihood of such an event would be approximately 0.0324%, or 1 in 3086. Therefore, there is a high probability that the mother and grandmother were afflicted with a hereditary form of the disease. If this is the case, then, assuming an autosomal dominant transmission, the patient has a 50% chance of carrying the genetic abnormality.

Third, both the patient's mother and grandmother were diagnosed with cancer at a significantly younger age than the average age of 61 years seen in the general population. Although this is not a conclusive finding of hereditary ovarian cancer, characteristically hereditary ovarian cancer has a much younger average age of onset than the general population. The relative risk for a patient with one first-degree relative diagnosed with ovarian cancer prior to age 45 has been reported as 14.2. The fact that both relatives were diagnosed at a young age lends support to this being a hereditary ovarian cancer.

The patient also has two maternal aunts who developed breast cancer at a fairly young age. This is significant for several reasons. First, such a pedigree lends further support to the existence of a breast/ovarian cancer syndrome in this family. Second, merely having a strong family history of premenopausal breast cancer would approximately double the patient's risk of ovarian cancer. Third, the patient's risk for breast cancer is significantly increased. Her relative risk from having a first-degree relative diagnosed with ovarian cancer prior to age 55 is 2.2. The lifetime risk of breast cancer in a patient with one first-degree relative with ovarian cancer and one first-degree relative with breast cancer diagnosed before age 50 is 34%, and this patient's risk (with two second-degree relatives with breast cancer) may be similar.

All together, the patient's family history is highly suggestive of hereditary ovarian cancer. Numerous recent studies using linkage analysis have found a strong association between the BRCA1 gene and breast or ovarian cancer in women with a significant family history. Narod et al., in a collaborative report that included members of the Gilda Radner Familial Ovarian Cancer Registry, demonstrated that in a group of 81 families with two or more ovarian cancer cases and two or more breast cancer cases diagnosed prior to age 60, 92% of all cases were linked to BRCA1 gene. BRCA1 defects appear to be transmitted in an autosomal dominant fashion, with a penetrance thought to be around 85%. Thus, knowledge of this patient's carrier status would be ideal, as she would probably be at little or no increased risk if she did not carry a BRCA1 abnormality. Unfortunately, at the present time, such information is only available using linkage analysis, an expensive technique requiring accessibility to a large number of affected and nonaffected family members. This approach is simply not practicable for clinical testing. The BRCA1 gene is being intensely studied for the development of a mass screening test for abnormalities. Although 38 distinct mutations among 80 studied patients have been reported as of February 1995, 3 of these appear to be relatively common, and mutations resulting in a truncated protein accounted for 86% of all mutations identified. Thus, a screening test that would detect a large percentage of BRCA1 abnormalities may be available in the relatively near future.

Until BRCA1 testing is available, management will have to be based on history alone. Naturally, this patient should have annual mammography and perform monthly breast self-examination. Unfortunately, there are no good screening tests for the early detection of ovarian cancer. Routine transvaginal ultrasound and CA-125 testing has too high a false-positive rate, especially in premenopausal women, to justify its use in the general population. However, when screening by ultrasonography is restricted to women with a family history of ovarian cancer, the yield (diagnosing stage I ovarian cancer) may be high enough to justify the false-positive cases. Bourne et al. reported that of 1601 women with at least one first- or second-degree relative with a history of ovarian cancer, 61 had a positive screening ultrasound result; of these, 6 had ovarian cancer (5 at stage IA and 1 at stage III). No ovarian cancers developed within 24 months of the last scan. However, 2 peritoneal carcinomas did develop 2 and 8 months after the last scan, both with normal ovaries at surgery. Thus, the reported sensitivity for ovarian cancer was 100% and the positive predictive value was 10%. Whether 10 surgical explorations are justified to diagnose one case of ovarian cancer is open to debate, but we feel that the yield is acceptable. Obviously, further study is needed to confirm the high sensitivity and reasonable specificity and, most importantly, to document improved survival benefit of routine screening.

At the present time, we are recommending that all women with two or more first- or second-degree relatives undergo prophylactic oophorectomy at the completion of childbearing, ideally before age 35, when the risk of ovarian cancer begins to rise. Therefore, we would recommend that this patient start and complete her family as soon as possible. Hopefully, in several years a screening test for BRCA1 abnormalities will be available, and she may not require prophylactic oophorectomy if she is found not to be a carrier of a BRCA1 abnormality. In the interim, we would recommend pelvic examination, transvaginal ultrasound, and CA-125 testing every 6 months.

References

Bourne TH, Campbell S, Reynolds KM, et al. Screening for early familial ovarian cancer with transvaginal ultrasonography and colour blood flow imaging. Br Med J. 1993; 306:1025–1029.

Claus EB, Risch N, and Thompson WD. The calculation of breast cancer risk for women with a first-degree family history of ovarian cancer. Breast Cancer Res Treat 1993; 28:115–120.

Houlston RS, Bourne TH, Collins WP, et al. Risk of ovarian cancer and genetic relationship to other cancers in families. Hum Hered 1993; 43:111–115.

Narod S, Smith S, Ponder B, et al. An evaluation of genetic heterogeneity in 145 breast-ovarian cancer families. Am J Hum Genet 1995; 56:254–264.

Piver MS, Baker TR, Jishi MF, et al. Familial ovarian cancer: A report of 658 families from the Gilda Radner Familial Ovarian Cancer Registry (1981–1991). Cancer 1993; 71:582–588.

Shattuck-Edens D, McClure M, Simard J, et al. A collaborative survey of 80 mutations in the BRCA1 breast and ovarian cancer susceptibility gene. JAMA 1995; 273:535–541.

PHYSICIANS' RESPONSE

DAVID ALBERTS
LOIS LOESCHER

The early age (i.e., 44 years) of diagnosis of her mother's advanced ovarian cancer, the breast cancers in her two maternal aunts at relatively young ages, and her grandmother's early death (which had the "earmark" of advanced ovarian cancer) suggest strongly that this 25-year-old woman comes from a breast/ovarian cancer family. The lifetime risk of ovarian cancer in women with such a strong family pedigree may be as high as 40% (1). Now that the BRCA1 gene has been identified and can be tested for in this patient, it should be possible to determine definitively if she suffers from this familial syndrome (although 15% who test positive for the gene will never develop cancer).

Let us assume that this young woman tests positive for the BRCA1 gene. Although she would be at extremely high risk for developing breast or ovarian cancer and might benefit from bilateral subtotal subcutaneous mastectomies and bilateral oophorectomy, she has recently married and wants to bear children. Under these conditions, I would recommend the following:

1. In-depth discussion with the patient and husband/family of the risks of breast and ovarian cancers, including all of the surgical approaches.
2. If, after this discussion, the patient still wishes to have children, the following surveillance program should be followed:
   a. Monthly breast self-examination
   b. Twice yearly mammography
   c. Twice yearly serum CA-125 and bimanual rectovaginal pelvic examination
   d. Yearly transvaginal ultrasound (and consideration of Doppler flow studies of both ovaries)

The pregnancies should be completed by the patient's early 30s. Since her mother developed ovarian cancer at age 44, the patient is at greatest risk during the 10 years preceding her 44th birthday (i.e., ages 34 to 44). Once childbearing has been completed, the patient should again undergo genetic counseling concerning her high risks for both breast and ovarian cancers. Detailed pedigree analyses show a vertical transmission pattern of autosomal dominant inheritance with a 0.74 to 0.79 lifetime probability of penetrance (for ovarian cancer) (2).

A bilateral salpingo-oophorectomy and total abdominal hysterectomy (BSO/TAH) should be recommended by age 35. If the patient rejects this surgery, she should continue to undergo twice yearly bimanual rectovaginal pelvic exams and serum CA-125 determinations as well as yearly transvaginal ultrasound. Additionally, bilateral ovarian Doppler flow scans might be included in the screening process as a research procedure. The rationale underlying a bilateral subcutaneous mastectomy is somewhat less strong than that for BSO/TAH, mainly because all glandular breast tissue, especially under the areola and in the deep axillae, cannot be removed. Of course, any remaining tissue would continue at risk and mammograms of the remaining tissue would be virtually worthless. Additionally, the subsequent breast reconstruction procedures would make breast self-examination even more difficult. Thus, the patient would have to see a well-qualified physician frequently for intensive physical exams of the chest wall areas.

Regardless of her ultimate decisions regarding surgery, the patient should be given specific and ongoing psychosocial and socioeconomic counseling and nutritional/physical exercise advice. Although the latter two approaches will have limited effects in the setting of a BRCA1-positive person, a diet low in fat (i.e., < 20% calories in fat each day)/high in fiber (i.e., > 30 g of dietary fiber each day), and high in fruits and vegetables (i.e., > 5 to 8 servings per day) would be healthful and might decrease the potential phenotypic expression of the BRCA1 gene. Furthermore, it has been shown that 4 to 6 hr of exercise per week can reduce the risk of breast cancer by 25% in the general population.

Obviously, no matter what decisions the patient makes, her daughters, should she have any, would, at the appropriate time (again dependent on patient counseling), have to undergo BRCA1 testing so that rational decisions could be made concerning family planning and ovarian and breast cancer surveillance.

References

1. Averrette HE, Nguyen HN. Gynecol Oncol 1994; 55:538–541.
2. Lynch HT, Conway T, Lynch J. Hereditary ovarian cancer pedigree studies: Part II. Cancer Genet Cytogenet 1991; 52:161–183.

PHYSICIANS' RESPONSE

HOLLY H. GALLION
HENRY T. LYNCH

Since a family history of ovarian cancer is now recognized as perhaps the strongest risk factor for ovarian cancer, this patient is appropriately concerned. For women who are members of true hereditary ovarian cancer families (i.e., breast/ovarian, site-specific ovarian and hereditary nonpolyposis colorectal cancer or Lynch type II syndrome), the risk of ovarian cancer can be quite high. In these families, the susceptibility to cancer is transmitted as an autosomal dominant trait with a high degree penetrance. Accordingly, the sisters and daughters of a woman with hereditary ovarian cancer have a 50% chance of inheriting the disease gene and a lifetime risk of ovarian cancer approaching 40%.

Unfortunately, the majority of women with a family history of ovarian cancer have only one or two affected family members, making assessment of risk more difficult. Compared to the lifetime risk of ovarian cancer in the general population, which is 1.4%, the risk for women with only a single affected first-degree relative is increased to 5%; in women with two or more affected relatives, the risk is increased to 7% (1). However, some of families with two or more ovarian cancer cases actually have a true hereditary ovarian cancer syndrome, and for them the ovarian cancer risk can be much greater than 7%.

A comprehensive, well-documented family history of cancer is needed to accurately assess cancer risk in this patient. This should include a complete family history of ovarian, breast, endometrial, and colon cancer; age of onset of disease; and confirmation of disease by pathology reports or death certificate. If she truly has only one first-degree relative with ovarian cancer—her mother— then her ovarian cancer risk is approximately 5%. However, her maternal grandmother may have had ovarian cancer. This, in combination with the fact that her mother and maternal aunt were both premenopausal when they developed cancer, suggests that this family may well be a hereditary breast/ovarian cancer (HBOC) family. If so, this patient's lifetime risk for ovarian cancer would approach 40%.

A confirmatory diagnosis of HBOC syndrome in this family could be accomplished through genetic testing. Clinical testing for germ-line mutations in the BRCA1 gene, which appears to be responsible for disease in the majority of HBOC and site-specific ovarian cancer families, is in its infancy. However, if appropriate DNA samples could be obtained from at least two affected family members, this could be accomplished. If this patient inherited the disease gene, she could then be counseled about available screening modalities and prophylactic oophorectomy at the completion of childbearing. Alternatively, if she did not inherit the disease gene, she could be reassured and undergo routine cancer screening as recommended by the American Cancer Society.

Based on the available family history alone, a conservative estimate of the patient's lifetime risk of ovarian cancer is 5%. However, if BRCA1 testing could not be done in this family, one might err on the side of caution and assume that she is at risk for HBOC.

Although the benefits of screening for ovarian cancer are unproven, potentially useful surveillance modalities include bimanual pelvic examination, CA-125 testing, and transvaginal ultrasound (TVS). Historically, pelvic examination has been ineffective in detecting early-stage disease. Unfortunately CA-125 is elevated in only half of patients with stage I ovarian cancer. Since the detection of early, potentially curable stage I disease is the goal of ovarian cancer screening, CA-125 alone is inadequate. Although TVS is capable of detecting many small ovarian tumors, metastatic disease can be present at the time of detection (2). In addition, both TVS and CA-125 can be abnormal in the presence of benign disease, and this may lead to unnecessary surgical intervention.

Despite the limitations of screening, we would recommend that this patient begin surveillance with annual pelvic examinations, TVS, and serum CA-125 testing. In addition, as her risk of breast cancer is also increased, she should be instructed in monthly breast self-examination, and mammography should be obtained annually. Finally, the patient should consider prophylactic oophorectomy at the completion of childbearing or at age 35, whichever occurs first.

References

1. Kerlikowske K, Brown JS, Grady DG. Should women with familial ovarian cancer undergo prophylactic oophorectomy? Obstet Gynecol 1992; 80:700–707.
2. DePriest PD, Buckley SL, Bailey C, et al. Transvaginal sonography as a screening method for the detection of early ovarian cancer. Gynecol Oncol. In press.

PHYSICIANS' RESPONSE

JOHN CARLSON
CHARLES DUNTON

This 25-year-old nulligravida has a family history that is suspicious for the hereditary breast/ovarian cancer syndrome. As such, her risk of acquiring breast or ovarian cancer may be inherited as an autosomal dominant gene with variable penetrance. A complete family history with an extended pedigree of males should be performed and could identify Lynch type II family syndrome. A consultation with a geneticist may be appropriate for this family.

A major concern for this patient is that at-risk members of such families tend to be diagnosed at younger ages with each successive generation. Since most previous cancers in this family have been diagnosed between 42 and 49 years of age, our patient may enter into her risk period as early as age 32 to 35 years.

Since our patient may have less than 10 years before entering into a high-risk range, we think this would be a very reasonable time for her to begin childbearing after having a normal baseline CA-125 and transvaginal sonogram of the ovaries. If she decides to defer pregnancy, we believe that semiannual physical exams with serum CA-125 testing and transvaginal ultrasound imaging of the ovaries would be appropriate. If there were no medical contraindications, we would recommend ovarian suppression with oral contraceptives. Although none of these measures has been proven effective in high-risk women, this combination of chemoprevention and maximum monitoring offers our patient the best strategy. We would encourage her to complete childbearing by age 30 or 32 and then have prophylactic oophorectomies. She must also become skilled at regular breast self-examination and should begin mammography at an early age, approximately age 30.

While BRCA1 gene testing is still investigational and not commercially available, this family could well be a carrier of the BRCA1 gene and we would recommend that all surviving female family members be tested if possible. If prior cancer cases have confirmed BRCA1, then our patient's risk of future cancer may be estimated based on whether or not she also carries the BRCA1 gene. Certainly, if the BRCA1 gene is evident in all cancer-afflicted family members but is not present in our patient, she has no increased genetic risk and can be monitored routinely. If she also carries the BRCA1 gene, intensive management and prophylactic measures are in order. Alternatively, if none of the afflicted family members harbor the BRCA1 gene, then the patient's risk remains high because of the family profile.

PHYSICIAN'S RESPONSE

MICHAEL HOPKINS

This is an increasingly common problem and, because of recent publicity, the best way to approach it is a very common clinical question. This patient fits the classic pattern for an autosomonal dominant genetically inherited predisposition to develop epithelial ovarian cancer. Two or more first-degree relatives are necessary to establish this possibility. They can be on either the paternal or maternal side. The patient's maternal grandmother most likely had ovarian cancer, and she would be the person with the identifiable gene. This family pedigree also fits the classic autosomonal dominant inheritance pattern with the development of the malignancy in the fifth decade of life. Recently, breast, ovarian, bowel, and uterine cancer have also been linked.

I would counsel this patient that the gene appears to be expressed in the family and that, with an autosomonal dominant pattern, she has approximately a fifty-fifty chance of developing malignancy. I would try to obtain verification that the malignancies were epithelial ovarian in nature.

I would discuss the patient's plans for childbearing. If she does not want to conceive, then an oral contraceptive would be the best appropriate birth control method. The incidence of ovarian cancer is decreased in women who have taken oral contraceptives. The incidence of nulliparity is higher in women with ovarian cancer. It is not known if this is an early sign of ovarian dysfunction or if incessant ovulation increases the risk. There is currently an unknown risk for a woman who uses ovulatory inducing agents. The risk is probably minimal, but recently it has been suggested to increase risk. I would caution her that, if she cannot conceive and begins infertility evaluation eventually resulting in the use of ovulatory inducing agents, continued ongoing screening is absolutely mandatory.

Once she has completed her family or in her middle to late thirties, I would recommend to her that she undergo bilateral salpingo-oophorectomy. At that time, I like to skeletonize the ovarian pedicle for approximately 5.0 to 10.0 cm. This skeletonization removes extra tissue along the embryologic tract of ovarian migration and ensures complete removal of the ovary. In the interim, a CA-125 tumor antigen level and ultrasound can be obtained on a yearly basis. At the patient's present age of 25, I would expect this to be normal. This test may be of more value as she becomes older.

Prophylactic oophorectomy unfortunately is not a guarantee against developing an ovarian cancer–like syndrome. Malignancy can develop in a small ovarian remnant if the ovary is not completely removed. A papillary peritoneal cancer can also develop, which involves the peritoneal surface of the pelvis and abdomen.

3

Familial Breast/Ovarian Cancer

CASE

A 44-year-old woman has a mother and sister who were diagnosed in their forties as having high-grade papillary serous carcinoma of the ovary. The patient's sister, at age 49, has just been diagnosed with breast cancer. The patient is extremely worried and has come to your office requesting that her ovaries be removed. Past history: No previous operations, no previous medical illnesses, and no allergies. Physical exam: The patient is 5 ft, 4 in tall, weighs 151 lb, and appears to be in good health. Physical exam is within normal limits. All blood tests are normal except the patient's cholesterol is 268 with an above-normal LDL fraction.

PHYSICIANS' RESPONSE

ANDREW K. SALTZMAN
LINDA F. CARSON

This case concerns the issues of familial ovarian cancer and the risks and benefits of prophylactic oophorectomy. The patient in question is 44 years old and has two first-degree relatives (mother and sister) who had ovarian cancer in their forties. In addition, the patient's sister developed breast cancer at age 49. The patient requests oophorectomy.

The first step in counseling such a patient is to obtain a thorough family history, with documentation by reviewing pathology reports, medical records, and death certificates as appropriate. The case states that "the patient's sister . . . has just been diagnosed with breast cancer." We *might* assume that this is the same sister that had previously had ovarian cancer, although this is not clear. Perhaps this is another sister. Additionally, perhaps other family members have other cancers; construction of a detailed pedigree would allow a more precise estimation of this patient's cancer risk.

There are three syndromes that make up "hereditary ovarian cancer." From the most to the least common they are hereditary breast-ovarian carcinoma syndrome, Lynch type II syndrome, and site-specific ovarian cancer. The fact that a given patient with ovarian cancer might have other family members with ovarian cancer does not necessarily mean she has *familial ovarian cancer.* One review estimates that hereditary ovarian cancer is responsible for less than 1% of all cases of ovarian cancer (1). In any pedigree, the greater the number of affected family members, the greater the likelihood that a currently unaffected family member is at risk for hereditary ovarian cancer. In the breast/ovarian syndrome, affected family members have either breast cancer, ovarian cancer, or both. The patient in this case might belong to such a family. The second most common syndrome responsible for hereditary ovarian cancer is Lynch type II syndrome. Initially describing families afflicted by colorectal cancer, Lynch coined the term *hereditary nonpolyposis colorectal cancer* (HNPCC) to differentiate this entity from familial adenomatous polyposis. HNPCC was then subdivided into (a) Lynch type I syndrome (or hereditary site-specific colonic cancer), which is characterized by early onset of colorectal cancer, predominance in the proximal colon, and an excess of multiple primary colonic cancers; and (b) Lynch type II syndrome, (or the cancer family syndrome), which has all of the characteristics of Lynch type I as well as susceptibility to other forms of cancer, particularly of the endometrium and ovary. In the least common hereditary ovarian cancer syndrome, site-specific ovarian cancer, affected family members have ovarian cancer alone.

Kerlikowske et al. analyzed existing studies and estimated odds ratios and lifetime probabilities for the development of ovarian cancer in women with a family history of ovarian cancer (1). The comparison group, women without a family history, had an assigned odds ratio of 1.0 and a lifetime probability of 1.6% that a 35-year-old would develop ovarian cancer. For women with one affected relative, the odds ratio was 3.1 and with two or three relatives, 4.6; the lifetime probabilities were 5.0 and 7.2%, respectively. If a woman was truly a member of a hereditary ovarian cancer syndrome family, the lifetime probability that she would develop ovarian cancer was approximately 50%.

For the patient in this case scenario, we would agree with her desire for bilateral oophorectomy, and she would be a good candidate for laparoscopy. We would discuss any indications for perhaps performing a laparoscopic-assisted hysterectomy in addition to the oophorectomy. We would do a thorough exploration with the laparoscope, including the upper abdomen and subdiaphragmatic spaces. We would obtain cytological washings from multiple areas and would request that the pathologist perform more than the usual number of sections on the removed ovaries. Familial ovarian cancer seems to occur at an earlier age than spontaneous cases, and prophylactic surgery should be performed by the time a woman is in her forties if not earlier (1). If a similar patient presented for counseling and did *not* want an oophorectomy, we would then discuss the possible protective effects of oral contraceptives, tubal ligation, and dietary and lifestyle alterations (low-fat, high-fiber diet and no use of perineal talc) as well as the issues of prospective screening. When we consent a patient about to undergo prophylactic oophorectomy, we inform her of the sporadic case reports of primary peritoneal carcinomatosis following oophorectomy (2) and the health mainte-nance–related concerns regarding surgical menopause. These are also "risks" of the procedure in addition to the usual surgical risks.

The patient in this case *is* at modest risk following surgical menopause: she is overweight and has an elevated serum cholesterol. A 64-in woman ideally weighs 136 lb, and when this patient's body-mass index is calculated, it also confirms her to be overweight but not obese. Additionally, current recommenda-tions are for dietary intervention in patients with a serum cholesterol above 200 and for intensive efforts at lowering cholesterol when the level is above 240. Finally, the risk of osteoporosis in a menopausal woman should always prompt the consideration of hormonal replacement. When this particular patient un-dergoes menopause, she will not only face the risk of osteoporosis but her lipid profile will be even less favorable unless she has received estrogen replacement. Whatever benefits a particular patient might realize by undergoing prophylactic oophorectomy are offset by risks, although many of these risks can be ameliorated by hormone replacement. Speroff et al. have elegantly shown the risks of noncompliance with estrogen replacement (3). While these calculations were made for patients undergoing routine oophorectomy (as opposed to "indicated" surgery, as for a patient with familial ovarian cancer), the conclusions are important nonetheless. Without elaborate genetic marker studies, the majority of patients who have undergone prophylactic oophorectomy would not have devel-oped ovarian cancer; but unless they are scrupulously compliant with estrogen replacement therapy, they *will* be at risk for a variety of other conditions.

References

1. Kerlikowske K, Brown JS, Grady DG. Should women with familial ovarian cancer undergo prophylactic oophorectomy? Obstet Gynecol 1992; 80:700–707.
2. Piver MS, Jishi MF, Tsukada Y, Nava G. Primary peritoneal carcinoma after prophy-lactic oophorectomy in women with a family history of ovarian cancer: A report of the Gilda Radner Familial Ovarian Cancer Registry. Cancer 1993; 71:2751–2755.
3. Speroff T, Dawson NV, Speroff L, Haber RJ. A risk-benefit analysis of elective bilateral oophorectomy: Effect of changes in compliance with estrogen therapy on outcome. Am J. Obstet Gynecol 1991; 164:165–174.

PHYSICIAN'S RESPONSE

DAVID GERSHENSON

This patient is probably a member of a breast/ovarian cancer family. She has two first-degree relatives who developed papillary serous ovarian cancer at a relatively early age, one of whom also has breast cancer. Using estimates based on information from breast/ovarian cancer families, this patient would theoretically have up to a 50% probability of developing epithelial ovarian cancer and up to a 21% chance of developing breast cancer. Linkage analysis studies of several large breast/ovarian cancer families have focused on a gene located on chromosome 17q21. Recently, the BRCA1 breast and ovarian cancer susceptibility gene, a tumor suppressor gene, has been identified. Women with germ-line BRCA1 mutations may have an 85 to 90% lifetime risk of breast cancer and a 20 to 50% risk of ovarian cancer. BRCA2, the second susceptibility gene for breast cancer, has recently been localized to chromosome 13 and may account for up to 70% of cases of inherited breast cancer that are not related to BRCA1 mutations.

I would advise this patient to have a transvaginal sonogram and a serum CA-125 determination. I would also recommend that this patient be tested for the presence of a germ-line BRCA1 mutation if the test is available to her. If not, based on current estimates, I would recommend that she have a prophylactic oophorectomy. Even if she does undergo such a procedure, she is at risk for developing a primary peritoneal tumor. Based on the work of Piver and associates, however, it appears that this risk is less than 5%.

A confounding factor in this patient is the presence of an elevated blood cholesterol and LDL fraction. Current information suggests that replacement progesterone in conjunction with replacement estrogen therapy will decrease the risk of endometrial cancer but may increase the LDL fraction, decrease the HDL fraction, and even increase the risk of breast cancer. Of course, we do not yet know the relative influences of these hormonal manipulations in patients in breast/ovarian cancer families or with genetic mutations compared with the normal population. Therefore, based on current information, I would recommend that this patient consider a laparoscopically assisted vaginal hysterectomy and bilateral salpingo-oophorectomy so that the concern about future endometrial cancer, breast cancer, or further increase in LDL fraction associated with the use of progesterone would not be an issue. I would recommend that she take estrogen replacement therapy (with Premarin, 0.625 mg daily) after the surgery, although controversy exists regarding the possible association of estrogen replacement therapy and breast cancer. In addition, I would recommend that she follow a low-fat diet to control her cholesterol and triglyceride levels and to decrease her risk of breast cancer, although we do not yet know if such dietary manipulation has any impact on women with a genetic mutation. If diet does not normalize her cholesterol and lipids, I would recommend that she consider drug therapy.

The other issue that should be addressed in this patient is that of prophylaxis against the development of breast cancer. Data are lacking regarding the risk reduction associated with prophylactic mastectomy or subcutaneous mastectomy. I would refer her to a breast cancer expert to discuss options for management of the breasts. If she elects not to undergo prophylactic breast surgery, mammography every 6 months would be recommended.

References

Miki Y, Swensen J, Shattuck-Eidens D, et al. A strong candidate for the breast and ovarian cancer susceptibility gene BRCA1. Science 1994; 266:66–71.

Shattuck-Eidens D, McClure M, Simard J. et al. A collaborative survey of 80 mutations in the BRCA1 breast and ovarian cancer susceptibility gene: Implications for pre-symptomatic testing and screening. JAMA 1995; 273:535–541.

PHYSICIAN'S RESPONSE

ROBERT C. WALLACH

Although it has been suggested that there may be environmental factors such as talc, asbestos, other carcinogens, or decreased sunlight and that there may be some endogenous factors such as incessant ovulation that lead to the development of ovarian carcinoma, none of these factors is a clearly identifiable carcinogen which can be eliminated, with subsequent protection from the development of ovarian cancer. That an inherited trait predisposes some women to an increased risk for ovarian cancer has been considered for many years (1), and the recognition by physicians of a tendency to familial carcinoma was reported over a century ago (2). Allelic differences in the BRCA1 gene may lead to increased risk for breast or breast and ovarian cancer. Also, the Lynch type II syndrome will include women who are at risk for colon, breast, ovarian, endometrial, stomach and urinary tract carcinoma.

Even without the family history of breast cancer, the presence of ovarian carcinoma in the mother and sister leave this woman at risk for ovarian cancer that is probably greater than 50%.

I would strongly subscribe to the patient's request for removal of the ovaries, but she must be made aware that this is not an absolute guarantee against the development of a related disease, either from some ectopic ovarian tissue or from the pelvic or abdominal peritoneal surfaces, which have probably given rise to this disease in some of the cases reported in the literature. In addition, I would strongly suggest that the surgery be performed with hysterectomy because of the probable increased risk for an endometrial carcinoma and a relatively small difference in surgical morbidity. The patient should also have very close surveillance with clinical, radiologic, and endoscopic evaluation of the breasts and colon.

Problematic is the issue of estrogen replacement after removal of the ovaries. With conflicting information available on the subject and without a conclusive demonstration of added risk for breast cancer, the patient should receive hormone replacement after removal of the ovaries.

References

Liber AF. Ovarian cancer in mother and 5 daughters. Arch Pathol 1950; 49:280–290.
Broca PP. Traite Des Tumeurs. Vols. I and II. Paris: P. Asselin, 1866–1869.

PHYSICIANS' RESPONSE

D. SPICER
F. MUGGIA

This 44-year-old woman is at a very substantial risk for the development of ovarian cancer on the basis of a family history of two first-degree relatives with ovarian cancer, although the age at diagnosis of these two relatives is not stated. Further, the recent diagnosis of early-onset (< 50 years of age) breast cancer in a sister may indicate an increased risk of both neoplasms. Prophylactic bilateral oophorectomy and hysterectomy have been advocated for the prevention of ovarian cancer in individuals from families with a well-documented familial (genetic) predisposition to ovarian cancer (1,2). It would be prudent for this woman to undergo surgery if she has completed childbearing.

It has been suggested that the mode of inheritance in such families is autosomal dominant with carriers of the yet unidentified gene developing a high rate of ovarian cancer at a young age. Oophorectomy would be expected to substantially decrease the risk of ovarian cancer; the risk may not be totally eliminated, however, as occurrences of abdominal carcinomatosis have been described (1). Bilateral oophorectomy would best be done transabdominally, since occasionally ovarian tissue might not be totally resected by the vaginal route and such tissue can still give rise to cancer (1).

The medical consequences of surgical menopause must be carefully considered and long-term management planned. In order to prevent osteoporosis, signs and symptoms of the menopause, and a rise in cardiovascular disease risk, such oophorectomized women are given estrogen replacement therapy (ERT). In some families an increased risk of breast cancer has been described (3), and in some the increased risk will be linked to the BRCA1 gene (4). Although oophorectomy would be predicted to reduce the risk of breast cancer in these women, the ERT is predicted to slightly decrease this benefit, although it will not return breast cancer risk to nonoophorectomized rates (5). It has been suggested that a progestogen, given with the ERT, may provide a protective effect against breast cancer (2). However, the bulk of available data concerning the etiology of breast cancer suggest that the addition of a progestogen may actually increase breast cancer risk above that of oophorectomy and ERT and that it is unjustified in women without a uterus. It would be imprudent to consider oophorectomy for the prevention of breast cancer under most if not all other circumstances.

There is irrefutable evidence that ovarian hormones are intimately involved in the genesis of breast cancer. In the large case-control study of Trichopoulos et al. (6), women with artificial menopause (surgical oophorectomy or radiation ablation) prior to age 35 were found to have a 64% reduction in breast cancer risk compared to women with menopause at ages 45 to 54. Even thirty or more years later, breast cancer risk was reduced by two-thirds in women with menopause induced before age 35 (6). After oophorectomy and hysterectomy and baseline mammograms, this patient should be placed on 0.625 mg of Premarin daily. A careful discussion of the possible increase in the risk of breast cancer should ensue. If the BRCA1 gene is subsequently found in the family, an enhanced risk of breast cancer from this dose of exogenous estrogens is possible but currently not yet established. One might consider employing lower doses as long as lipid abnormalities and other risks for osteoporosis (thin body habitus) are not manifest.

References

1. Tobacman J, et al. Intra-abdominal carcinomatosis after prophylactic oophorectomy in ovarian-cancer-prone families. Lancet 1982; 2:795–797.
2. Cruickshank D, et al. The multidisciplinary management of a family with epithelial ovarian cancer. Br J Obstet Gynaecol 1992; 99:226–231.
3. Lynch H, et al. Familial association of breast/ovarian cancer. Cancer 1978; 41:1543–1548.
4. Schattuck-Eidens D, et al. A collaborative survey of 80 mutations in the BRCA1 breast and ovarian cancer susceptibility gene: Implications for presymptomatic testing and screening. JAMA 1994; 2723:535–541.
5. Spicer DV, Pike MC. The prevention of breast cancer through reduced ovarian steroid exposure. Acta Oncol 1992; 31:167–174.
6. Trichopoulos D, MacMahon B, Cole P. Menopause and breast cancer risk. J Natl Cancer Inst 1972; 48:605–613.

PHYSICIAN'S RESPONSE

THOMAS J. RUTHERFORD
PETER E. SCHWARTZ

A more detailed history must be obtained. We do not know the patient's parity, whether she breast-fed children, or whether she has used oral contraceptives, all of which are protective against ovarian cancer, presumably through suppression of ovulation.

The family history suggests that this woman may have an inherited susceptibility to ovarian or breast cancer. In a population-based study of 493 patients with ovarian cancer, 34 (6.9%) women had a family history of ovarian cancer; however, only 1 (3%) of the 34 patients with ovarian cancer had a hereditary ovarian cancer syndrome. These studies may underestimate the true incidence of familial carcinoma in patients whose relatives have not demonstrated the disease process as yet. Since these are female reproductive malignancies, mother-to-daughter transmission is easily recognized. Therefore a complete family cancer history must be obtained.

If this patient fits into a hereditary ovarian cancer syndrome with two or more affected first-degree relatives, her risk of developing ovarian cancer may be as great as 50%, as estimated from the Gilda Radner Familial Cancer Registry. The probability of hereditary cancer syndrome will increase with the number of affected first-degree relatives, total relatives, generations affected, and the development of ovarian malignancy at a young age.

For women with a family history of ovarian cancer, the effect of prophylactic oophorectomy would reduce the lifetime risk from 5 to 50% (the exception being peritoneal carcinoma). Another major benefit of prophylactic oophorectomy is breast cancer protection. The younger the patient is at prophylactic oophorectomy, the more beneficial the effects of breast cancer reduction. This patient is at risk for breast cancer because of her family history and obesity.

Arguments against prophylactic oophorectomy include surgical risks, osteoporosis, and cardiovascular complications. When lack of compliance with hormone replacement therapy is an issue, the increased risks of cardiovascular disease and osteoporosis could outweigh the benefits of ovarian and breast cancer protection. A 35-year-old woman without a familial risk of ovarian cancer undergoing a prophylactic oophorectomy would lose 1.4 years from her total life expectancy if estrogen replacement therapy were not instituted. This patient presents with an elevated cholesterol of 268 with an abnormal LDL fraction and obesity and therefore is already at significant risk for cardiac disease. We do not know whether she uses tobacco; if she does, this could further increase her cardiac risk.

It would be reasonable to offer the patient a prophylactic oophorectomy after consideration of a more complete family history. If there is evidence that the patient has a familial hereditary ovarian cancer syndrome, prophylactic oophorectomy is warranted. If the pedigree demonstrates a nonhereditary ovarian cancer with baseline risks, the decision for prophylactic oophorectomy depends on the patient's preference and her ability to comply with estrogen replacement. If the patient does not want surgical castration, she may be enrolled into an ovarian screening clinic and closely followed by transvaginal sonograms, CA-125 levels, and routine examinations, although the value of this approach remains unproven.

Reference

Nguyen, HN, Averette HE, Janicek M. Ovarian carcinoma: A review of the significance of familial risk factors and the role of prophylactic oophorectomy in cancer prevention. Cancer 1994; 74:545–554.

4

Familial Ovarian Cancer

CASE

Two sisters, 44 and 28 years of age, arrive at your office seeking advice as to their future risk of ovarian cancer. They report that their mother has just been diagnosed with an ovarian cancer. Their mother has two sisters who are alive and well, but their grandmother may have had breast cancer shortly before she died at age 77.

PHYSICIANS' RESPONSE

GUNTER DEPPE
VINAY MALVIYA

Recommendations

A complete family history should be taken to determine whether the patients belong to a family with hereditary ovarian cancer syndrome. This includes a history of ovarian cancer, breast cancer, endometrial cancer, and nonpolyposis colorectal cancer. An attempt should be made to verify the diagnosis by obtaining pathology or autopsy reports. A family pedigree by a physician or a genetic counselor should be requested.

The 28-year-old patient should undergo an annual gynecological examination that includes pelvic and breast examinations. She should have a baseline mammogram at the age of 40 and repeat mammograms annually after the age of 50. If she desires contraception, oral contraceptives should be the preferred method of birth control. The 44-year-old patient should undergo a screening examination that includes pelvic and abdominal examinations, CA-125 testing, transvaginal ultrasound, and color-flow Doppler imaging of the ovarian vascular tree. Regular semiannual gynecological evaluation should be performed as well as transvaginal ultrasonography if clinically indicated.

Discussion

Women with one relative with ovarian cancer have an estimated 5% lifetime probability of developing ovarian cancer (1). The lifetime probability of developing breast cancer in patients at no familial risk for breast cancer is approximately 10%. Whether a lifetime probability of 5% is sufficiently high to warrant oophorectomy depends upon patients' attitudes concerning the risks of surgery and long-term hormone replacement. Estrogen replacement therapy is associated with a decreased risk for fractures and coronary heart disease. Long-term therapy may also be associated with a small increase in breast cancer risk.

The protective effect of oral contraceptive pills appears to increase with the duration of use and to persist for 10 to 15 years after the oral contraceptives have been discontinued. Pooled estimates of ovarian cancer risks in patients who take oral contraceptive pills suggest that a 35-year-old woman with one relative with ovarian cancer, whose estimated lifetime probability of ovarian cancer is 5%, can reduce this probability risk to about 3% if she takes oral contraceptive pills for 5 to 9 years and to 2.5% if she takes oral contraceptives for 10 or more years (2) (see Table 1).

Table 1 Lifetime Probability of Ovarian Cancer and Life Expectancy in Women with Familial Ovarian Cancer

Family History of Ovarian Cancer	Estimated Odds Ratio (95% Cl)	Lifetime Probability of Ovarian Cancer in a 35-Year-Old Woman	Life Expectancy (years) of a 35-Year-Old Woman
No family history of ovarian cancer	1.0 (comparison group)	1.6%	82.4
One relative with ovarian cancer	3.1 (2.2–4.4)	5.0%	82.1
One first-degree relative with ovarian cancer	3.4 (1.1–4.5)	5.0%	82.1
Two or three relatives with ovarian cancer	4.6 (1.1–18.4)	7.2%	81.8
Hereditary ovarian cancer syndrome	NA	50%	74.7

Source: Adapted from Ref. 1.

To my mind the risk is not sufficiently high to recommend prophylactic oophorectomy in these patients. They should be informed that although there is some evidence that the screening of postmenopausal women by transvaginal sonography may decrease the stage at diagnosis and mortality of ovarian cancer, no controlled trial has been conducted to determine whether any screening test or combination of tests prolong life. Therefore routine surveillance tests for women with a family history of ovarian cancer are of questionable value. Women with a family history of ovarian cancer who request screening should be informed that the risk of screening may include unnecessary laparotomy. In addition, women who request screening should be encouraged to participate in controlled clinical trials.

References

1. Kerlikowske K, Brown JS, Grade DG. Should women with familial ovarian cancer undergo prophylactic oophorectomy? Obstet Gynecol 1992; 80:700–707.
2. Steinberg K, Thacker S, Smith S, et al. A meta-analysis of the effect of estrogen replacement therapy on the risk of breast cancer. JAMA, 1991; 265:1985–1990.

PHYSICIAN'S RESPONSE

HARRISON G. BALL

These sisters are concerned about their risk of developing ovarian cancer after the diagnosis of ovarian cancer in their mother. On the basis of their ages, it is reasonable to assume that their mother is about age 60. The only other family information regards a grandmother who may have had breast cancer at the age of 77. Are these sisters at increased risk for developing ovarian cancer? Is there a defined cancer syndrome in this family? If they are at increased risk, what is the magnitude of the risk and can we do anything about it?

Most women with epithelial ovarian cancer have the sporadic form of the disease. A small number (< 5%) will have an inherited form of the cancer. Several hereditary cancer syndromes associated with epithelial ovarian cancer have been defined, including site-specific ovarian cancer, breast/ovarian cancer syndrome, and Lynch type II syndrome.

Current information on gene mutations is promising but does not yet allow us to identify a high-risk group. Pedigree analysis is the best approach to identifying high-risk patients. An adequate family history must contain at least three generations. Caution should be exercised in relying on hearsay information, and every attempt should be made to obtain the relevant hospital records, pathology reports, and autopsy records.

Site-specific ovarian cancer syndrome where ovarian cancer occurs in multiple generations is uncommon and can be ascertained by a careful family history.

Breast/ovarian cancer syndrome involves multiple generations with relatives having one or both cancers. It is not unusual to see bilateral breast cancers and early age of onset of both the breast and ovarian cancers. Since both syndromes are transmitted as autosomal dominant traits with variable penetrance, 50% of the female offspring may develop the disease. Lynch type II syndrome is defined by multiple generations developing colon, breast, endometrial, and ovarian cancers.

Lacking a defined cancer syndrome and with a single first-degree relative diagnosed as having epithelial ovarian cancer, the lifetime risk of developing ovarian cancer for each of our patients is no greater than 1 in 20. The estimated cumulative risk by 29 years of age is 1 in 400; by 49 years of age, it is 1 in 200. Having a single first-degree relative with epithelial ovarian cancer is not associated with an earlier age of onset of the cancer in the offspring.

If pedigree analysis suggests site-specific ovarian cancer or breast/ovarian cancer syndrome, the lifetime risk of developing ovarian cancer may be as high as 1 in 2; in such cases, prophylactic oophorectomy should be considered when childbearing has been completed. The risk of developing ovarian cancer for family members with Lynch type II syndrome is harder to define but may be as high as 1 in 10. Since these family members are also at risk for developing endometrial cancer, if prophylactic oophorectomy is considered, then hysterectomy also should be performed in this group of women.

If there are no additional family members with ovarian, breast, endometrial, or colon cancers, these sisters are only at a slightly increased risk of developing epithelial ovarian cancer over their lifetimes. I would not recommend prophylactic oophorectomy for them unless their level of anxiety after counseling and reflection resulted in their asking for this procedure. I do not believe there is a role for periodic screening with CA-125. I would recommend annual screening with transvaginal ultrasonography, since this appears to offer the greatest likelihood of detecting ovarian cancer while it is confined to the ovary in high-risk patients.

References

Cohen CJ, Jennings TS. Screening for ovarian cancer: the role of noninvasive imaging techniques. Am J Obstet Gynecol 1994; 170:1089–1094.

Offit K, Brown K. Quantitating familial cancer risk: A resource for clinical oncologists. J Clin Oncol 1994; 12:1724–1736.

PHYSICIANS' RESPONSE

GINI FLEMING
OLUFUNMILAYO OLOPADE

It is important to get as complete a family history as possible from patients who are seeking counseling regarding a hereditary risk of cancer. Details regarding all cancers on both the maternal and paternal sides of the family should be solicited. Patients may mistakenly believe that a risk for cancers affecting women, such as breast and ovarian cancers, can be transmitted only through their mothers.

The most common familial ovarian cancer syndrome is probably the breast/ovarian cancer syndrome associated with defects in the BRCA1 gene on chromosome 17. Male carriers of the mutant gene may have an increased risk of prostate and colon cancer (1). The other two relatively common syndromes are the hereditary nonpolyposis colon cancer syndrome (Lynch type II syndrome), in which early-onset colon cancer is associated with a variety of other cancers, including those of the endometrium, ovary, breast, pancreas, and urothelial system, and the site-specific ovarian cancer syndrome. It is estimated that these four syndromes together account for 5 to 10% of all ovarian cancer.

Factors suggesting a familial cancer syndrome include two or more affected first-degree relatives, unusually early age of onset of the cancers, bilaterality (for breast cancer), and multiple affected generations. Assuming that these sisters have no important family history other than that noted, it is unlikely that they have any hereditary ovarian cancer syndrome. Having a mother with ovarian cancer and a grandmother with breast cancer might make one think of a hereditary breast/ovarian cancer syndrome. However, the relatively late ages of onset for both the mother and grandmother make this less likely. Breast cancer is exceedingly common, and the lifetime risk of breast cancer for North American women of about 1 in 8 is only slightly increased by having one second-degree relative with postmenopausal breast cancer. The lifetime risk for ovarian cancer for a North American women is about 1 in 70, and this is increased to a lifetime risk of about 1 in 20 for women with one affected first-degree relative. The actual risks that these sisters will develop breast or ovarian cancer are lower than the lifetime risks quoted since some of that lifetime risk has been used up—they have survived this long with no cancer (2).

Currently available diagnostic techniques do not have sufficient sensitivity or specificity for use as screening tools in this group of patients. For example, one group reported screening 386 (largely premenopausal) women with one affected first-degree relative for ovarian cancer using CA-125 measurements and transvaginal ultrasound with color-flow Doppler. Eleven percent of patients had a CA-125 over 35 U/mL. Nineteen surgical procedures were performed, and no cases of ovarian cancer were found. Only one of the programs in the United States for women with at least one first-degree relative with ovarian cancer has reported the diagnosis of a case through screening (3).

Our approach would be to reassure these sisters that it is highly unlikely that they carry any breast or ovarian cancer-susceptibility gene and to explain that no special testing or screening for ovarian cancer has proven to be of any benefit at this point, while screening tests may lead to unnecessary surgery. We would encourage them to enroll in any available clinical screening trials. Should there not be any clinical trials available and should they very much desire some sort of screening, we would discuss the possibility of annual transvaginal ultrasound examinations and CA-125 measurement, preferably after menopause. Both sisters should, of course, have routine annual gynecological exams and annual mammography starting by age 50.

References

1. Ford D, Easton DF, Bishop DT, et al. Risks of Cancer in BRCA1-mutation carriers. Lancet 1994; 343:692–695.
2. Brown K, Offit K. Quantitating familial cancer risk: A resource for clinical oncologists. J Clin Oncol 1994; 12:1724–1736.
3. Westhoff C. Current status of screening for ovarian cancer. Gynecol Oncol 1994; 44:S34–S37.

PHYSICIAN'S RESPONSE

DAVID MOORE

Perhaps the two greatest risk factors for epithelial ovarian cancer are (a) age and (b) family history. To better assess genetic risk, pedigrees should encompass cancers of the ovary, breast, and colon in both female and male relatives. Whenever possible, malignant disease should be verified by obtaining medical records. A hasty risk assessment followed by recommendations based on incomplete information—as in this case—can have dire physical and emotional consequences for the patient.

Accepting the case presentation as both accurate and complete, the two sisters have an approximate 7% lifetime risk of developing ovarian cancer, which is three to four times the risk of the general population. The risk that either of these two sisters will develop breast cancer is much greater than the risk that they will develop ovarian cancer; they should closely follow published breast cancer screening guidelines.

Addressing their future potential for developing ovarian cancer, there are three options: (a) ovarian cancer screening, (b) prophylactic oophorectomy, and (c) preventive measures. There is no cost-effective method for detecting early-stage ovarian cancer in asymptomatic individuals. A combination of transvaginal ultrasonography to assess ovarian volume and morphometry with serum CA-125 is a rational screening approach untested by a large, prospective, multicenter trial. Recent cloning of the BRCA1 gene will lead to the exciting possibility of genetic testing. Referral to a research laboratory to assess whether either of these women possesses a BRCA1 mutation is a consideration. Laboratory quality control, the large number of described mutations within the BRCA1 gene with undefined risk associations, the ethical dilemma of possessing a genetic mutation, and other complex issues must be resolved before genetic testing becomes a clinical standard.

Prophylactic oophorectomy likewise is a rational yet unproven approach. Cases of an ovarian cancer–like syndrome have been seen following prophylactic oophorectomy, suggesting that the inheritable disease in truly high-risk subjects may in fact be a primary adenocarcinoma of the peritoneal cavity. The decision to perform a prophylactic oophorectomy only after extensive counseling is often made for subjective reasons. In my experience, third-party payers do not reimburse patients for this procedure. However, after the completion of childbearing, bilateral oophorectomy is strongly recommended if either of these women were to undergo an abdominal operation for other reasons (cholecystectomy for gallstones, appendectomy for appendicitis, and so on).

Recognizing the significant risk reduction with hormonal methods of contraception, it is strongly recommended that the younger sister be started on oral contraceptives. Among all possible interventions, this is perhaps the most cost-effective.

References

DePriest PD, Van Nagell JR, Gallion HH, et al. Ovarian cancer screening in asymptomatic postmenopausal women. Gynecol Oncol 1993; 51:205–209.

Piver MS, Jishi MF, Tsukada Y, Nava G. Primary peritoneal carcinoma after prophylactic oophorectomy in women with a family history of ovarian cancer. Cancer 1993; 71:2751–2755.

Shattuck-Eidens D, McClure M, Simard J, et al. A collaborative survey of 80 mutations in the BRCA1 breast and ovarian cancer susceptibility gene: Implications for pre-symptomatic testing and screening. JAMA 1995; 273:535–541.

PHYSICIAN'S RESPONSE

JOE YON

Here we have two sisters, one 44 years of age and the other 28, whose mother was just diagnosed as having ovarian cancer. First of all, I think we can assume that the mother is probably over age 60, and therefore falls into the expected range for random occurrence of ovarian cancer. It is noted that the mother had two sisters who are alive and well, but we do not know whether they are older or younger than the mother, and that a grandmother may have had breast cancer at age 77, but again, this is not further defined. It would be worthwhile to get more information on the family history and even to try to establish some sort of pedigree, although it does require three generations with fairly complete data in order to establish any sort of familial connection.

So the first thing that I would do in this case is to try to establish some sort of pedigree if possible, but I would not go to the extent of having a geneticist do a formal consult unless my preliminary investigation indicated that there was more likelihood of a familial association than is suggested by the history given. Both daughters should be examined if they have not been examined recently, and if all of this proves to be within normal limits, we have to assume that the mother is a random case of ovarian cancer and that the daughters assume a slightly increased risk over that of the general population. If one assumes that the risk to the general population of women is 1.4%, then having a mother with ovarian cancer who is over the age of 50 at the time of diagnosis would probably increase that risk to somewhere between 3 and 5%.

Past history of the use of oral contraceptives, full-term pregnancies, and/or breast feeding can all decrease the risk to the daughters. A lifetime use of oral contraceptives up to about 10 years could reduce the risk to about 40% of that faced by the general population and, interestingly enough, this does not have to be consecutive, but the protection appears to be cumulative.

Recommendations might be that the 28-year-old daughter could consider going on oral contraceptives if she is not on them already and that, if the 44-year-old daughter is not a cigarette smoker, she might consider low-dose oral contraceptives as well. The risks here do not appear high enough to justify prophylactic surgery in the form of interval oophorectomy; but if either one of these patients were to undergo pelvic surgery, particularly hysterectomy, for other reasons, she should seriously consider undergoing oophorectomy at the same time. One of the biggest problems with prophylactic oophorectomy is that the patients may subsequently fail to take their estrogen replacement therapy, thereby increasing their risk of other complications such as osteoporosis, coronary artery disease, and so on. These risks may well outweigh the risk of the ovarian malignancy for which the prophylactic oophorectomy was done. Therefore, when prophylactic oophorectomy is being planned, either as an interval or with other pelvic surgery, it must be ascertained preoperatively that the patient is willing to take replacement therapy and has a history of being able to tolerate it.

Otherwise, these women should be counseled that nothing more than annual examination is indicated and that, at the present time, the use of CA-125 and/or pelvic ultrasound as a screening test has not been shown to reduce the morbidity or mortality from ovarian cancer. These procedures are therefore not recommended. However, if these patients are overly concerned, then possibly ultrasound examinations and CA-125 determinations after menopause might be considered, although the patients must be warned that these tests are not recommended, are not cost-effective, and are not very efficacious.

References

NIH Consensus Conference, "Ovarian Cancer." JAMA 1995; 273:491–497.

PHYSICIANS' RESPONSE

EDWARD PODCZASKI
RODRIGUE MORTEL

The lifetime risk of ovarian carcinoma for women in the United States is approximately 1.2%. Several factors that may increase the risk of ovarian cancer include nulliparity, age, use of fertility drugs, and a family history of ovarian cancer. A positive family history is one of the strongest independent risk factors for ovarian cancer. Although not clearly defined in the literature, the term *familial ovarian cancer* is used to describe ovarian cancer in a woman with one or more relatives with ovarian cancer or a woman with a hereditary ovarian cancer syndrome.

At least three well-described hereditary ovarian cancer syndromes exist: the hereditary site-specific ovarian cancer syndrome, the hereditary breast/ovarian cancer syndrome with a mixture of first- and second-degree relatives affected by either or both of these cancers; and the Lynch type II syndrome, characterized by nonpolyposis colorectal cancer and an increased risk of endometrial and ovarian cancer. The hereditary ovarian cancer syndromes are. rare and account for less than 1% of ovarian epithelial cancers. These syndromes have an autosomal dominant pattern of inheritance with variable degrees of penetrance and usually affect clusters of women in two to four generations of the same family. Furthermore, the ovarian cancers due to these syndromes occur at a younger age than those in the general population.

It may be difficult to differentiate a hereditary ovarian cancer syndrome from nonhereditary ovarian cancer as well as to assign the correct syndrome involved. The family pedigree is the main diagnostic tool. Unfortunately, this method is often limited by incomplete information, small family sizes, missed paternity, or a predominance of male family members. In an Australian cancer screening program, 240 women with a first-degree relative with ovarian cancer participated. Although 34% of all women gave a history of at least one other first-degree relative with either breast, bowel, or endometrial cancer, a hereditary ovarian cancer syndrome was suspected in only two families.

The majority of women with a family history of ovarian cancer are not from families with hereditary ovarian cancer syndromes. Approximately 7% of women with ovarian cancer have a positive family history for the disease; of these women, over 90% have only one relative with ovarian carcinoma. Women with one relative with ovarian cancer have an estimated 5% lifetime risk of ovarian cancer, as opposed to a 1.6% lifetime risk of ovarian cancer in a 35-year-old women without such a history. There is also no evidence that women with a positive family history develop ovarian carcinomas at a younger age than those without such a history.

In the clinical scenario presented, the patients have a first-degree relative with ovarian cancer without clear evidence of a hereditary ovarian cancer syndrome. As such, they have an approximately 5% lifetime risk of ovarian cancer as opposed to an approximately 10% lifetime risk of breast cancer. A 5% lifetime risk of ovarian cancer may prompt some women to seek prophylactic oophorectomy after completion of childbearing. However, prophylactic oophorectomy must be weighed against the risks of surgery and anesthesia as well as the complications of estrogen deprivation if the patient does not use hormonal replacement.

While patient's preferences should be considered, we do not believe the risk of ovarian cancer is high enough in this case to recommend prophylactic oophorectomy. We would also not recommend yearly or twice yearly screening with CA-125 and/or transvaginal ultrasound. Although there is evidence that the screening of asymptomatic women can detect early ovarian carcinomas, no randomized trials have been conducted to determine the efficacy of such screening. However, young patients with such a clinical history may benefit substantially from the use of oral contraceptives, and this should be considered in the case of the 28-year-old sister described. Ten years of oral contraceptive use by women with a positive family history reduced their risk of ovarian cancer to a level below that of women whose family history was negative and who never used oral contraceptives.

References

Grover S, Quinn MA, Weideman P. Patterns of inheritance of ovarian cancer: An analysis from an ovarian cancer screening program. *Cancer* 1993; 72:526–530.

Gross TP, Schlesselman JJ. The estimated effect of oral contraceptive use on the cumulative risk of epithelial ovarian cancer. Obstet Gynecol 1994; 83:419–424.

Kerlikowske K, Brown JS, Grady DG. Should women with familial ovarian cancer undergo prophylactic oophorectomy? Obstet Gynecol 1992: 80:700–707.

5

Stage 1 High-Grade Fallopian Tube Cancer in a Young Woman

CASE

A 35-year-old woman presents to her local emergency room with what is believed to be an ectopic pregnancy. At surgery the patient is found to have a cancer involving the right fallopian tube; it appeared to be localized to that organ. As the procedure was performed on an emergency basis, a complete exploration was not attempted. However, the gynecologist who performed the surgery stated there was no gross evidence of disease outside the fallopian tube. The tumor was high grade and washings obtained at the time of surgery were negative.

PHYSICIAN'S RESPONSE

PETER ROSE

Two principal questions must be addressed: First, should the patient receive further therapy? And, second, is there any role for reoperation?

The management of patients with fallopian tube carcinoma is very similar to that for those with ovarian carcinoma (1). However, because of the rarity of fallopian tube cancer, no controlled clinical trials have been performed. In contrast to ovarian carcinoma, only a limited number of patients with stage I disease have been treated with surgery alone. In view of the fact that the patient had a high-grade tumor that is at least stage IA, adjuvant therapy would be advocated, which would be consistent with the management of ovarian cancer in the National Cancer Institute/Gynecologic Oncology Group (NCI/GOG) protocols (7602, 95). These studies have randomized patients to chemotherapy or radioactive chromic phosphate (^{32}P). Since the patient has not been comprehensively staged and, specifically, the retroperitoneum has not been evaluated, based on the published experience in ovarian cancer, the patient should not receive ^{32}P. With respect to chemotherapy, again, no randomized studies exist in tubal cancer. Cisplatin-based combination chemotherapy has been utilized with an overall response rate of 60%, which is similar to the case in ovarian cancer. Small retrospective studies in tubal carcinoma have found no difference in response rates comparing cisplatin, doxorubicin, and cyclophosphamide to cisplatin and cyclophosphamide or cisplatin to carboplatin. A baseline CA-125 level should be obtained, since, if this is elevated, it will be helpful in evaluating response to therapy.

Is there any role for reoperation either immediately or following the completion of therapy? Surgical therapy for fallopian tube cancer should be the same as for ovarian cancer. In cases grossly confined to the tube, a careful staging procedure should be performed that includes peritoneal washings and systematic inspection and palpation of the peritoneal surfaces. Omentectomy and bilateral pelvic and paraaortic lymphadenectomy should be performed and peritoneal biopsies obtained. Maxon et al. reported that in two of five patients who had nodal sampling at primary surgery, the results were positive. However, one recent study examining routine lymphadenectomy found no cases of nodal metastasis in a small series of patients with disease grossly confined to the adnexa (2). A computed tomography (CT) scan of the abdomen and pelvis should be obtained. However, since this patient had a high-grade tumor, she will require treatment, and reoperation would be advised only if nodal enlargement were seen on her CT scan. As with ovarian cancer, in the absence of clinically evident or progressive disease, disease status following therapy is difficult to assess. Second-look laparotomy (SLL) has been shown to be of prognostic importance in tubal cancer, and survival for the patients who are pathologically disease-free is significantly different than it is for those who are clinically disease-free. Nodal evaluation is essential and paraaortic nodal metastasis have been detected as the only evidence of persistent disease at second-look laparotomy. As with ovarian cancer, recurrences following negative SLL have occurred.

In summary the recommendation would be to obtain a CT scan of the abdomen and pelvis to exclude nodal disease and to obtain a baseline CA-125 level. Treat the patient with platinum-based therapy and consider second-look laparotomy or observation.

References

1. Rosen AC, Sevelda P, Klein M, et al. A comparative analysis of management and prognosis in stage I and II fallopian tube carcinoma and epithelial ovarian cancer. Br J Cancer 1994;; 69:577–579.

2. Kein M, Rosen A, Lahousen M, et al. Radical lymphadenectomy in the primary carcinoma of the fallopian tube. Arch Gynecol Obstet 1993; 253:21–25.

PHYSICIAN'S RESPONSE

HOWARD W. JONES, III

Because of the difficulty of diagnosing carcinoma of the fallopian tube prior to exploratory laparotomy, it is not at all unusual for these patients to be incompletely staged (1). This patient appears to have a poorly differentiated carcinoma confined to the right fallopian tube with negative washings and no clinically observed evidence of any metastatic disease. The data on carcinoma of the fallopian tubes are limited, but since this entity behaves in a fashion similar to ovarian cancer, it is reasonable to assume that perhaps as many as 33% of such patients will have microscopic metastatic disease in the omentum, on the diaphragm, in retroperitoneal nodes, or elsewhere.

Because this patient has a poorly differentiated cancer, I would recommend that she be treated with chemotherapy postoperatively, even if no other disease is present. Therefore I do not recommend reoperation for formal surgical staging biopsies. I think it *would* be reasonable to get a CT scan of the abdomen and pelvis as a baseline study to be sure there are no unsuspected abnormalities identified and then to treat her with platinum-based chemotherapy such as carboplatin (250 mg/m^2) and paclitaxel (Taxol) (135 mg/m^2). Other active combinations that have been reported include platinum, doxorubicin (Adriamycin), and cyclophosphamide or platinum and cyclophosphamide.

Reexploration for definitive staging might be considered, but since it would not change my management, I do not recommend it. If, because of the patient's reluctance to undergo chemotherapy, the option of no postoperative therapy was being strongly considered, then reoperation for comprehensive surgical/pathological staging would be absolutely indicated. There is a moderate risk of persistent unrecognized metastatic disease in this incompletely staged patient.

There are almost no data available concerning radiotherapy in carcinoma of the fallopian tubes. However, a retrospective analysis of 115 patients showed some benefit of pelvic radiation (2).

References

1. Norden AJ. Primary carcinoma of the fallopian tube: A 20-year literature review. Obstet Gynecol Survey 1994; 49:349–361.
2. Klein M, Rosen A, Lahousen M, et al. The evaluation of adjunctive therapy after surgery for primary carcinoma of the fallopian tube. Arch Gynecol Obstet 1994; 255:14–24.

PHYSICIAN'S RESPONSE

LEO LAGASSE

This patient requires reexploration to stage the tumor and complete the operation. Prior to surgery, posteroanterior and lateral chest films and a CA-125 are required. Some surgeons would obtain an abdominal pelvic CT to help identify any enlarged lymph nodes, but this evaluation can be made at surgery. The groins should be clinically examined carefully with a plan to excise any suspicious or enlarged inguinal nodes.

After complete bowel preparation, surgery should be carried out through a midline incision and should include the following:

Repeat cytologic washings from pelvis, right paracolic gutters, right diaphragm

Hysterectomy (bilateral salpingo-oophorectomy)

Bilateral pelvic and paraaortic lymphadenectomy to the level of the renal arteries

Omentectomy, appendectomy

Removal of any suspicious groin node masses

Removal of all resectable metastatic nodules

Cauterization or argon beam coagulation of all nonresectable metastases

Random peritoneal biopsies from pelvis, small and large intestine, diaphragm

Careful clinical evaluation of entire small and large intestine

All patients with high-grade carcinoma of the fallopian tube require post operative chemotherapy. While not specifically studied in tubal cancers, results in patients with ovarian cancer suggest that paclitaxel (Taxol) combined with either cisplatin or carboplatin offers the best treatment results. Cyclophosphamide would be an acceptable substitute for Taxol. Chemotherapy is given every 4 weeks for six courses.

During chemotherapy, monitoring of disease status consists of monthly abdominal and pelvic examination and CA-125 measurements. During the first posttreatment year, these same follow-up procedures would be carried out every 2 months. The value of routine abdominal pelvic CT is not clearly established but it is reasonable to recommend it at 1-year follow-up.

The value of routine second-look operative restaging has not been demonstrated, though many experimental treatment protocols require surgical reassessment to document response. A second-look procedure may be laparotomy or laparoscopy. When the second look is positive, salvage therapy can be begun immediately. Even with a negative second look, many patients ultimately will have a recurrence of cancer, but the addition of consolidation therapy has not yet been found useful in decreasing these later recurrences.

The management of patients who show evidence of recurrence during follow-up either by clinical exam or rising CA-125 is controversial. Some will suggest watching for further progression, some will resume chemotherapy without surgery, while others will carry out surgery with maximal tumor removal and then follow with chemotherapy.

While there are only a few studies which address this point, results in ovarian cancer suggest longer survival in recurrent patients who have maximal tumor removal before resuming chemotherapy. Restarting chemotherapy without pathological proof of recurrence might expose some patients who did not have recurrence to cytotoxic treatment. Following patients with evidence of recurrence without therapy will presumably make successful treatment later less likely. Thus, many believe that surgery followed by chemotherapy is the most logical approach to recurrent disease.

PHYSICIAN'S RESPONSE

R. F. OZOLS

Although it is stated that this 35-year-old woman underwent emergency surgery for presumed ectopic pregnancy and was found to have an apparently localized fallopian carcinoma, it is unclear exactly what surgery was performed other than presumably removal of the involved ovary and tube. The histology of the tumor was that of a poorly differentiated fallopian carcinoma. It should be pointed out, however, that it is frequently difficult to establish the origin of tumors found in the fallopian tube and that many are the result of metastases, most commonly from the ovary. Fallopian tumors are much less frequent than ovarian tumors. They have many biological similarities to the much more common epithelial ovarian carcinomas. However, they also appear to have some clinically significant differences. These tumors can spread throughout the abdonominal cavity and lead to widespread intraabdominal carcinomatosis. However, in contrast to ovarian cancer, fallopian tube carcinomas are more frequently diagnosed at an earlier stage than ovarian cancer because, as the tumor grows in the fallopian tube, it frequently leads to acute symptoms of abdominal pain and vaginal bleeding or discharge. For patients who do present with metastatic disease throughout the abdomen, the overall prognosis is similar to that of ovarian cancer. Most but not all studies have reported similar sensitivity to platinum-based chemotherapy, which had represented the standard of care for advanced-stage fallopian tube carcinomas after debulking surgery. Consequently, for advanced disease, the principles that apply to the management of ovarian cancer likewise pertain to fallopian tube carcinomas.

There appear to be some clinical differences between early-stage ovarian cancer and early-stage fallopian tube carcinomas. Pelvic and paraaortic lymph nodes are frequent sites of unsuspected metastases from fallopian tube primaries. In contrast to ovarian cancer, where in early stages the tumor's degree of differentiation has a marked impact upon survival and is a primary determinant in the selection of postoperative therapy, it appear that the histologic grade has less impact on prognosis in early-stage fallopian tube carcinomas. Recently, in retrospective studies, it has also been demonstrated that patients with apparently localized fallopian tube carcinomas have a significantly worse prognosis than those with early-stage ovarian carcinoma. In a European study, the 5-year survival for early-stage ovarian cancer was > 75%, compared with 50.8% for fallopian tube carcinoma of equal stage.

This particular patient had not undergone a comprehensive staging laparotomy. She does not appear to have gross disease on the basis of a less than optimal visual inspection at the time of the emergency surgery. Furthermore, even if she had undergone a comprehensive staging laparotomy including a hysterectomy, bilateral salpingo-oophorectomy, lymph node sampling, exploration of the diaphragm, and multiple blind biopsies of peritoneal surfaces, which would have possibly established the fallopian tube to be the primary site of the tumor and have failed to show any other sites of disease, she would still be a candidate for some type of adjuvant therapy since, as noted, patients with early-stage fallopian tube carcinomas are at a high risk for recurrence. The optimum form of postoperative adjuvant therapy, however, has not been established for these rare tumors of the gynecological tract. Parallel to the situation with ovarian cancer, treatment options would include combination chemotherapy or pelvic and abdominal radiotherapy.

My specific recommendations for this patient would be to undergo a comprehensive staging and therapeutic laparotomy as described above. Following such a procedure, I would recommend a course of chemotherapy depending upon the extent of disease. It has recently been demonstrated that paclitaxel plus cisplatin is superior to cisplatin plus cyclophosphamide in the treatment of patients with advanced suboptimal stage III and IV ovarian cancer. Consequently, since fallopian tube carcinomas have the same sensitivity to platinum compounds as epithelial carcinomas, I would also recommend paclitaxel plus a platinum compound to be used as the postoperative chemotherapy for this patient. The choice of dose and schedule of paclitaxel and the selection of which platinum compound to use (i.e., carboplatin or cisplatin) are issues that are being tested in epithelial ovarian cancer in prospective randomized trials by the Gynecologic Oncology Group (GOG). The GOG separates it clinical trials in ovarian cancer on the basis of stage and residual disease into three distinct categories: early-stage disease, optimal stage III, and suboptimal stages III and IV. If, after a comprehensive laparotomy, this patient were found to have small volume residual stage III disease, I would recommend six cycles of cisplatin plus paclitaxel. If, however, she were found to have early-stage fallopian tube carcinoma, my chemotherapy would likewise be tailored to the GOG studies. In previous studies it has been demonstrated that there was no difference between melphalan and intraperitoneal chromic phosphate (^{32}P) in patients with poor-prognosis early-stage epithelial ovarian carcinomas, and ^{32}P was selected for further evaluation against a combination of cisplatin plus cyclophosphamide because it had a more favorable toxicity profile than did melphalan. The results of this latter comparison have not yet been published. The GOG now will be evaluating three versus six cycles of paclitaxel plus carboplatin in early-stage ovarian carcinoma with poor prognostic features. Since there is a very high predilection for spread to retroperitoneal and inguinal lymph nodes, I would not recommend the use of ^{32}P in this patient. My recommendation would be for her to receive postoperative carboplatin plus paclitaxel if the laparotomy were to demonstrate localized fallopian tube carcinoma. I would treat her with six cycles of carboplatin dosed to an area under the curve of 7.5 together with paclitaxel at a dose of 175 mg/m^2 in a 3-hr infusion. After six cycles of chemotherapy, I would not perform a second-look procedure and merely follow the patient. If the patient did not accept the recommendation to undergo a formal staging laparotomy prior to initiation of chemotherapy, I would recommend that she receive chemotherapy with six cycles of paclitaxel plus either cisplatin or carboplatin as outlined above and then undergo a total abdominal hysterectomy and bilateral salpingo-oophorectomy (TAH/BSO).

References

Rosen AC, Sevelda P, Klein M, et al. A comparative analysis of management and prognosis in stage I and II fallopian tube carcinoma and epithelial ovarian cancer. Br J Cancer 1994; 69:577–579.

Hellström A-C, Silfverswärd C, Nilsson B, Pettersson F. Carcinoma of the fallopian tube: A clinical and histopathologic review. The Radiummhemmet series. Int J Gynecol Cancer 1994; 4:395–400.

PHYSICIAN'S RESPONSE

JAMES ROBERTS

Fallopian tube carcinoma is one of the rarest cancers, occurring in less than 1 in 1600 women. In spite of the fact that most of these women present, as did this woman, with pelvic pain, the condition is rarely diagnosed preoperatively. More often, the preop diagnosis is ectopic pregnancy, pelvic inflammatory disease, or an adnexal mass (1). Therefore, this case represents a rather typical preoperative presentation.

Due to the rarity of this entity, there are few clinical studies available to direct the course of care for these women. Instead, most physicians will approach this disease as if it were ovarian cancer. Its pathophysiology is very similar to that of ovarian cancer. Therefore, under optimal circumstances, this woman should be subjected to a complete surgical staging. This should include resection of the uterus, tubes, ovaries, omentum, pelvic lymph nodes, paraaortic lymph nodes, and as much tumor as is possible. In addition, washings and biopsies should be obtained from the pelvis, both colic gutters and subdiaphragmatic space. It can be expected that up to 20% of women undergoing such staging will be found to have additional disease in their abdomens.This staging can be done either via a laparotomy or laparoscopy.

Since this woman has recently undergone an operative procedure, it may be difficult to subject her to another for the same pathological process. The staging can be foregone, but under that circumstance one must assume one of two conditions. First, it could be assumed that there is no additional disease present and that therefore no additional therapy would be required. This would result in the clinical recurrence of cancer in at least 20% of the cases. While it is my experience that fallopian tube carcinomas respond to chemotherapy slightly better than ovarian cancer, those women who are left to recur will be advanced when diagnosed. At this point, they will be unlikely to respond completely to any therapy. Second, it can be assumed that there is residual cancer present. Under this situation, it would be necessary to treat this woman with chemotherapy. Once again, there are no clinical studies to support the use of any particular regimen. Most oncologists recommend the same regimens used for the treatment of ovarian cancer. Therefore, this woman should be started on cisplatin 75 mg/m^2 and paclitaxel 175 mg/m^2 every 3 weeks for a total of six courses.

This decision can be simplified by reviewing the pathology. It is usual to treat high-grade ovarian cancer with chemotherapy, even early-stage disease. Thus, staging may not be needed for this woman if high-grade disease is present. In addition, it has been shown that the depth of invasion of a fallopian tube carcinoma correlates with the chance of recurrence (2). The facts regarding this should be obtained from the pathologist. These two factors make it easy to decide that this woman should be treated with chemotherapy.

Since formal surgical staging will not be done, a second-look laparotomy or laparoscopy should be considered once the chemotherapy has been completed. This will serve to check the status of the disease as well as to complete the staging. This information can then be used to plan consolidation therapy.

References

1. Roberts JA, Lifschitz SG. Primary adenocarcinoma of the fallopian tube. Gynecol Oncol 1982; 13:301–308.
2. Peters WA III, Anderson WA, Hopkins MP, et al. Prognostic features of carcinoma of the fallopian tube. Obstet Gynecol 1988; 71:757–762.

6

Vaginal Cancer: Stage I Bulky Squamous Cell Carcinoma

CASE

A 68-year-old woman arrives in your office, appearing older than her stated age. She has been experiencing some vaginal bleeding for the past 6 months and now presents for examination. She is moderately obese and appears to be sitting with a great deal of discomfort. The chest is clear. The heart shows a regular rate and rhythm. No abdominal masses or suspicious inguinal nodes are palpable. On examination of the vulva, it is found to be quite moist and the lower third of the vagina is filled with a bulky squamous cell carcinoma attached to the right lateral and posterior vaginal walls. Abdominal pelvic computed tomography (CT) shows no evidence of metastatic disease. Chest x-ray is normal. Complete blood count and chemistries are normal.

PHYSICIANS' RESPONSE

RICHARD REID
GARTH D. PHIBBS

To complete the workup of this patient, sigmoidoscopy should be done to rule out infiltration of the rectal mucosa.

As in this instance, most patients are diagnosed with Fédération Internationale de Gynecologie et d'Obstétrique (FIGO) stage II disease. Spread is principally by direct extension into the paracolpium and by lymphatic embolization from the rich lymphatic anastomosis within the vaginal muscularis. Because of embryologic factors, tumors from opposite ends of the vagina display different patterns of local invasion and lymphatic drainage. During embryogenesis, vaginal epithelium is formed by ingrowth of cloacal endoderm into the solid cord of mesoderm that represents the future vagina. Hence, there are no intrinsic differences between vaginal intraepithelial neoplasias. However, when invasion occurs, the differences in muscularis derivation between the upper two-thirds (mullerian) and lower one-third (urogenital sinus) have important clinical implications. First, upper vaginal lesions drain to the pelvic nodes; lower vaginal lesions are primarily directed to the inguinofemoral nodes. Second, direct anterior or posterior invasion in lesions of the upper two-thirds is limited by the presence of two well-defined barriers: the vesicovaginal and rectovaginal spaces. However, there are no planes of cleavage separating the lower third of the vaginal muscularis from urethra (anteriorly), pubococcygeus muscle (laterally), and perineal body/ lower rectum (posteriorly). Thus, for lower vaginal tumors, direct urethral or rectal invasion is more common, clear margins of surgical resection are more difficult to attain, and surgery following radiation therapy carries a higher risk of fistula formation. In addition, lower-third lesions carry a significant risk of inguinofemoral nodal involvement, which is best managed by dissection prior to radiation therapy.

The preferred treatment for vaginal cancer is radiation therapy, with surgery being reserved for failures or recurrences. As such, this patient would normally receive external beam teletherapy to the pelvis and inguinal areas as needed, along with full fall-off fields to cover the vagina and posterior vulva. Once tumor volume shrinks, usually following 5000 cGy, additional 1000- to 2000-cGy fields should be considered. In general, large tumor beds should be boosted by *brachytherapy* using either *intracavitary* or *interstitial* techniques. If facilities exist, interstitial application using a Seyed implant is preferred (1). As pioneered by Boronow et al. (2), radiation can be combined with wide excision of the tumor bed. In such instances, closure by transposition of a suitable myocutaneous flap (e.g., gluteus maximus or gracilis) will improve local blood supply, thereby offering some protection against fistula formation. Plastic reconstruction is also more likely to preserve good cosmetic appearance and effective sexual function (3).

By analogy with standard chemoradiation regimens for head and neck squamous cancers and, more recently, advanced vulvar cancers (4), consideration could be given to concurrent infusional 5-fluorouracil as a radiation sensitizer. While there have been no formal protocols extending this principle to the management of vaginal carcinoma, potential advantages are obvious. Standard radiation therapy for bulky tumors (perhaps requiring a dose of 7500 cGy) is always limited by the proximity of bladder and bowel. Tailored interstitial implants using open or endoscopic assistance along with mobilization of intestine and omental interposition are often helpful in achieving tumoricidal doses in these instances.

References

1. DiSaia PG, Creasman W. Clinical Gynecologic Oncology, 4th ed. St. Louis: Mosby-Year Book, 1993.
2. Boronow RC, Hickman BT, Reagan MT, et al. Combined therapy as an alternative to exenteration for locally advanced vulvovaginal cancer: II. Results, complications, and dosimetric and surgical considerations. Am J Clin Oncol 1987; 10:171.
3. Achauer BM, Braly P, Berman ML, DiSaia PG. Immediate vaginal reconstruction following resection for malignancy using the gluteal thigh flap. Gynecol Oncol 1984; 19:79.
4. Thomas G, Dembo A, DePetaillo A, et al. Concurrent radiation and chemotherapy in vulvar carcinoma. Gynecol Oncol 1989; 36:181.

PHYSICIAN'S RESPONSE

JOHN MIKUTA

The major considerations in this case involve the appropriate management of this lesion in order to produce optimal control of the tumor with a minimal amount of morbidity. The case presentation does not clarify several important issues. The first is whether the lesion is a primary vaginal lesion and not one that has arisen secondary to a cancer of the cervix or upper portion of the vagina. Second, because of its location, it is important to determine whether the lesion is mobile or whether it is fixed to the perivaginal tissues, and to what exact extent. This would decide the stage of the cancer. Much of this can be determined by a thorough rectovaginal examination and, of course, a proctosigmoidoscopy along with a complete colon examination should be a part of the evaluation. Absent any obvious further lesions, as suggested, the choices of management would depend on the following:

The patient's age and obesity and the fact that she appears older than her stated age would be factors in the decision against a surgical approach. It appears that the ideal choice of management would accomplish the desired result without altering the patient's functional anatomy and that would avoid the performance of a colostomy. In view of the absence of local or distant metastases, I would favor managing the patient by external radiation therapy, covering all of the pelvis and including the inguinal areas, followed by local implantation of either iridium or a vaginal mold with cesium. This may be combined with a preoperative sensitizing dose of a chemotherapeutic agent such as cisplatin. It is important that all of the vagina and external portion of the vulva be covered by the external radiation fields.

This treatment provides roughly a 50% chance of cure, depending, once again, on the extent and sensitivity of the tumor. If the treatment fails to accomplish the desired result, there still is the option of a posterior exenteration.

One might question whether pretreatment biopsy of inguinal and retroperitoneal nodes would be of any value. In the presence of a normal abdominal/pelvic CT scan and nonpalpable or nonsuspicious inguinal nodes, I think pretreatment biopsy, particularly prior to radiation, would only delay the treatment and increase morbidity without accomplishing anything substantial.

PHYSICIANS' RESPONSE

MANUEL A. PENALVER
LOREN SIMOVITCH

The 68-year-old woman in this case presents with 6 months of vaginal bleeding, appearing somewhat ill, and with what is assumed to be a biopsy-proven primary squamous cell carcinoma of the lower third of the vagina. This patient presents with the most common symptom associated with this disease, and since she is symptomatic, her presentation is suggestive of invasive disease. In an asymptomatic stage, careful physical examination with the help of Pap smear and Lugol's solution can identify abnormal areas of tissue in a preinvasive form.

Primary malignant tumors of the vagina constitute only 1 to 2% of all gynecological malignancies, and squamous cell carcinoma is the most common histological type. Vaginal cancer is most often found in the seventh or eighth decade but is not limited to this age group. Generally, exophytic growth is seen and the disease spreads locally and invades the underlying mucosa and muscularis. Due to its anatomic location, extension to the bladder or rectum is a key pattern to detect. After local spread, lymphatic invasion and metastases account for mode of spread. This patient presents with a posteriorly located tumor in the lower third of the vagina, so that lymphatic drainage will be primarily to the inguinal nodes and subsequently to the pelvic nodes.

To date the patient's abdominopelvic CT scan, chest x-ray, CBC, and blood chemistries are negative. The cancer workup, however, should include an evaluation for local or distant spread analogous to that of cervical carcinoma. A thorough history and physical exam would include rectovaginal examination, chest x-ray, intravenous pyelogram, cystoscopy, proctosigmoidoscopy, and possibly a lymphangiogram and barium enema. A negative endocervical curettage and endometrial biopsy in the absence of a cervical target lesion adequately assures a primary vaginal squamous cell carcinoma rather than a metastasis from a primary cervical cancer. Carcinoembryonic antigen (CEA) and squamous cell carcinoma (SCC) antigen tumor markers may also aid in subsequent surveillance if they are elevated.

From the information provided, this patient most likely has stage II disease with carcinoma limited to the vaginal mucosa and submucosa without extension toward the pelvic side walls. With extension to the pelvic walls, the lesion would be stage III; with involvement of the rectum or bladder or bullous edema of the bladder, stage IVA; and with involvement of organs outside the true pelvis, stage IVB.

The curability of vaginal squamous cell carcinoma is primarily a function of the stage of the disease at the time of presentation. Less important contributing factors include the location of the tumor within the vagina and the tumor grade. Radiation has evolved to be the most common mode of therapy, although surgery can provide equivalent cure rates in early disease. Often the patients are elderly, with associated medical problems, making surgery less desirable. Depending on the location of the tumor—with proximity to bladder or rectum—the ability to obtain clear surgical margins makes surgery a more difficult choice.

When patients are amenable to surgical therapy, the operation includes removal of the exophytic lesion with radical hysterectomy, pelvic lymphadenectomy, and partial or complete vaginectomy. Vaginal grafting to preserve function may be required. Surgery is most often used for upper vaginal lesions; since in this case the lesion is noted to be in the lower vagina, this patient would be more amenable to radiation therapy. Radiation for this patient should entail whole pelvic external radiation of 4000 to 5000 cGy with concomitant intercavitary radiation to deliver 3000 to 4000 cGy to the vaginal area. The 5-year disease-free survival period following this treatment is in the range of 32 to 58% according to various reports. Recurrences are most commonly locally and occur primarily within 2 years of therapy. Recurrent or persistent vaginal carcinoma requires ultraradical surgery, which has a response rate of approximately 40%.

PHYSICIANS' RESPONSE

TALLY LEVY
ROBERT GIRTANNER
ALAN KAPLAN

Primary carcinoma of the vagina is a rare tumor representing 1 to 2% of all gynecologic malignancies. Some 80 to 90% of these lesions are squamous cell cancers, which usually occur in older women in the seventh and eighth decades of life and are most frequently located on the upper posterior wall of the vagina. Although some few asymptomatic early lesions may be found by abnormal cytology, most patients present with abnormal bleeding. Other less frequent presenting symptoms are vaginal discharge, dysuria, and pelvic pain.

The international staging scheme for vaginal cancer is clinical. The described pelvic findings suggest that this is a bulky stage I lesion, as no mention is made of extension into the paravaginal tissues. The evaluation thus far has included an abdominal pelvic CT scan and chest x-ray, both of which were negative. Proctoscopy should also be done, as the cancer involves the posterior vaginal wall.

Pretreatment measurements of serum tumor markers such as CEA and squamous cell carcinoma (SCC) antigen can be helpful in surveillance if they are elevated (1). The primary regional nodes for a lesion arising from the lower third of the vagina are the inguinal nodes, and these were noted to be clinically negative.

The treatment of carcinoma of the vagina is highly individualized contingent primarily on the age and medical status of the patient and stage, size, and location of the lesion. In general, we lean toward surgery in the young patient if this is feasible. The appropriate regional nodal treatment is determined by location. Size, stage, and proximity to the bladder or rectum are critical factors in selecting surgery or radiation as primary therapy. The limiting factor in the use of vaginectomy for early lesions is the proximity of the lesion to the bladder or rectum. The vesicovaginal and rectovaginal septa are quite thin, and this compromises the surgical margins. Ultraradical or exenterative surgery with removal of the bladder and/or rectum is not indicated as primary therapy for early lesions, as these patients do equally well with radiation. An exenteration is occasionally considered for an advanced lesion that responds poorly to external radiation.

The case presented is a 68-year-old woman with a bulky, apparently stage I squamous cell carcinoma of the lower third of the posterior and right lateral vaginal walls. A radical vaginectomy can be considered for small stage I lesions; however, we do not think this would be an adequate operation for this patient. Radiation thus becomes the treatment of choice.

The first step in the radiation program should be external radiation. This is given to shrink the tumor mass and to treat the appropriate regional lymph nodes. The standard pelvic field should be enlarged to include the lower portion of the vagina and the inguinal nodes. After completion of the external radiation, highly individualized local therapy is given. The most important part of the local therapy is the interstitial implant because of the necessary depth dose. This is usually done with a template of interstitial needles. Intracavitary implants and transvaginal cone therapy may be used to augment the dose, but these are rarely used alone except for small stage I lesions confined to the surface of the vagina. If shrinkage is not adequate after the external radiation to allow effective local therapy, we consider exenterative surgery.

References

1. Maruo T, Shibata K, Kimura A, et al. Tumor-associated antigen TA-4 in the monitoring of the effects of therapy of squamous cell carcinoma of the uterine cervix. Cancer 1985; 56:302–308.

7

Recurrent Granulosa Cell Tumor of the Ovary

CASE

A 55-year-old patient undergoes a staging laparotomy and is found to have a stage I granulosa cell tumor of the ovary. No postoperative adjuvant therapy is administered.

The patient remains symptom-free. However, on a routine follow-up pelvic examination performed 24 months after the patient's initial surgery, a left-sided pelvic mass is detected. Computed tomography reveals no disease other than the recurrent mass in the pelvis. Laboratory evaluation is unremarkable.

PHYSICIANS' RESPONSE

EDWARD J. KAPLAN
DATTA NORI

Granulosa cell tumors are sex-cord stromal tumors that account for 2 to 3% of all ovarian neoplasms and, along with theca cell tumors, constitute the majority of functioning ovarian malignancies. Both frequently secrete estrogen, but—in contrast to thecomas, which are benign—granulosa cell tumors carry a malignant potential of approximately 25%. Most granulosa cell tumors, like the one in our patient, are stage I at presentation and are treated surgically with excellent results. The long-term survival rate for stage I patients exceeds 90%. Because of the rarity of these tumors, there have been no randomized trials regarding adjuvant treatment. Postoperative pelvic irradiation is frequently given empirically.

Failures often occur more than 5 years after initial treatment, and salvages are anecdotal. Most recurrences are intraperitoneal, although nodal and distant metastases have been reported. In an early report on five patients with recurrent granulosa tumors, results were mixed. Radiotherapy was delivered to one patient postoperatively and two patients at the time of failure, but the interval between recurrences tended to be long and the impact of radiotherapy is uncertain (1). In Sweden, where the incidence of ovarian cancer is the highest in the world, the recurrence rate among more than 300 cases in the literature has been reported at between 9 and 21%, with no documented salvages. Patients there have received postoperative radiotherapy for decades.

Our patient has a local recurrence in the pelvis, and despite its being isolated, this is usually an ominous sign in most gynecological malignancies. Optimal therapy for recurrent lesions in general and side wall disease in particular has not been determined. The disease-free interval was shorter than expected for this tumor, which may signify an especially aggressive recurrence. Even assuming that all gross disease has been removed, there is no way to resect this lesion without leaving behind microscopic residual.

Since granulosa cell tumors are known to be radioresponsive, it is reasonable to integrate irradiation into the salvage regimen. This recurrence cannot be approached with intracavitary high- or low-dose brachytherapy. Other options include external beam therapy, which she did not receive at the time of her initial surgery, and/or interstitial brachytherapy.

Our recommendation is exploratory laparotomy to rule out intraperitoneal disease and assess the extent of her side-wall disease, debulk it, release any bowel adhesions, and perhaps insert a bowel sling or tissue expander to separate the bowel from the area of the recurrence. For an isolated side-wall recurrence that is incompletely resected, a permanent iodine-125 (^{125}I) volume implant is required, while, following gross total resection, a single-plane implant embedded in Gelfoam is positioned over the tumor bed, covering an area out to 1 cm beyond the tumor margins in both cases (2). A pelvic wall plasty using an omental pedicle graft may then be brought down to act as an additional buffer, reducing the bowel and bladder doses to < 25%. We would give 130 to 160 Gy minimum peripheral dose to the tumor residuum via a ^{125}I implant followed by 45 Gy whole pelvis irradiation. We would expect 15 to 30% local control at 5 years using this approach.

References

Simmons RL, Sciarra JJ. Treatment of late recurrent granulosa cell tumors of the ovary. Surg Gynecol Obstet 1967; 124:65–70.

Nori D, Hilaris BS, Kim HS, et al. Interstitial irradiation in recurrent gynecological cancer. IJROBP 1981; 7:1513–1517.

PHYSICIAN'S RESPONSE

EDWARD PARTRIDGE

This 55-year-old patient very likely has recurrent granulosa cell tumor of the ovary. Although it is not clear that she was adequately staged at the original laparotomy, it would certainly have been appropriate to recommend no adjunctive therapy to a patient with an apparent stage I granulosa cell tumor.

Other than a preoperative serum Inhibin level, no further workup is indicated at this time in this otherwise healthy patient. Serum Inhibit level has been reported to be a useful tumor marker in this disease (1).

In the absence of ascites or other evidence of intraabdominal or extraabdominal disease, laparotomy with resection of this lesion is indicated. This laparotomy will not only confirm the suspected diagnosis of recurrent disease but may also, again, render the patient clinically disease-free.

At laparotomy, extent of disease should be determined and complete resection attempted if technically possible. If apparent disease is limited to the one area noted on CT scan and is resected completely, it would be appropriate to surgically stage the patient. This surgical assessment should include pelvic and paraaortic node biopsies, omentectomy, washings, and perhaps peritoneal biopsies. Surgical staging would be particularly important if complete staging were not performed at the original surgical procedure.

If the recurrent disease is incompletely resected or surgical staging reveals residual microscopic disease, postoperative chemotherapy is definitely indicated. However, if a single isolated recurrence is completely resected and no evidence of disease elsewhere is noted, the role of adjunctive chemotherapy is not clear. Follow-up with serum inhibin levels with institution of chemotherapy only in the event of rising levels or other evidence of subsequent recurrence would be a very reasonable approach.

In the event that chemotherapy is indicated, the most effective therapy would appear to be a combination of bleomycin, etoposide, and platinol (cisplatin) (BEP). Although radiation and other combinations of chemotherapy have been utilized in the past, their relative value is unclear. The promising report by Colombo (2) of 6 Cr and 3 PR in 11 patients treated by Platinol, Velban (vinblastine), and bleomycin (PVB) led to the adoption of BEP as the combination of choice by the Gynecologic Oncology Group for their current study of patients with this disease. This study is still open for accrual and all patients with recurrent disease including this one should be treated on this protocol if eligible.

In the absence of convincing evidence that radiotherapy or other combination are effective, BEP is the current treatment of choice for nonprotocol patients.

References

1. Lapbohn RE, Burger HG, Bohma J, et al. Inhibin as a marker for granulosa-cell tumors. N Engl J Med 1989; 321:790.
2. Colombo N, Sessa C, Landon F, et al. Cisplatin, vinblastine, and bleomycin combination chemotherapy in metastatic granulosa cell tumor of the ovary. Obstet Gynecol 1986; 67:265.

PHYSICIAN'S RESPONSE

C. R. HARRISON

Granulosa cell tumors occur at a mean age of 53, are stage I in 90% of patients, and are bilateral in less than 5%. Postmenopausal women account for 50% of all patients with this disease, and evidence of endocrine activity is present in over 75%. Superficial cells are noted in 80% of Pap smears; endometrial hyperplasia or polyps have been reported in 50% with an associated history of postmenopausal or abnormal uterine bleeding, and 5 to 15% have endometrial adenocarcinoma. Survival is related to stage, size, mitotic activity, and age. Five- and 10-year survival is 95% with stage I disease. Recurrent disease may appear as late as 20 to 30 years following diagnosis. The risk of recurrence is low for lesions less than 5 cm, 20% for lesions 5 to 15 cm, and over 30% for larger lesions. Tumors with more than two mitotic figures per 10 high-power fields and those with a diffuse (sarcomatoid) appearance also have a greater risk of recurrence. The slow rate of growth and relative indolence of the disease has led to the watchful management recommended to this patient. There is no proven beneficial role for adjuvant chemotherapy or radiation therapy in patients with stage I disease.

A review of this patient's report would be of interest. What precisely was observed at surgery, and what was performed? It is possible that only her involved ovary was removed and that the pelvis was inspected visually. If she had an emergent operation for a hemoperitoneum, which complicates this disease 5 to 20% of the time, she may have had an exploration, removal of the involved ovary, and only a gross inspection of the pelvis, resulting in the impression that she had stage I disease. In that situation, rupture and peritoneal reaction may lead to an incorrect assessment regarding stage. Was the recurrent mass on the same side as the original tumor or in the contralateral ovary? If the uterus was left in situ, was an endometrial biopsy accomplished to exclude a carcinoma? Could the mass represent metastatic endometrial cancer? For the sake of the remainder of this discussion, it will be assumed that the "staging laparotomy," in light of her age, included washings for cytology, a total abdominal hysterectomy, bilateral salpingo-oophorectomy, peritoneal biopsies, an omentectomy, pelvic and periaortic lymph node sampling, and biopsies of any suspicious peritoneal, mesenteric, or serosal bowel lesions.

The original pathological material additionally must be reviewed, particularly as the recurrence is relatively early for a granulosa cell tumor. The less well differentiated forms of this disease, such as the diffuse pattern, must be distinguished from a small-cell carcinoma, metastatic endometrial stromal sarcoma to the ovary, or undifferentiated carcinoma. An elevated serum inhibin would support the diagnosis of a recurrent granulosa cell tumor.

The optimal therapy of recurrent or advanced-stage disease is not known. The volume of residual disease appears to correlate with chemotherapy response and survival and provides a basis for surgical re-exploration and debulking. Subsequent therapy has been influenced by intraoperative findings, metastatic spread pattern, volume of residual disease and the histopathology of the mass. In localized disease, postoperative radiation therapy has been employed, with some long-term survivors reported. Colombo et al. treated 11 women with stage III to IV or recurrent granulosa cell tumors with cisplatin, vinblastine, and bleomycin. There were 6 pathologic complete responses and 3 partial responses. All of the complete responders had residual disease of less than 2 cm. Median follow-up of the complete responders was 14 months. Five patients remained NED, and 1 died of disease at 22 months. Of the 3 partial responders, 2 succumbed to a "toxic death." The third patient had 2- to 5-cm residual disease noted at the time of recurrence 8 years following initial diagnosis, had persistent disease noted at second look, and was clinically NED 34 months later. Gershenson et al reported on 5 patients with recurrent or stage II to III granulosa cell tumors treated with cisplatin, doxorubicin, and cyclophosphamide following surgical resection. Of these, 4 patients had microscopic residua, and 3 were re-explored at completion of chemotherapy (the fourth patient had progressive disease and died at 4 months). Two of the three patients had pathologically complete responses and remained NED for 17 and 48 months. The third patient had stable disease documented, received whole abdominal radiotherapy, and was clinically NED at 13 months. The fifth patient in the series had residual disease greater than 2 cm and died of disease at 36 months.

As this patient has not received any adjuvant therapy, I would recommend surgical exploration, particularly if the clinical exam and CT scan permitted a conclusion that the disease could be optimally debulked. In light of the proven capacity of this tumor to recur, if it is indeed the same disease, adjuvant therapy, ideally governed in a protocol setting, should be offered.

References

Colombo N, Sessa C, Landoni F, et al. Cisplatin, vinblastine, and bleomycin combination chemotherapy in metastatic granulosa cell tumor of the ovary. Obstet Gynecol 1986; 67:265.

Gershenson, DM, Copeland, LJ, Kavanagh JJ, et al. Treatment of metastatic stromal tumors of the ovary with cisplatin, doxorubicin, and cyclophosphamide. Obstet Gynecol 1987; 70:765.

Morrow CP, Curtin JP, Townsend DE, eds. Gonadal stroma and germ cell ovarian tumors. In: Synopsis of Gynecologic Oncology, 4th Ed. New York: Churchill Livingstone 1993.

Scully RE. Sex Cord–Stromal tumors, In: Tumors of the Ovary and Maldeveloped Gonads. Washington, DC: Armed Forces Institute of Pathology, 1982.

Williams SD, Gershenson DM, Horowitz CJ, Scully RE: Ovarian germ cell and stromal tumors. In: Principles and Practice of Gynecologic Oncology. Philadelphia: Lippincott, 1992.

Young RH, Scully RE: Sex cord–Stromal, steroid cell, and other ovarian tumors with endocrine, paraendocrine, and paraneoplastic manifestations. In: Blaustein's Pathology of the Female Genital Tract, 3d ed. New York: Springer-Verlag, 1987.

PHYSICIAN'S RESPONSE

HUGH R.K. BARBER

This tumor belongs to the gonadal stromal group of tumors. Recurrences are usually local and characteristically recur 5 or more years after the initial therapy. The overall malignancy rate is 25 percent and the bilaterality rate is 5 percent. It is unusual in that the histological appearance of a granulosa cell tumor is no index of its final behavior.

Since the patient was 53 years of age at the time of initial treatment, it is assumed that there was removal of the uterus, tubes, and ovaries and biopsies of any suspicious areas. Some 25% of granulosa cell tumors function, but there is no evidence that this is so in this case.

The two significant features of this tumor—indicative in this patient of a poor prognosis—are the age of the patient (over 40 years of age) and tumors measuring 15 cm or more, as well as the early recurrence in this patient. The size of the tumor is not given, but the patient has two findings pointing to a poor prognosis. However, in general, stage has proved to be more important than histological or the nuclear grade.

The patient ideally should be seen in follow-up every 3 months during the first year by careful pelvic examination. The patient should be instructed to take an enema before the examination so that a proper pelvic examination can be carried out (i.e., vaginal, rectovaginal, and rectal examinations). Sonograms are ordered as clinical judgment indicates.

Tumor markers—such as CA-125, CEA, NB/70K, and LASA-P—have limited value in following patients with granulosa cell tumors. However, serum inhibin provides an excellent tumor marker for following patients who have had a diagnosis of granulosa cell tumor. Inhibin is an ovarian hormone that inhibits the secretion of follicle-stimulating hormone by the anterior pituitary gland.

Women with granulosa cell tumors of the ovary have elevated serum inhibin concentrations. This provides a wonderful way for following up and monitoring any treatment.

Currently, this patient has a left-sided mass. After a workup that includes an intravenous pyelogram and a barium enema, a bowel prep is indicated, followed by an exploratory laparotomy. Ideally, the tumor should be excised in its entirety; if not, clips should be used to outline the tumor, because granulosa cell tumors are usually very responsive to irradiation therapy. The external radiation therapy should be given from L5 to the symphysis and should include the field between the heads of the femur (protecting the neck of the femur). Having marked the site where tumor was left, the irradiation therapist can give a booster dose to this area. The decision about chemotherapy will depend on the findings of spread outside the pelvis. The first-line therapy recommended is cyclophosphamide and Platinol, with paclitaxel (Taxol) given as a second-line drug. Creatinine clearances must be evaluated before Platinol therapy is given.

The patient should have careful follow-up examinations at 3-month intervals during the first year and, following this, at 6-month intervals. Serum inhibin concentrations are very important in monitoring therapy for granulosa cell tumor. Since granulosa cell tumors may recur up to 15 years or more following treatment, the follow-up must be carefully planned for long-term evaluation.

References

Healy DL, Bulzer HG, Mannes P, et al. Elevated serum inhibitor concentrations in postmenopausal women with ovarian tumors. N Engl J Med 1993; 1539:329.

Barber HRK (ed). Ovarian Carcinoma Etiology: Diagnosis and Treatment, 3d ed. New York: Springer-Verlag, 1993.

8

Completely Resected Stage III Granulosa Cell Tumor of the Ovary

CASE

A 42-year-old woman presents to her gynecologist with abdominal pain of 3 weeks duration. Physical examination reveals a left-sided pelvic mass. Computed tomography (CT) reveals an enlarged left ovary.

At exploratory laparotomy the patient is found to have an ovarian mass with several pelvic implants and nodules in the omentum. There is no ascites or evidence of gross disease in the upper abdomen and all lymph node regions appear normal. All macroscopic disease is resected.

Pathology reveals a granulosa cell tumor. Washings are negative.

PHYSICIANS' RESPONSE

JUDY CHENG
WILLIAM MANN

Granulosa cell tumors are rare ovarian sex cord–stromal tumors, constituting 1 to 2% of all ovarian malignancies. Typically, these patients present with abnormal uterine bleeding, abdominal pain, or abdominal distension. Peak incidence for adult-type granulosa tumors is between 50 and 55 years of age. More than half of all granulosa cell tumors are associated with estrogen production, which increases a given patient's risk of concurrent endometrial hyperplasia or carcinoma. Ordinarily, endometrial biopsy would be included as part of the patient's preoperative evaluation.

Traditionally, granulosa cell tumors have been considered low-grade malignancies, with the majority of patients presenting with stage I disease. In this situation, total abdominal hysterectomy and bilateral salpingo-oophorectomy appears to be adequate treatment, with an anticipated survival rate in the area of 90%. When childbearing is an issue, unilateral salpingo-oophorectomy is adequate therapy. Appropriate staging procedures (omentectomy, pelvic and paraaortic node biopsies, peritoneal biopsies) are also performed.

With more advanced disease, however, survival approaches 25 to 50% at 5 years. Recurrences, even in patients presenting with early disease, may appear many years distant from initial presentation.

In early disease, it has been suggested that initial tumor size, stage, mitotic rate, the S-phase fraction, nuclear area, and nuclear perimeter are prognostic factors. However, in advanced disease, it is not clear that any of these factors are significant.

In the patient under discussion, we agree with the approach of total abdominal hysterectomy, bilateral salpingo-oophorectomy, omentectomy, and resection of all visible disease. It is our custom to sample pelvic and paraaortic lymph nodes or to resect enlarged nodes if encountered. If ascites is not present, washings are taken.

Experience with this tumor in advanced stages is so rare that there are no data to support cytoreductive surgery. However, we continue to pursue aggressive surgical cytoreduction, as this tumor is often indolent and slow-growing. Postoperatively, we believe that this patient will require adjuvant therapy. While there have been some suggestions that this tumor may be radiosensitive, our personal view is that whole abdominal irradiation in a patient who has undergone cytoreductive surgery is fraught with complications, including bowel obstruction and fistula. Therefore, we would prefer adjuvant chemotherapy. Again, no great clinical experience exists to favor one regimen over another. Our preference is for VAC (vincristine, actinomycin-D, and cyclophosphamide), but we recognize that others favor VBP (vinblastin, bleomycin, cisplatin) and other regimens. Even progestational therapy has been shown to benefit selected patients.

At this time we do not feel that there is a role for second-look surgery, and we would plan a course of therapy of approximately six cycles. We would then follow the patient expectantly. There has been some very preliminary evidence to suggest that inhibin may serve as a marker for granulosa cell tumors, although this assay is difficult to obtain. Recurrences would be treated with reexploration and resection and reinstitution of chemotherapy. Should progression occur during initial chemotherapy, an alternative regimen would then be instituted. Overall, one would expect this particular patient to have a guarded prognosis. We have, in a very few patients, obtained prolonged survival with secondary attempts at cytoreduction when recurrence was documented clinically.

References

Malmstrom H, Hogberg T, Risberg B, Simonsen E. Granulosa cell tumors of the ovary: Prognostic factors and outcome. Gynecol Oncol 1994; 52:50–55.

Young RE, Scully RE. Ovarian sex cord stromal tumors: Recent progress. Int J Gynecol Pathol 1980; 1:153–162.

PHYSICIANS' RESPONSE

WILLIAM A. CLIBY
MARY M. GALLENBERG
JOHN H. EDMONSON

This patient with stage III granulosa cell tumor has significant risk of recurrence based on the tumor's extraovarian spread. Although more indolent in its course, the granulosa cell tumor, when adjusted for stage of disease (1), eventually causes death in about the same proportion of its victims as does epithelial ovarian carcinoma. Thus, we would attempt to utilize our most promising and active therapeutic options aimed at the elimination of this cancer.

As undoubtedly had already been done in this case, we would perform a total abdominal hysterectomy/bilateral salpingo-oophorectomy and omentectomy with the excision of all visible disease and selective sampling of lymph nodes, peritoneal sites, and diaphragm. Postoperatively, we would introduce adjuvant chemotherapy for this patient, most likely offering her a regimen similar to that in the current Gynecologic Oncology Group adjuvant chemotherapy protocol (GOG 115), which employs bleomycin, etoposide, and cisplatin. Although this approach must still be considered investigational in a disease which recurs late, early reports of the effectiveness of this regimen in advanced granulosa cell tumor seem very promising (2). Indeed, the complete regression of advanced disease in about half of the treated patients has been observed using a combination cytotoxic drug regimen (3). Because we cannot say with certainty that adjuvant chemotherapy will prolong the life of this patient, she would have the alternative reasonable option of observation without additional treatment following her primary surgery if she preferred, with later treatment at the time of relapse.

During treatment and afterward, we would follow the patient's progress by physical examination and abdominopelvic CT scanning; also, serum inhibin levels would be observed (4). One might also measure the serum follicle regulatory protein (FRP) level if available. Ordinarily estrogen would not be used as a tumor marker, but estrogen replacement therapy would be instituted immediately after surgery and given continuously in the absence of some specific contraindication. We would follow this patient for any evidence of recurrence for at least 15 years with progressively longer intervals between visits.

References

1. Malmstrom H, Hogberg T, Risberg B, Simonsen E. Granulosa cell tumors of the ovary: Prognostic factors and outcome. Gynecol Oncol 1994; 52:50–55.
2. Jones WB. "Sex cord–stromal tumors ovary," In: Markman M, Hoskins WJ, eds. Cancer of the Ovary. New York: Raven Press, 1993: 385–405.
3. Colombo N, Sessa C, Landoni F, et al. Cisplatin, vinblastine, and bleomycin combination chemotherapy in metastatic granulosa cell tumor of the ovary. Obstet Gynecol 1986; 67:265–268.
4. Llappöhn RE, Burger HG, Bouma J, et al. Inhibin as a marker for granulosa-cell tumors. N Engl J Med 1989; 321:790–793.

PHYSICIANS' RESPONSE

MARCUS E. RANDALL
JIANAN GRAYBILL

Granulosa cell tumor of the ovary is the most common type of ovarian stromal tumor, with a peak incidence in the sixth decade. Although published data regarding this tumor in its pure form with adequate treatment and follow-up information is limited, this tumor is thought to have an indolent natural history in many cases. However, Fox et al., in a detailed review of 92 cases, determined a number of factors associated with an unfavorable outcome, including age over 40, presentation with abdominal symptoms, a palpable mass, a solid large tumor, bilateral tumors, extraovarian spread, and a high mitotic rate (1).

The patient presented herein has most of these adverse prognostic factors, probably the most important being the finding of gross serosal and omental disease. In the review of Evans et al. of 118 patients, advanced-stage patients had a recurrence rate of 30% (2). The risk of recurrence in the patient presented is likely to be even greater. While metastatic disease is seen with granulosa cell tumors, the predominant failure pattern is locoregional, and salvage rates after recurrence are very low. Therefore, in this patient, a strong case for adjuvant therapy exists, assuming that effective treatment is available.

Adjuvant therapies that have been administered in this disease include chemotherapy and radiation therapy (RT). Although its use continues to be studied by the Gynecologic Oncology Group and others, the role of chemotherapy of granulosa cell tumors is not well defined at present. While responses in patients with measureable disease are seen, clear curative potential remains to be demonstrated. Furthermore, toxicities of the aggressive germ-cell regimens frequently employed may be prohibitive, particularly in these patients, who tend to be older than those having true germ-cell ovarian tumors. Radiation therapy has been commonly used in this rare tumor; however, it should be pointed out that controlled data do not exist in the adjuvant setting that compare RT to no further treatment.

Support for the adjunctive use of RT in this patient comes from the documented radiosensitivity of granulosa cell tumor—data that confirm the authors' own experience, suggesting that these tumors are considerably more radiosensitive than epithelial ovarian tumors (3,4). It is generally accepted that whole abdominal radiotherapy is the optimal radiation technique due to the tendency of these lesions to disseminate intraperitoneally, as was the case in this patient.

Following adequate recovery from surgical staging and optimal debulking, this patient should receive whole abdominal radiotherapy with the open-field technique. Care should be taken to include the entire peritoneal cavity in the radiation fields. Appropriate kidney localization and blocking should be undertaken to make sure that tolerance is not exceeded. A midplane dose of 2550 cGy at 150 cGy/day is reasonable and would have a low complication rate, although other fractionation schemes have been used successfully. The use of a pelvic boost is controversial unless gross disease remains or there is a close or positive margin.

Additional work is needed to better estimate prognosis and recurrence rates as well as to determine the respective roles of chemotherapy and RT. In view of the somewhat unpredictable clinical course of these patients, controlled trials with large numbers of patients will be required to answer these questions—a difficult task in view of the rarity of granulosa cell tumors.

References

1. Fox H, Agrawal K, Langley FA. A clinicopathologic study of 92 cases of granulosa cell tumor of the ovary with special reference to the factors influencing prognosis. Cancer 1975; 35:231–241.
2. Evans AT III, Gaffey TA, Malkasian GD, Annegers JF. Clinicopathologic review of 118 granulosa and 82 theca cell tumors. Obstet Gynecol 1980; 55:231–238.
3. Kalavathi N. Granulosa cell tumour: Hormonal aspects and radiosensitivity. Clin Radiol 1971; 22:524–527.
4. Kumar P, Good R, Linder J. Complete response of granulosa cell tumor metastatic to the liver after hepatic irradiation: A case report. Obstet Gynecol 1986; 67:95S–98S.

PHYSICIAN'S RESPONSE

JOANNA CAIN

Granulosa cell tumors—because of their rarity, the variety of surgical management, and the variety of treatment—have been difficult to set standard therapies for. Recently, Malmstrom et al. (1) have pointed out that stage for stage, the behavior of this tumor is more like that of epithelial ovarian cancers than was appreciated in the past. Stage III tumors, in particular, have a poor prognosis if there is residual disease > 2 cm. Thus, aggressive initial surgical resection is important in this stromal cancer as well. Also, survival seems to be related to the mitotic rate of the tumor, with a decrease in survival to less than 4 years if there are > 10 mitoses per 10 high-power fields (1). Since this is relatively inexpensive, an estimate of the mitoses would be helpful in assessing this particular tumor's behavior.

It may be of value at this time to draw a serum inhibin level. Inhibin is a hormone made in the ovary that inhibits the secretion of follicle-stimulating hormone (FSH) by the anterior pituitary gland. The inhibin secreted by granulosa cell tumors seems to be functionally different than that in other epithelial ovarian cancers, as its ability to suppress FSH is greater. Typically, preoperative levels are elevated up to seven times normal premenopausal follicular phase levels, and they can be meaningful markers for recurrent or persistent disease (2). A baseline level could be of long-term value in following this patient and for comparison when questions of recurrence or failure to respond to treatment arise.

Because this patient is at high risk for recurrence or persistence of disease, she requires therapy. Radiation therapy has been used in various small case reports but without significant long-term response rates particularly in a salvage mode. Multiple types of chemotherapy have been tried, with combinations including cisplatin (+ doxorubcin, cyclophosphamide, and hexamethylmelamine in various combinations), and there have been encouraging partial responses. The best responses were seen with cisplatin, vinblastine, and bleomycin in untreated but advanced patients (3). The Gynecologic Oncology Group, building on these data, designed a trial of bleomycin, etoposide (VP-16) substituted for vinblastine, and cisplatin for malignant tumors of the ovarian stroma. This protocol (#115) is ongoing and accrual of additional patients will advance our knowledge of these diseases as well as treat this patient with the most promising combination of chemotherapy available at present. This protocol also includes a second-look assessment. While we cannot assume that this would affect the survival of any one patient, it will allow us to assess the value of this therapy for granulosa cell cancers of the ovary more rapidly overall.

References

1. Malmstrom H, Hogberg T, Risberg B, Simonsen E. Granulosa cell tumors of the ovary: Prognostic factors and outcome. Gynecol Oncol 1994; 52:50–55.
2. Jobling T, Mamers P, Healy DL, et al. A prospective study of inhibin in granulosa cell tumors of the ovary Gynecol Oncol 1994; 55:285–289.
3. Colombo N, Sessa C, Landoni G, et al. Cisplatin, vinblastine, and bleomycin combination chemotherapy in metastatic granulosa cell tumor of the ovary. Obstet Gynecol 1986; 67:265–268.

PHYSICIAN'S RESPONSE

F. J. MONTZ

Before rendering my consultative opinion, I would have preferred to have the following information if available:

1. At time of presentation, did the patient have any signs or symptoms of hyperestrogenism (abnormal vaginal bleeding, breast tenderness, etc.)?
2. At the time of the surgery, what procedures were actually performed?
   a. Was the uterus and the contralateral adnexa removed?
   b. Was a thorough operative staging as per GOG guidelines and including selective pelvic and paraaortic node sampling performed?
   c. If the uterus was not removed, was endometrial sampling performed?
3. What were the final histopathological characteristics of the granulosa cell tumor (subtype, size, atypia, mitotic count, presence of lymph vascular space invasion, etc.)?
4. Is there any preoperative serum available that could be used for estradiol and inhibin determinations? If this is not available, have postoperative determinations been completed? If so, what are they?

On the assumption that *none* of this information is available and that only an adnexectomy, resection of evident implants/nodules, and omentectomy with removal of all nodules has been performed, I would recommend the following:

1. A chest x-ray and a CT of the abdomen if they were not performed in conjunction with the preoperative pelvic CT.
2. An office hysteroscopy and complete endometrial sampling.
3. Measurement of serum estradiol and inhibin levels.
4. The patient is not a candidate for GOG protocol 115 as she does not have residual disease or positive cytology. However, I would treat her in an ad hoc fashion using the same chemotherapy regimen as recommended in that protocol (bleomycin 20 Un/m^2 (maximum of 30 Un) on day 1, repeated every 3 weeks for four courses; etoposide 75 mg/m^2 on days 1, 2, 3, 4, and 5 every 3 weeks for four courses; and cisplatin 20 mg/m^2 on days 1, 2, 3, 4, and 5 every 3 weeks for four courses).
5. If the perioperative estradiol and/or inhibin levels were elevated or unknown, I would follow the patient with serial estradiol and/or inhibin determinations. In the setting where the serum estradiol is markedly elevated and the contralateral ovary was left in situ, I would suppress the endogenous production of estrogen with a gonadotropin releasing hormone (GnRH) antagonist so as to limit fluctuations of serum estradiol levels due to the normal physiological changes found in a premenopausal

woman. I would perform these determinations monthly during the chemotherapy and quarterly thereafter. I would add back low levels of oral hormone replacement (estrogen and progesterone on a continuous basis), as this regimen would have little effect on serum estradiol determinations. Transdermal estrogen should not be administered as it is more likely to elevate serum estradiol levels.

6. I would stress to the patient the need for long-term diligence in follow-up in light of the reported delayed recurrences (> 20 years) in similar patients.

References

Colombo N, Sessa C, Landoni F, et al. Cisplatin, vinblastine, and bleomycin combination chemotherapy in metastatic granulosa cell tumor of the ovary. Obstet Gynecol 1986; 67:265.

Jobling T, Mamers P, Healy D, et al. A prospective study of inhibin in granulosa cell tumors of the ovary. Gynecol Oncol 1994; 55:285.

9

Granulosa Cell Tumor:
Emergency Surgery

CASE

A 28-year-old woman was returning from the supermarket late one evening when she developed acute abdominal pain. She was driven to her local emergency room, where she was diagnosed as having an acute abdomen. Her blood pressure was 70/30 and her hematocrit 32. Her pulse was 138. She was taken to the operating room, where a lower abdominal midline incision was made and a ruptured hemorrhagic right ovarian mass was removed. It was difficult to tell what the size of the mass would have been in the unruptured state, but the best guess was approximately 14 cm. On gross inspection, the mass appeared to be predominantly blood clot. A right salpingo-oophorectomy and an appendectomy were performed. The left tube, ovary, and the uterus looked normal. There was a great deal of blood clot spread throughout the abdomen. The abdomen was irrigated thoroughly and the incision closed. Three days postoperatively the final pathology identified a granulosa cell tumor of mixed microfollicular and diffuse type. The patient's postoperative course was smooth and she was discharged from the hospital on her third postoperative day.

The patient is quite anxious about any other recommendations for follow-up, since her husband is in the military and is being transferred out of the country in approximately 6 weeks.

PHYSICIAN'S RESPONSE

MAUREEN JARRELL

Although the case presented lacks information that might be helpful, it is clear that this premenopausal patient has been found to have an unstaged granulosa cell tumor of the ovary. Her presentation with cyst rupture and hemoperitoneum prompted a speedy exploration. Apparently the surgical team was not suspicious of an ovarian malignancy, as frozen section was not performed at the time of surgery. It is not stated whether a gynecological surgeon was present or consulted. The tumor size was approximately 14 cm and the abdomen was grossly full of clot. The remaining pelvic organs were described as normal.

The gravidity and parity of the patient are pertinent as well as her desire for future pregnancies. Her menstrual status prior to the diagnosis is also important because of the well-known association with endometrial hyperplasia and endometrial cancer found in women with granulosa cell tumors. In some studies the association with hyperplasia is as high as 50%, with a 5 to 15% incidence of endometrial cancer (1).

Granulosa cell tumor is considered a low-grade malignancy with a favorable prognosis when it presents as stage IA disease. Other, more advanced stages of disease have a higher recurrence rate and necessitate adjuvant therapy. Although the histological pattern of the tumor has not been shown to be a prognostic indicator, the mitotic index is important and should be determined for this patient.

The first step in the management of this patient is to determine her goals in terms of future pregnancies. The second step is to adequately stage her tumor.

If the patient has completed childbearing, exploratory laparotomy with cytological washings, total abdominal hysterectomy, and left salpingo-oophorectomy should be recommended. At the time of surgery, a pathologist should inspect the removed ovary and uterus and perform frozen section studies if indicated. If a concurrent endometrial cancer is found, it should be staged surgically with nodal dissection based on the depth of myometrial penetration. In addition, lymph nodes should be sampled from the right paraaortic distribution as well as the entire pelvis. The pelvic and abdominal peritoneum should be inspected, including the surfaces of the bowel. The peritoneum over the diaphragm and capsule of the liver should be inspected, with biopsy of any suspicious areas. Any adhesive disease should be sampled. If the tumor was described as adherent to the pelvic side wall by the initial surgeon, this peritoneum should be carefully excised.

Alternatively, if the patient wishes to retain her fertility, the approach would be different. Endometrial sampling should precede exploratory laparotomy. If endometrial hyperplasia or grade I adenocarcinoma is present, the patient should be counseled about her risks and need for hormonal manipulation and close follow-up. In this area her future plans and medical follow-up are critical in a decision to retain the uterus. Exploratory laparotomy should follow the guidelines outlined above. If disease is found on the contralateral ovary and confirmed by biopsy, the uterus, left tube, and ovary should also be removed.

If the staging laparotomy confirms the diagnosis of stage IA disease, the patient may be followed without further therapy. Any more advanced disease, including stage IB disease, should be treated with chemotherapy. In an adjuvant setting such as this, a platinum-containing drug plus etoposide is an excellent choice. Although platinum, vinblastine, and bleomycin have been shown to have activity against granulosa cell tumors, unexplained deaths due to bleomycin make this combination unacceptable for adjuvant treatment.

The patient should be advised of the need for long-term follow-up, as granulosa cell tumors often recur more than a decade after initial presentation. Inhibin has been shown to be a valuable tumor marker for this disease (2,3). Also, follicle regulatory protein (FRP) has recently been shown to parallel the clinical course of patients with granulosa cell tumors (4).

References

Greene JW Jr. Feminizing mesenchymomas (granulosa and theca-cell tumors) with associated endometrial carcinoma: Review of the literature, and a study of the material in the Ovarian Tumor Registry, Am J Obstet Gynecol 1957; 74:31–41.

Jobling T, Mamers P, Healy D, et al. A prospective study of inhibin in granulosa cell tumors of the ovary, Gynecol Oncol 1994; 55:285–289.

Lappohn R, Burger H, Bouma J, et al. Inhibin as a marker for granulosa cell tumors. N Engl J Med 1989; 321:790–793.

Montz FJ, Rodgers KE, diZerega GS, et al. Follicle regulatory protein (FRP): A new tumor marker for granulosa cell tumors (GCT) of the ovary, ASCO Proc 8(589): 1989.

PHYSICIANS' RESPONSE

JOHN L. LOVECCHIO
DAVID GAL

Spontaneous rupture of a granulosa cell tumor is an uncommon gynecological cause of hemorrhagic shock in women of reproductive age. Such a clinical event is usually associated with bleeding from either a ruptured ectopic pregnancy or corpus luteum cyst. Granulosa cell tumors vary widely in appearance. They may vary in size from being clinically undetectable to large pelvic abdominal masses and may be entirely cystic, mixed cystic and solid, or uniformly solid in nature. They are often hemorrhagic and have a propensity to rupture spontaneously. Like epithelial tumors, they can spread transperitoneally and also involve retroperitoneal lymph nodes. Relevant clinical facts in this case suggest that this mass ruptured and its contents spilled. It was estimated to be approximately 14 cm in size, and there were no signs of regional intrapelvic spread, abdominal carcinomatosis, or retroperitoneal involvement.

The literature suggests that 90% of granulosa cell tumors are stage I at the time of diagnosis and that less than 5% are bilateral (1). Unquestionably surgical staging is required to determine if this patient truly has disease confined to the ovary.

Unfortunately this was not done. In lieu of this, one must examine other factors that may be of prognostic value. Some observers suggest that the size of the lesion may be influential in predicting prognosis; however, most of these studies are uncontrolled for surgical staging. Similarly, only scant clinical evidence is available in the literature to assess the prognostic influence of uncontrolled rupture of these nonepithelial lesions. Therefore no overwhelming adverse factors can be identified in this particular case that would dictate the need for surgical reexploration.

If one assumes that this patient has stage I disease and that the disease is entirely resected, no further adjuvant therapy is advocated. Computed tomography of the abdomen and pelvis is strongly suggested as a baseline study. Continued long-term gynecological surveillance is indicated, since late recurrences, even years after diagnosis, are not uncommon. Pregnancy is not contraindicated.

Reference

Bjorkholm E, Silfversward C. Prognostic factors in granulosa cell tumors. Gynecol Oncol 1981; 11:261.

PHYSICIANS' RESPONSE

DANIEL TOBIAS
CAROLYN D. RUNOWICZ

This is a challenging case. Should the clinician reoperate on this patient? Is there a need for a full-staging laparotomy? Does the patient require a total abdominal hysterectomy and right salpingo-oophorectomy? Is there a role for adjuvant chemotherapy or radiotherapy?

Unfortunately, with respect to this particular patient, review of the literature does not provide a wealth of information. In the majority of reported cases, the patients are postmenopausal and have been treated with total abdominal hysterectomy and bilateral salpingo-oophorectomy, with or without adjuvant radiation therapy and, less commonly, chemotherapy. A poor prognosis is associated with large tumor size, advanced stage of disease, age > 40, and tumors with a high mitotic rate. Of all of these factors, it would appear that stage of disease is the most predictive of prognosis and overall survival. Most studies do not find a consistent correlation with histopathological type and prognosis.

In reviewing the available literature, it is important to remember that most published reports use the 1974 staging system of the Fédération Internationale de Gynécologie et d'Obstétrique (FIGO), since they represent retrospective reviews. With that staging system, the patient would have been classified as a presumed stage Iaii (growth limited to one ovary, with capsule ruptured). A revised FIGO surgical staging system was implemented in 1987. Using this classification, the patient would be classified as at least a stage IC and perhaps higher, as a full staging laparotomy was not performed. In the 1974 FIGO surgical staging system, stage IC is defined as comprising patients with ascites or positive peritoneal washings. Since most reports are retrospective reviews that report series of patients prior to the revised surgical staging, the patient's prognosis will be best calculated by classifying her as a Iaii, rather than a IC, when reviewing the older literature. The reported 10-year survival rate for stage Iaii is approximately 90%, but according to one small study, it decreases to 60% at 25 years.

With respect to this patient, her risk factors include abdominal pain with tumor rupture and a tumor size of 14 cm. Due to the patient's young age as well as the indolent nature of these tumors and their unilaterality, we would not recommend further surgery. The available literature supports the contention that this disease is unilateral in more than 95% of the cases. The data for epithelial ovarian cancer suggest that 30% of patients with disease apparently confined to the ovary at initial surgery will have disease spread beyond the ovary at repeat staging laparotomy. However, granulosa cell tumors differ biologically from epithelial tumors, and these data may not apply to them. Granulosa cell tumors tend to have a more indolent course. Although recurrences may appear within 5 years, they are often not evident until after a much longer postoperative interval. Removal of the uterus and remaining tube and ovary after completion of child-bearing in a patient treated conservatively is controversial.

Additional studies that might be helpful in this patient include the mitotic index, degree of nuclear atypicality, S phase, and ploidy status. This patient, like all patients with granulosa cell tumors, will require lifelong follow-up because of the propensity for late recurrences. Serum estradiol and inhibin levels may be useful in the follow-up of this patient.

References

Bjorkholm E, Silfversward C. Prognostic factors in granulosa-cell tumors. Gynecol Oncol 1981; 11:261.

Fox H, Agrawl K, Langley FA. A clinicopathologic study of 92 cases of granulosa cell tumor of the ovary with special reference to the factors influencing prognosis. Cancer 1975; 35:231.

Malmstram H, Hogberg T, Risberg B, Simonsen E. Granulosa cell tumors of the ovary: Prognostic factors and outcome. Gynecol Oncol 1994; 52:50.

PHYSICIAN'S RESPONSE

RICHARD R. BARAKAT

In view of this patient's age and probably desire to maintain fertility as well as her critical status at presentation, the appropriate conservative surgical procedure was performed. The majority of patients diagnosed with granulosa cell tumors of the ovary will present with disease confined to the ovary. These tumors are bilateral in only 3% of cases. In very rare cases, the patient will present with advanced metastatic disease. Isolated recurrences in the paraaortic lymph node chain suggest that appropriate staging at the initial surgery may be important. In view of the small number of such cases, there would be minimal benefit from reoperating on this patient to perform a formal staging procedure.

A baseline CT scan of the abdomen and pelvis should be performed to be certain that there is no evidence of metastatic disease. In addition, a blood sample should be obtained to determine the level of the polypeptide hormone inhibin (follicular regulatory protein), which may be a useful tumor marker in granulosa cell tumors. Approximately 75% of granulosa cell tumors produce estrogen. This may result in endometrial changes ranging from hyperplasia to frank carcinoma in up to 13% of cases. Since the patient did not have endometrial sampling performed at the time of surgery, she should undergo such a procedure, which in all likelihood can be performed in the office setting.

The majority of patients with granulosa cell tumor limited to the ovary will be cured of their disease by resection. Several prognostic factors may be important in such tumors. These include a tumor diameter greater than 15 cm, rupture at the time of surgery, and high tumor grade. There is no evidence that any form of adjuvant therapy, including chemotherapy or radiation, is effective in reducing the risk of recurrence in patients with completely resected adult granulosa cell tumor. Since the risk of relapse is very low in patients with apparent stage I disease, most physicians would not recommend adjuvant therapy.

Any patient with a completely resected granulosa cell tumor should be carefully followed after her initial surgery. This follow-up should include a pelvic examination every 3 months for the first 2 years following surgery, every 6 months for an additional 3 years, and annually thereafter. Prolonged follow-up is necessary as these tumors have a tendency to behave in an indolent manner and recurrences as late as 30 years following primary surgery have been reported. In patients whose serum inhibin levels are elevated at the primary surgery, follow-up levels should be obtained at each visit, since they may serve as useful markers of recurrence.

PHYSICIAN'S RESPONSE

THOMAS F. ROCERETO

Granulosa cell tumors are the most common stromal tumors of the ovary. They are considered as a low-grade malignancy with a favorable prognosis. These tumors make up less than 5% of all ovarian malignancies and are rarely bilateral. Their peak incidence is in the first postmenopausal decade. The patient usually presents with vague lower abdominal symptoms, abdominal distension, and/or a pelvic mass. Rupture of the tumor either prior to or at the time of surgery is not uncommon. As in this case, rupture with an acute abdomen may be the reason for surgery. Unfortunately, at the time of emergency surgery, the nature of the mass was not recognized and adequate staging surgery was not performed.

Stage of disease at the initial surgery is a very important prognostic factor in this disease. Granulosa cell tumors have a propensity to spread to the pelvic and paraaortic lymph nodes, with the latter spread being more common. In the patient who has completed her childbearing, the proper operative procedure should include at least a total abdominal hysterectomy, bilateral salpingo-oophorectomy, pelvic and paraaortic lymph node sampling, and an infracolic omentectomy. In the patient who wishes further childbearing, conservative surgery usually consists of a unilateral oophorectomy along with the node sampling and omentectomy. Conservative surgery may be considered in those patients with stage IA disease, recognizing a potential increase risk for recurrence. In stage IA, the recurrence rate after a total abdominal hysterectomy/bilateral salpingo-oophorectomy (TAH/BSO) has been reported at 6%, while the rate with less than a TAH/BSO is reported at 25%. Recurrence in the latter case usually appears in the remaining pelvic organs. Some 75% of patients who develop a recurrence die from their tumor.

Patients whose tumor ruptures before or at the time of surgery have a worse prognosis than those whose tumor is removed unruptured. Patients with large tumors have a greater risk of dying from their tumor. Unfortunately patients who are symptomatic from their tumor usually have large tumors that rupture prior to or at the time of surgery. Multiple histological patterns of growth have been described in these tumors, with most having a mixture of these patterns, which have not been shown to have prognostic value. Nuclear atypia and the mitotic rate are more important for prognosis. The survival rate with a mitotic rate of less than 5 per 10 per high-power fields is close to 100%. The median survival with a mitotic rate of 5 to 9 per 10 per high-power fields is reported as 9 years, while that of a higher rate is only 4 years.

Removal of all tumor at the time of surgery is the most important aspect of the overall treatment of these patients. In the more advanced stages, survival correlates best with tumor debulking. Even in the patient with recurrence, surgical removal of all the tumor gives the best prognosis.

Postoperative pelvic radiation has not been shown to improve survival in the patient with stage I disease who has been adequately staged. Radiation, although used widely in the past, in general seems to have a minimal role in the postsurgical treatment. Chemotherapy is more commonly used in these patients as well as in those with recurrences. Alkylating agents, either singly or in combination, were widely used in the past. More recently the combination of cisplatin, vinblastine, and bleomycin has been shown to produce a good response. In newer regimens, vinblastine is replaced with etoposide.

One of the special aspects of this tumor are recurrences long after initial treatment. Recently the polypeptide hormone inhibin has been reported to be a tumor marker for granulosa cell tumors. This hormone has been reported to be elevated months before recurrences have been detected. The hormone estradiol may also be elevated before evidence of recurrence. Both of these hormones may be useful in the follow-up of these patients.

Granulosa cell tumors have a significant chance of being hormonally active. Endometrial hyperplasia has been reported in up to 50% of cases. More importantly, endometrial carcinoma has been associated with 10 to 13% of these tumors. If the uterus is left for future childbearing, dilation and curettage (D&C) must be performed in order to evaluate the status of the endometrium.

In the present case, a 28-year-old woman has had an emergency operation with the removal of what is postoperatively found to be a large granulosa cell tumor that had ruptured. Because the mass was probably thought to be a ruptured hemorrhagic cyst at the time of surgery, further staging surgery was not performed. Now it is known that she had a granulosa cell tumor with at least two poor prognostic factors, size and rupture. The recommendation at this time should be reexploration with a total abdominal hysterectomy, left salpingo-oophorectomy, right salpingectomy, sampling of the pelvic and paraaortic lymph nodes, infracolic omentectomy, and pelvic and abdominal washings. This recommendation is based on the fact that this patient has greater then stage IA disease. A dilemma would be posed if the patient wanted further childbearing. Surgical staging with nodes and an omentectomy should still be performed. Leaving the remainder of the reproductive organs in situ potentially increases the patient's risk for recurrence and thus her risk of dying from her tumor. Recommendation could be made not to perform this conservative surgery, but the decision must be made by the patient. If the uterus is not removed, then a D&C must be part of the second procedure.

References

Bjorkholm E, Silfversward C. Prognostic factors in granulosa-cell tumors. Gynecol Oncol 1981; 11:261–274.

Evans AT, et al. Clinicopathologic review of 188 granulosa and 82 theca cell tumors. Obstet Gynecol 1980; 55:231–238.

Hoskin WJ, Perez CA, Young RC, eds. Principles and Practices of Gynecologic Oncology. Philadelphia: Lippincott, 1992:727–728.

Malmstrom H, et al. Granulosa cell tumors of the ovary: Prognostic factors and outcome. Gynecol Oncol 1994; 52:50–55.

Piura B, et al. Granulosa cell tumor of the ovary: A study of 18 cases. J Surg Oncol 1994; 55:71–77.

10

Ovarian Fibrosarcoma in a Young Woman

CASE

A 32-year-old woman presents with the sudden onset of abdominal pain. Physical exam reveals a left ovarian mass, which is confirmed on ultrasound. At surgical exploration, performed by a gynecological oncologist, the patient is found to have an enlarged left ovary (three times normal size), which is removed. There is no other evidence of pathology in the pelvis or abdominal cavity. Pathology reveals the patient to have an ovarian fibrosarcoma.

Chest x-ray and abdominal and pelvic computed tomography (CT) scans are normal.

PHYSICIANS' RESPONSE

BOB TAYLOR
ROBERT PARK

This 32-year-old patient has Fédération Internationale de Gynécologie et d'Obstétrique (FIGO) stage IA ovarian fibrosarcoma, according to the criteria established for the surgical staging of the more common epithelial ovarian carcinoma.

Ovarian fibrosarcoma is an extremely rare malignancy and differs from the common ovarian fibroma and cellular fibroma by demonstrating nuclear pleomorphism and a mitotic rate of greater than 3 mitoses per 10 high-power fields (1). Ovarian fibromas are benign lesions and cellular fibromas are thought to possess a low malignant potential, having a 20% recurrence rate. Ovarian fibrosarcomas are highly malignant and are associated with an extremely poor prognosis, due to their tendency for early hematogenous and lymphatic metastasis.

Despite the rather small size of this lesion (6 cm), we may still suspect subclinical metastases. This notion is based on the general predilection of sarcomas to metastasize early in their disease course. Obviously, this patient's best chance for long-term survival is predicated on the absence of such metastases. It would therefore be reasonable to initiate a metastatic survey, knowing that a dedicated search for metastatic disease can unfortunately miss small-volume lesions, particularly if they are less than the size resolution of our current imaging modalities.

Given the lack of prospective data on postoperative therapy for ovarian fibrosarcomas, treatment options range from observation to pelvic radiotherapy to systemic chemotherapy. Several phase II trials have investigated radiotherapy for uterine sarcomas (pure and mixed mesodermal), generally finding a benefit in local control without affecting survival. We would caution on the use of pelvic radiotherapy in ovarian sarcomas as it would not cover all of the major lymphatic and venous drainage pathways, nor are there any data on the basis of which whole-abdomen radiotherapy could be recommended in such patients.

Applicable data on chemotherapy come from the literature on uterine corpus sarcoma as reviewed by Hannigan et al (2). The Gynecologic Oncology Group (GOG) has phase II data from patients treated for advanced or recurrent uterine leiomyosarcoma showing an increased response rate to doxorubicin (Adriamycin) without affecting survival. Another GOG study evaluated Adriamycin as an adjuvant to surgery in early-stage disease, finding no effect on recurrence or survival.

Given the rarity of ovarian fibrosarcoma, its inclusion into clinical trials is precluded. In the absence of applicable clinical trials and the absence of clinical data showing any significant survival advantage to either adjuvant radiation or chemotherapy, we would recommend observation for this patient.

References

Pratt J, Scully RE. Cellular fibromas and fibrosarcomas of the ovary: A clinicopathologic review of 17 cases. Cancer 1981; 47:2663.

Hannigan E, Curtin JP, Silverberg SG, et al. Corpus mesenchymal tumors, In: Hoskins WJ, Perez CA, Young RC, eds. Principles and Practice of Gynecologic Oncology. Philadelphia: Lippincott, 1992:695.

PHYSICIAN'S RESPONSE

ALEXANDER W. KENNEDY

This patient presents a most unusual clinical situation. As is so frequently the case in rendering gynecological oncology consultations, expert pathological consultation is essential to properly advising this patient regarding her status. While ovarian fibromas are commonly encountered, the malignant variety, fibrosarcoma, is a most rare tumor to arise within the ovary, particularly in a premenopausal patient. As in the case of cellular uterine leiomyomas, pathologists have recognized a cellular variety of these tumors. Ovarian fibromas are characterized by increased cellular variety with a low level of mitotic activity and pleomorphism. Mitotic activity is less than 4 mitoses per 10 high-power fields. The prognosis for patients with these lesions is excellent, although a small minority of patients may experience recurrence. In contradistinction to cellular fibromas, ovarian fibrosarcomas have a higher mitotic rate with increased cellularity and pleomorphism. The prognosis for the malignant variety is very grave, with most patients experiencing a rapidly progressing malignancy with diffuse intraperitoneal involvement or pulmonary metastases.

Therefore, the initial step in the management of this patient should be an expert review of her pathology materials to confirm that she does indeed have a fibrosarcoma and not a cellular fibroma. If the patient is felt to have a primary ovarian sarcoma, consideration for adjuvant therapy would be in order. Her radiological studies as well as an apparently careful intraoperative exploration by a gynecological oncologist were negative and would not be repeated. The patient should understand that she has a rare tumor without adjuvant therapy that has been proven to be effective. I would recommend that she consider prophylactic cytotoxic chemotherapy, including the most active currently available agent. Presently, I would advise three courses of ifosfamide (3-day infusion) and then careful clinical and radiological follow-up examinations.

Reference

Pratt J, Scully RE. Cellular fibromas and fibrosarcomas of the ovary: A comparative clinical pathologic analysis of 17 cases. Cancer 1981; 47:2663–2670.

PHYSICIAN'S RESPONSE

JOHN MALFETANO

This young woman appears to have an uncommon malignancy of the ovary. Although the patient was not optimally staged, there is intraoperative information indicating no apparent gross disease outside of the ovary.

Ovarian sarcomas account for less than 1% of all ovarian malignancies. The histogenesis of ovarian sarcomas is debatable and there is no current universally accepted classification. Many pathologists feel that these sarcomas should be classified as nonspecific tumors of the ovary, while others believe they arise from specialized ovarian stromal cells or unspecialized fibroblasts. The most common "fibrous" tumors of the ovary are benign fibromas, which account for 4% of all ovarian neoplasms. The criteria for distinguishing benign cellular fibromas from malignant fibrosarcomas are credited to Pratt and Scully (1), who, in 1981, reported 17 cases and defined pathological criteria to differentiate these two lesions on the basis of their degree of mitotic activity. Those neoplasms with 1 to 3 mitotic figures per 10 high-power fields were considered benign (cellular fibroma), and those with 4 or more mitotic figures per 10 high-power fields were considered malignant (fibrosarcoma). Six out of their 17 patients had 4 or more mitotic figures per 10 high-power fields, and these lesions were designated fibrosarcomas. The average age of the 6 patients was 58, and 3 had FIGO stage I disease. All 6 patients developed recurrence; 4 within the first 6 months, 1 at 18 months, and 1 at 44 months. At the time of Pratt and Scully's publication, 4 of the 6 patients had died of recurrence. One patient with recurrence died of intercurrent disease and a second had distant metastasis at 13 months but was lost to follow-up.

Since the exact pathological diagnosis is crucial in this young woman, the slides should be sent to a referee pathologist to confirm the diagnosis of fibrosarcoma. Few data are available on ovarian fibrosarcomas other than that they recur rapidly and have a poor prognosis.

After the pathological confirmation, I would present to the patient and her family the available literature regarding her condition. No further diagnostic studies are necessary at this time. The treatment options are (a) to prescribe no further adjuvant therapy at this time and to follow the patients clinically at 2-to 3-month intervals for recurrence, or (b) to prescribe adjuvant chemotherapy. With no surgical staging specimens other than the left ovary and an extremely aggressive neoplasm with an ultimately poor prognosis, I would encourage the patient to receive adjuvant systemic chemotherapy. I would utilize platinum, Adriamycin (doxorubicin), and cytoxan (PAC) or our present phase II combination of VIP (VP-16, ifosfamide, and platinum). Therapy would be given every 21 to 28 days for a total of 9 months.

References

Prat J, Scully RE. Cellular fibromas and fibrosarcomas of the ovary: A comparative clinicopathologic analysis of seventeen cases. Cancer 1981; 47:2663–2670.

11

Vulvar Cancer: Stage IV Squamous Cell Carcinoma

CASE

A 75-year-old woman, gravida IV, para IV, who is diabetic has had approximately 1 year of vulvar itching and burning. She was treated with some steroid cream by her family physician approximately 8 months ago and never returned for a follow-up visit. Instead, she went to see her daughter's gynecologist, who immediately referred her to you. On examination, she is a healthy-appearing woman looking younger than her stated age. Her physical examination is quite normal except for findings limited to the vulva and groins. She has a 3-cm ulcerative lesion on the right interior labium majus with bilateral firm 1- to 2-cm inguinal nodes.

PHYSICIAN'S RESPONSE

NEVILLE HACKER

This patient is elderly and a diabetic, but I would expect that she would be fit enough to undergo definitive treatment for her vulvar cancer. However, before planning treatment, I would want to obtain a full blood count, renal function tests, chest x-ray, and cardiogram; I would also want to be certain that her diabetes mellitus was stabilized. I would also perform colposcopy of the cervix, vagina, and vulva to be certain that the remainder of her lower genital tract was normal for her age.

My recommendations for management are based on the assumptions that she is medically fit for surgery and that her lower genital tract is normal except for the 3-cm ulcerative lesion on the right anterior labium majus.

It is important to determine the best treatment for the primary tumor and the regional lymph nodes. As the patient has clinically suspicious groin nodes, she will most likely require a combination of primary surgery and postoperative radiation therapy. To further determine the best approach to the lymph nodes, I would obtain a computed tomography (CT) scan of the pelvis preoperatively to see whether or not she had any enlarged pelvic lymph nodes. Bulky pelvic nodes are very unlikely to be sterilized by external beam radiation therapy, so I would want to remove any bulky nodes surgically prior to offering her postoperative radiation.

The primary lesion would be well treated by a radical local excision, ensuring that all surgical margins were at least 1 cm wide. The depth of dissection should be to the deep fascia.

My recommendation for the management of the regional nodes would depend on whether or not they were proven histologically to contain metastatic carcinoma. I would approach both groins through a separate incision. I would initially remove all of the palpably suspicious nodes and send them for a frozen section. If the nodes were positive, I would not do a full groin dissection, as the patient would be best treated by postoperative pelvic and groin irradiation, and quite severe leg edema might result from full groin dissection and postoperative radiation. If there were any enlarged pelvic nodes on the preoperative CT scan, I would extend the groin incision cephalad and remove the enlarged pelvic nodes through an extraperitoneal approach. Should the frozen sections be negative, I would undertake full inguinofemoral lymph node dissection.

My indications for postoperative pelvic and groin irradiation would be two or more microscopic lymph node metastases, one grossly positive node, or any evidence of extranodal spread.

References

Heaps JM, Fu YS, Montz FJ, et al. Surgical-pathological variables predictive of local recurrence in squamous cell carcinoma of the vulva. Gynecol Oncol 1990; 38:309.

Homesley HD, Bundy BN, Sedlis A, Adcock L. Radiation therapy versus pelvic node resection for carcinoma of the vulva with positive groin nodes. Obstet Gynecol 1986; 68:733.

PHYSICIAN'S RESPONSE

HANS KREBS

With a 3-cm ulcerative vulvar lesion and bilateral firm 1- to 2-cm inguinal nodes suspicious of metastases, the patient is likely to have stage IVA vulvar carcinoma according to the revised Fédération Internationale de Gynécologie et d'Obstétrique (FIGO) staging from 1989. If this is confirmed, her prognosis must be regarded as unfavorable with an anticipated 5-year disease-free survival rate of only approximately 20 to 40%. The plan of management should include assessment and documentation of her disease and aggressive treatment by a combination of surgery, radiation, and possibly also chemotherapy.

Documentation of the cancer is achieved by biopsy of the vulvar lesion under local anesthesia in the office.

The assessment of tumor spread should include basic laboratory tests such as a complete blood count (CBC) and blood chemistry with serum electrolytes, creatinine, blood urea nitrogen (BUN), and liver function tests. A chest x-ray to rule out pulmonary metastases is advised. Computed tomography of the abdomen and pelvis, including the groin area, should be obtained to evaluate pelvic and paraaortic lymph nodes and to map enlarged groin lymph nodes. Cystoscopy and proctoscopy are not necessary in this case, with the vulvar lesion being distant from the bladder and the rectum.

The treatment is directed to controlling the disease while causing the least amount of morbidity. Being a diabetic, the patient is especially prone to develop complications related to surgery or radiation therapy. But she is a healthy-appearing woman who looks younger than her stated age, and the radicality of the treatment necessary to control the disease should not be compromised just to avoid complications.

Some 10 or 12 years ago, most gynecological oncologists would have elected to perform a radical vulvectomy, bilateral groin dissection, and, if positive inguinal nodes were encountered, also a retroperitoneal pelvic lymphadenectomy. This approach changed in 1986, when Homesley and colleagues reported a decreased incidence of groin recurrence and a significant survival advantage at 2 years in patients with one or more positive groin nodes who received postoperative radiation therapy to the inguinal and pelvic areas compared to those treated by groin and pelvic node dissection. This and other studies convincingly demonstrated that radiation therapy can control microscopic disease in lymph nodes and elsewhere. The complete eradication of gross disease by radiation, however, is far less reliable. Finally, clinical experience has shown that a modified radical vulvectomy, partial radical vulvectomy, radical hemivulvectomy, or even a radical wide local excision clearing the primary vulvar lesion with margins of at least 1 cm result in the same local control of the disease as the classic radical vulvectomy.

Hence, for the patient described in this case report, the following treatment plan emerges (1,2):

1. A bilateral selective groin lymph node dissection is carried out through separate incisions to remove only the enlarged, clinically suspicious superficial and deep lymph nodes. A complete ("radical") groin dissection is performed if

frozen-section diagnosis does not reveal tumor metastases to the selectively resected nodes.

2. Pelvic lymph nodes found to be enlarged on computed tomography (CT) are selectively removed through a retroperitoneal approach.

3. The primary vulvar carcinoma is resected by a radical hemivulvectomy or radical local excision with wide margins.

4. If one or more of the groin lymph nodes are—as anticipated in this case—positive for metastatic cancer, a full course of radiation therapy (50 to 55 Gy) is delivered to the inguinal and pelvic areas as soon as the groin incisions have healed.

5. Adjuvant chemotherapy with 5-fluorouracil alone or in combination with platinol or mitomycin-C may further enhance the effectiveness of the radiation therapy.

Contrary to a radical groin dissection, the selective excision of clinically suspicious lymph nodes followed by radiation is less likely to result in serious complications such as infection, tissue necrosis, and lymphedema. Preservation of much of the vulva achieved by radical local excision will result in fewer complications, quick recovery, and less distortion of the body image. As a result, there will be fewer psychological sequelae without compromising the chance for cure when compared to the classic radical vulvectomy.

References

1. Hacker NF, Eifel P, McGuire W, Wilkinson EJ. Vulva. In: Hoskins WJ, Perez CA, Young RC eds. Principles and Practice of Gynecologic Oncology. Philadelphia: Lippincott, 1992:537–566.
2. Thomas GM, Dembo AJ, Bryson SCP, et al. Review: Changing concepts in the management of vulvar cancer. Gynecol Oncol 1991. 42:9–21.

PHYSICIANS' RESPONSE

RICHARD REID
GARTH D. PHIBBS

The past history of this patient, who presents with locally advanced vulvar cancer plus clinically suspicious inguinal lymphadenopathy in both groins, is significant for the all too common phenomenon of undue diagnostic delay, reflecting both physician and patient error.

Confirmation of the diagnosis requires biopsy. Given the presence of a 3-cm epitheliomatous ulcer, histological confirmation would likely require only a simple punch biopsy. However, to avoid obtaining too much necrotic material from the ulcer surface and too little viable tumor from the ulcer base, we would prefer a 2-cm wedge from the lesion edge. A wedge biopsy is also more likely to

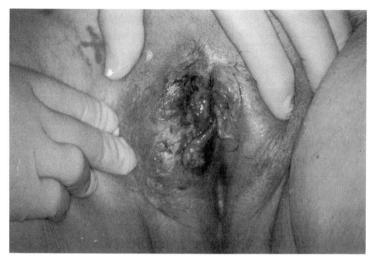

(A)

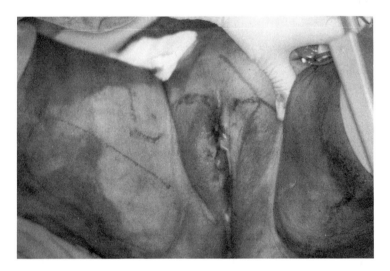

(B)

Figure 1   A 15 × 10 cm erythematous, hyperkeratotic plaque of Paget's disease. A
ulcer on the left anterior pilosebaceous line contains deeply invasive adenocarcinoma (A).
Skin marks outlining the proposed gluteal thigh flap. A robust versatile musculo-cutaneous
pedicle based on the inferior gluteal artery (IGA). As the IGA enters the buttock (just

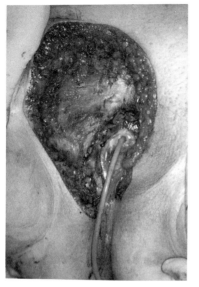

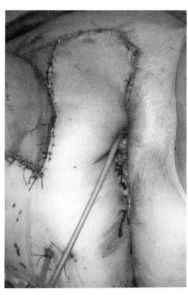

(C)   **(D)**

medial to the ischial tuberosity), it is accompanied (on its lateral side) by the posterior cutaneous nerve of the thigh. Hence, this flap is generally sensate. After sending muscular branches to caudal gluteus maximus, the IGA terminates in a long cutaneous ramus that runs all the way down the posterior thigh. Hence, the surgeon can raise an axial skin flap, having a width of up to 12 cm and a length extending to the popliteal fossa (if needed). Because the IGA is one of the terminal branches of the anterior division, this flap cannot be used for vulvar reconstruction after hypogastric ligation (B). Modified radical vulvectomy with extra wide cutaneous margins (Paget's disease) (C). The gluteus thigh flap can be directly transposed (as shown here), or raised as an island flap and tunnelled. Flap length must be generous (to avoid tension) and the points of rotation should be below the ischial tuberosity (to avoid kinking the IGA). For adequate mobility, the gluteus maximus must be partially transected. However, such transection must not extend above the posterior skin margin. With aggressive undermining, the donor site can generally be closed primarily (D).

provide such prognostically valuable information as depth of invasion, tumor differentiation, and involvement of vascular spaces.

Under the old (clinical) FIGO classification, this patient would be stage III (T_2,N_2,M_0) corresponding to a 66% risk of spread to the regional lymph nodes (1). Because the number of positive groin nodes is the single most important prognostic variable, the new FIGO classification is now surgical. Five-year survival for women with negative nodes is about 95%, falling to 80% for two positive nodes and below 20% for more than three positive nodes (2). Moreover, metastasis to the external iliac or obturator nodes is essentially limited to women with clinically suspicious (N_2) groin nodes or multiple microscopically positive nodes (2).

Lymphatic drainage from labium majus tumors is predominantly to the ipsilateral groin nodes. The presence of bilateral palpable groin nodes is therefore a poor prognostic sign, suggesting that this patient might fall into the (new) FIGO stage IVA. However, in a diabetic patient with an ulcerated cancer, clinically palpable nodes reflect lymphadenitis (rather than metastasis) in about one-third of cases. Additional preoperative workup should include chest x-ray and abdominal pelvic CT scan. Particular note should be made of the location of any suspicious pelvic nodes, since they may be removed in a retroperitoneal fashion with little morbidity at the time of primary inguinal dissection. Future follow-up is also facilitated by drawing a squamous cancer antigen titer.

Surgery remains the mainstay of treatment for vulvar cancer; however, over the last half century, surgical opinion has come full circle. In reaction to the < 25% cure rate from simple vulvectomy and bilateral inguinofemoral lymphadenectomy, sometimes extended further by extraperitoneal pelvic lymphadenectomy. The practice of widely undermining the wound edges and attempting primary closure carried a wound breakdown rate of at least 85%. Prolonged morbidity and even mortality resulted from problems such as local necrosis with secondary sepsis, cataclysmic hemorrhage from ulcerative erosion of the femoral vessels, bronchopulmonary or urinary tract infection, thromboembolism, and myocardial infarction. Over time, the pendulum has swung back to more conservative surgery, often bolstered by adjuvant radiation therapy. A major advance was the recognition that pelvic lymphadenectomy was unnecessary if the iliac nodes were negative, but "too little, too late" if the iliac nodes were positive. Hence, if the groin nodes are negative, modern protocols omit any therapy to the pelvic nodes. Conversely, for the patient with one or more positive groin nodes, postoperative radiation offers a significant survival advantage due to a decreased incidence of groin recurrence (24% versus 5%) (3). Modern protocols also favor groin dissection through separate incisions and individualization of the vulvar resection. In a younger woman with an otherwise healthy vulva, even a tumor of this size can be safely managed by hemivulvectomy as long as the surgeon obtains a 1-cm margin of resection. However, to a 75-year-old diabetic with chronic vulvar dystrophy, radical vulvectomy is often a profound relief.

In this specific case, we would recommend radical hemivulvectomy plus bilateral inguinofemoral lymphadenectomy, through separate incisions, to lessen the risk of postoperative leg edema and wound breakdown. We would send suspicious nodes for frozen section. If positive, we would be guided by Hacker's (4) recommendations for selective removal of large or fixed nodes, followed by up to 5000 cGy to the pelvic midplane at a rate of 180 to 200 cGy/day. Since attempted primary closure will likely result in wound breakdown, we would recommend vulvar reconstruction with a suitable flap. Despite its popularity, the gracilis flap has many unfavorable features (difficult dissection, morbid donor site, limited mobility, high risk of epithelial necrosis). Thus, if there is sufficient epithelial laxity, we would prefer a gluteus maximus myocutaneous flap (Fig. 1), based upon the terminal distribution of the inferior gluteal artery (5). Alternatively, if more skin is needed, the tensor fascia lata flap would be more suitable.

References

1. Iverson T, Elders JG, Christensen A, et al. Squamous cell carcinoma of the vulva: A review of 424 patients, 1957–1974. Gynecol Oncol 1980; 9:271.
2. Hacker NF, Berek JS, Lagasse LD, et al. Management of regional lymph nodes and their prognostic significance in vulvar cancer. Obstet Gynecol 1983; 61:408.
3. Holmesley HD, Bundy BN, Sedlis A, Adcock L. A randomized study of radiation therapy versus pelvic node resection for patients with invasive squamous cell carcinoma of the vulva having positive groin nodes (a Gynecologic Oncology Group study). Obstet Gynecol 1986; 68:733.
4. Hacker NF. Surgery for malignant tumors of the vulva. In: Gershenson DM, DeCherney AH, Curry SL. Operative Gynecology. Philadelphia: Saunders, 1993:173–200.
5. Achauer BM, Braly P, Berman ML, DiSaia PG. Immediate vaginal reconstruction following resection for malignancy using the gluteal thigh flap. Gynecol Oncol 1984; 19:79.

PHYSICIAN'S RESPONSE

A. ROBERT KAGAN

I will assume that this patient is a type II diabetic, with no diagnosis that would limit an operative procedure. Her workup should include a Pap smear, inspection of the vagina (with cytology if suspicious) chest roentgenogram, complete blood count (CBC), urinalysis, and liver function tests. If liver function tests are abnormal, a CT with contrast is recommended to look for enlarged lymph nodes and defects in the liver and kidneys.

Because the stage IV lesion, T_2,N_2, is anterior, I would recommend a radical vulvectomy. From the description, it appears to me that clearance of the symphysis pubis, inferior pubic ramus, vagina, anal canal, rectum, and urethra is very likely.

Let us turn our attention to the groins. Some would advocate only irradiation to the groins, but I would recommend inguinofemoral lymphadenectomy for both inguinal regions, which would usually include dissecting nodes just above the inguinal ligament. I would not recommend a pelvic lymphadenectomy or dissection of the deep groin nodes.

I will assume that both groins have positive nodes and consequently would recommend postoperative irradiation, since it is the patient with palpable metastatic nodes, not the one with occult metastasis, who experiences recurrence in the groin. An alternative would be a fine needle aspiration or single lymph node biopsy followed by irradiation. This management would not be my choice; the leg edema might be decreased with the lesser operative procedure, but the tolerance of the groin in this patient is not up to cancercidal doses. Irradiation with 5000 cGy by external beam, with a 1000-cGy electron boost, usually with 12 MeV or higher, is reaching above tolerance for most patients with 75-year-old skin. I will assume that the vulvar resection had 1 cm of normal tissue as a margin and that therefore the recurrence rate at the primary site would be very low. The patient's 5-year survival would be approximately 20%, the overall 5-year actual rate for 2598 operated patients being 52%.

PHYSICIANS' RESPONSE

TALLY LEVY
ROBERT GIRTANNER
ALAN KAPLAN

This 75-year-old woman with a 3-cm ulcerative lesion and bilateral firm, enlarged inguinal nodes is highly likely to have carcinoma of the vulva.

Vulvar cancer usually effects elderly postmenopausal women. In most of these patients, a history of long-term pruritus or a lump can be elucidated. Delay in diagnosis and treatment is still frequent, since most patients tend to put off seeking medical care and, in addition, many physicians treat these lesions with various steroid and antibacterial creams without performing a biopsy for definitive diagnosis.

The first diagnostic step in the present case should be a biopsy of the lesion, which can be done in the office under local anesthesia. Before any treatment is begun, the remaining segments of the lower genital tract must be evaluated, as lesions of the cervix and vagina are frequently associated with vulvar cancer. If the biopsy reveals a malignancy, treatment recommendations are then made.

In recent years the traditional performance of an en bloc radical vulvectomy and bilateral groin dissection has been replaced in most institutions by an individualized conservative resection of the primary tumor by either modified radical vulvectomy or radical local excision, with inguinal femoral lymphadenectomy done through separate incisions. This trend has resulted in better wound healing and reduced operative morbidity without compromising cure and survival rates. Patients with T_2 lesions (> 2 cm) and firm, palpable inguinal lymph nodes have a high likelihood of metastatic nodal involvement. In the past, such patients would have undergone pelvic lymphadenectomy after a full groin dissection. This procedure added further to the potential postoperative morbidity while adding only minimal potential survival benefit. Today, postoperative radiation to the groins and ipsilateral hemipelvis without pelvic lymphadenectomy is recommended based on the results of a Gynecologic Oncology Group (GOG) study, in which patients with positive groin nodes were randomized to either pelvic lymph node dissection or bilateral groin and pelvic irradiation (1). There is a significant survival advantage at 2 years to the group receiving radiation therapy, probably related to a significant decrease in the incidence of groin recurrence. Nevertheless, pelvic recurrence was higher in the group receiving pelvic radiation, possibly because radiation therapy is capable of sterilizing microscopic metastases in lymph nodes but incapable of eradicating bulky nodal disease.

Our approach to patients with clinically suspicious inguinal lymph nodes is to perform a preoperative CT scan of the pelvis to determine whether there are any enlarged pelvic nodes. During the surgery, we recommend removing the vulvar lesion by radical local excision, with surgically tumor-free margins of 1 to 2 cm. All enlarged groin lymph nodes are removed through a separate incision and sent for frozen section. If metastatic disease is found, we do not perform a full lymphadenectomy because this procedure, combined with groin irradiation, often produces severe leg edema. However, if the frozen section reveals no metastatic disease in the removed nodes, a full groin dissection is done. All enlarged pelvic nodes previously seen on CT scan should be removed by an extraperitoneal approach. Adjuvant groin and pelvic irradiation (45 to 50 Gy) should be given to patients with two or more positive lymph nodes as soon as the groin incisions heal.

References

1. Homesley HD, Bundy BN, Sedlis A, Adcock C. Radiation therapy versus pelvic node resection for carcinoma of the vulva with positive groin nodes. Obstet Gynecol 1986; 68:733–740.

12

Vulvar Cancer: Malignant Melanoma

CASE

A 52-year-old woman was recently found to have an asymptomatic pigmented lesion on the right labium majus at the time of a routine gynecological examination. She has no previous history of malignant disease or any serious medical illnesses and currently takes no medications. The 1-cm vulvar lesion was biopsied by a dermatologist and proved to be a malignant melanoma. The biopsy measured 2 by 1.5 cm and was approximately 0.5 cm deep. The lesion showed a depth of invasion of 2 mm and there also appeared to be some angioinvasion. The lesion was located approximately 2 cm to the right of the clitoris. Careful examination of the groins shows no evidence of palpable adenopathy. A chest x-ray is likewise negative.

PHYSICIANS' RESPONSE

SHARON SHEFFIELD
WELDON E. CHAFE

The management of vulvar melanoma in this patient provides an interesting challenge. This lesion, reported to be 1 cm in size, has been excised with a depth of invasion reported to be 2 mm, as well as showing evidence of angioinvasion. The system of the Fédération Internationale de Gynécolgie et d'Obstétrique (FIGO), used in the staging of carcinomas of the vulva, is not really applicable for melanomas, where the prognosis is mainly related to the tumor's depth of penetration.

Although numerous trials involving chemotherapy regimens and immunotherapy have been reported for cutaneous melanomas, surgery offers the only effective treatment with a reasonable prospect for control and potential cure of malignant melanoma.

The first question regarding surgical excision: What is the appropriate surgical procedure? Optimal surgical margins have not been defined for cutaneous melanomas. However, margins of at least 2 cm have been recommended for lesions 1 to 4 mm thick and margins of 3 cm for lesions greater than 4 mm. In this patient with a lesion 2 mm thick (both Chung and Breslow level III), a reexcision of the lesion site would make it possible to obtain these recommended margins and to spare the clitoris.

The second surgical question regarding surgical therapy: Is regional node excision indicated? In a prospective study by the Gynecologic Oncology Group reported in the journal *Cancer* (May 1994), patients with positive capillary lymphatic space invasion demonstrated a 31.8% incidence of positive regional lymph node involvement. Although elective lymph node dissection is not recommended for lesions with less than 1 mm of invasion (low risk of nodal metastasis) or greater than 4 mm of invasion (high risk of systemic hematogenous micrometastasis), there exists no recommendations for the lesion that is invasive from 1 to 4 mm. Theoretically, lymph node removal can potentially prevent systemic disease when tumor spread is confined to the regional lymph node group.

In this patient, we would recommend excision of the regional right groin nodes. We would also favor the en bloc resection of the lesion and nodes as opposed to the wide local excision of the lesion and a separate groin incision for the nodes. Of note, radical vulvectomy has offered no survival advantage over radical (2-cm margin) local excision.

In summary, we recommend radical wide local excision of the melanoma site with en bloc groin node dissection for this patient.

Reference

Phillips GL, Bundy BN, et al. Malignant melanoma of the vulva treated by radical hemivulvectomy: A prospective study of the Gynecologic Oncology Group. Cancer 1994; 73:2626–2632.

PHYSICIAN'S RESPONSE

JAVIER MAGRINA

This case involves a 52-year-old asymptomatic woman with a 1-cm melanoma, 2 mm of invasion and associated angioinvasion, located 2 cm to the right of the clitoris and with no palpable groin nodes. Because it is located 2 cm to the right of the clitoris, it is considered a cutaneous (not mucosal) melanoma.

There are two questions to address:

1. One is related to the presence of metastatic disease. In the presence of nonpalpable groin nodes and negative chest x-ray, it is unlikely that there is metastatic disease elsewhere, since these are the two most common sites for metastases. However, I would obtain a liver computed tomography (CT) scan to rule out hepatic metastases. We will assume that this scan proves negative.

2. The second question pertains to the surgical treatment. There are two issues to address: one pertains to the excision of the lesion and the other to the removal of the regional lymph nodes.

   a. In regard to the excision of the lesion, there are two issues to solve: is a radical vulvectomy preferable to local excision, and what size margins are necessary for this vulvar melanoma?

      Radical vulvectomy does not seem to improve local control as compared to wide local excision (1). Therefore a wide local excision would seem preferable.

      It appears that margins of 3 cm are necessary for lesions with a depth of invasion > 0.76 mm (2), and these would be adequate margins for this lesion. A local recurrence rate of 33% can be expected (1). Margins of 2 cm are appropriate for lesions with a depth of invasion of < 0.76 mm. Margins > 3 cm have not resulted in improved local control (2).

   b. Relative to the regional lymph nodes, since this is a lateral lesion, the ipsilateral nodes are at risk for metastatic disease, about 25% in this patient (3). Superficial and deep groin node dissections are necessary in this patient. The groin node dissection must be performed en bloc with the wide local excision for two reasons: vulvar melanoma can produce satellite lesions in transit, and additionally, this lesion contains angioinvasions, indicating that there may be metastatic cells in transit.

There is no need for pelvic node dissection in the presence of negative groin nodes (4). However, if the groin nodes are positive, a contralateral groin node dissection, en bloc with the wide local excision, is necessary, as well as a laparoscopic bilateral pelvic node dissection. If the pelvic nodes are positive, an aortic node dissection would be indicated.

References

1. Rose PG, Piver MS, Tsukada Y, Lau T. Conservative therapy for melanoma of the vulva. Am J Obstet Gynecol 1988; 159:52–55.
2. Aitkin DR, Clausen K, Klein JP, et al. The extent of primary melanoma excision—a re-evaluation—how wide is wide? Ann Surg 1983; 198:634–641.
3. Podratz KC, Gaffey TA, Symmonds RE, et al. Melanoma of the vulva: An update. Gynecol Oncol 1983; 16:153–168.

4. Jaramillo BA, Ganjei P, Averette HE, et al. Malignant melanoma of the vulva. Obstet Gynecol 1985; 66:398–401.

PHYSICIANS' RESPONSE

DUNCAN SAVAGE
HENRY KEYS

Vulvar melanoma is the second most common histology for vulvar malignancies (10% of all vulvar malignancies); traditional therapy has consisted of radical vulvectomy with inguinal lymph node dissection. However, recently published data have prompted clinicians to reconsider the efficacy of this aggressive surgical approach. Based upon a clinicopathological study from the Gynecologic Oncology Group (GOG), recurrence-free interval for vulvar melanoma is most closely related to melanoma the staging of the American Joint Committee on Cancer (AJCC) (based upon depth of cutaneous/dermal invasion) (1) (see Table 1). The conclusion of this report is that the biological behavior of vulvar melanoma is similar to that of other nongenital cutaneous melanomas. Surgical treatment for cutaneous melanoma usually consists of wide surgical resection of the primary tumor site.

Currently, the FIGO stage of vulvar melanoma is the same as for vulvar carcinoma (see Table 2).

Favorable prognostic factors for vulvar melanoma include lesions less than 3 mm thick, absence of clinically palpable inguinal lymph nodes, no ulceration, and no vascular invasion (2). These patients can be treated with a wide local excision without elective inguinal lymph node dissection. Most studies do not support performing elective inguinal node dissections without clinically palpable inguinal lymph nodes. Pelvic lymph nodes are virtually never involved unless there are clinically palpable inguinal lymph nodes. Poor prognostic features include lesions greater than 3 mm thick, palpable inguinal lymph nodes, and an ulcerative lesion. Some reports have suggested that a centrally located tumor is associated with a worse prognosis.

Table 1   AJCC Staging of Melanoma

Stage		
	IA	Localized melanoma < 0.75 mm
	IB	Localized melanoma 0.76 mm to 1.5 mm
	IIA	Localized melanoma 1.5 mm to 4 mm
	IIB	Localized melanoma > 4 mm
	III	Limited nodal metastases
	IV	Advanced regional metastases or distant metastases

Table 2 FIGO Staging of Vulvar Cancer

T_1	Tumor confined to the vulva, 2 cm or less in diameter
T_2	Tumor confined to the vulva, more than 2 cm in diameter
T_3	Tumor of any size with adjacent tumor spread to the urethra and/or vagina and/or anus
T_4	Tumor of any size infiltrating the bladder mucosa or rectal mucosa or bone fixation
N_0	No palpable lymph nodes
N_1	Palpable lymph nodes, mobile, not thought to contain tumor
N_2	Palpable lymph nodes thought to contain tumor
N_3	Fixed or ulcerated lymph nodes

A large series of patients with vulvar melanoma reported from the Sloan-Kettering Cancer Center in New York City correlated 10-year survival with tumor thickness. Ten-year survival for tumors less than 0.75 mm in diameter was 48%; and for those between 0.75 and 1.5 mm, it was 68%; 1.51 and 3.0 mm, it was 44%; while for tumors larger than 3.0 mm, it was 22% (3).

In this patient, the lesion measured 1 cm in diameter and the biopsy specimen measured 2 by 1.5 cm. There was a 2-mm depth of invasion with pathological evidence of vascular invasion. This would represent stage IIA disease according to the AJCC melanoma criteria and FIGO stage T_1N_0 for vulvar malignancies. If this represented a squamous cell carcinoma, survival for this patient would be favorable, with an excellent change of long-term survival. However, the depth of invasion in this melanotic tumor is associated with a significant risk of distant metastatic disease. The recommended treatment for this patient would be reexcision with a 2-cm margin. The lesion is lateralized, and an attempt to spare the clitoris should be made. Since she has no palpable lymph nodes in the inguinal regions, an inguinal lymph node dissection is not required. Close follow-up with careful examination of the primary site and inguinal regions is indicated. The patient should also be questioned about her general health status, since she is at substantial risk for future development of metastatic disease to the liver, brain, and bone.

References

1. Phillips GL, Bundy BN, Okagaki T, et al. Malignant melanoma of the vulva treated by radical hemivulvectomy: A prospective study of the gynecologic oncology group. Cancer 1994; 73:2626–2632.
2. Tasseron EWK, van der Esch EP, Hart AAM, et al. A clinicopathological study of 30 melanomas of the vulva. Gynecol Oncol 1992; 46:170–175.
3. Trimple EL, Lewis JL Jr, Williams LL, et al. Management of vulvar melanoma. Gynecol Oncol 1992; 45:254–258.

PHYSICIAN'S RESPONSE

GEORGE MORLEY

Melanoma of the vulva is a rare malignancy with fewer than 500 cases reported in the literature, according to a recent review (1). In spite of its rarity, it is still the second most common cancer occurring in this region. Most often, this lesion arises in the anterior labia minora or clitoris. In this case the lesion was located approximately 2 cm to the right of the clitoris. These patients usually complain of itching, the presence of a vulvar sore, and/or localized bleeding; however, this patient was totally asymptomatic prior to being seen by the dermatologist.

There are basically three types of melanoma of the vulva: (a) intraepithelial or lentigo maligna, (b) superficial spreading melanoma, and (c) nodular melanoma. Some 80% of the lesions are of the superficial spreading type, and these have a more favorable prognosis. Podratz et al. (2) in 1983, reported on 48 patients with melanoma of the vulva. The 5-year survival rate of the 30 patients with superficial spreading lesions was approximately 75%, compared to that of the 15 patients with nodular growths, which was approximately 45%.

The FIGO classification for carcinoma of the vulva (including the TNM system) does not appear to be applicable to the staging of these melanomas, since a more accurate differential relates to microstaging of these lesions through the Clark (3) levels of invasion (Table 1) or the Breslow (4) system (Table 2) of millimeter measurements of vertical thickness. Obviously, one must await the pathologist's report as to the histological type and depth of invasion after reviewing the *excised* specimen.

Until recently, the treatment of choice for malignant melanoma of the vulva had been radical vulvectomy and bilateral groin and pelvic lymphadenectomy. In fact, early in my own career, one of the very distinguished gynecologic oncologists in this country stated that the most radical procedure should be performed at the earliest possible moment and that local excisions and unilateral groin dissection had no place in the definitive treatment of this condition. Over time, however, this concept has been modified through collaborative experience, and

Table 1 AJCC Staging of Melanoma

Level I	Neoplastic cells confined to the epithelium
Level II	Lesion penetrating the basement membrane and extending into the papillary dermis
Level III	Melanoma invading through the papillary dermis and involving the reticular dermis
Level IV	Pigmented cells found in the deep reticular dermis
Level V	Melanoma invading the subcutaneous tissue

Table 2 Breslow's Staging System[a]

Stage I	Invasion 0.75 mm or less
Stage II	Invasion 0.76 to 1.5 mm
Stage III	Invasion 1.51 to 3.0 mm
Stage IV	Invasion greater than 3.0 mm

[a]The Breslow levels are measured from the surface of the lesion.

now individualization of treatment is considered more appropriate. The routine preoperative assessment includes an accurate measurement of the gross lesion as well as a chest x-ray, hemogram, urinalysis; on occasion, a CT scan and/or lymphangiogram may be indicated.

There are basically two options considered by most gynecological oncologists in the treatment of this specific lesion, and they are either radical wide local excision of the primary lesion or radical vulvectomy and bilateral groin lymphadenectomy. The bilaterality of the latter dissection reflects the fact that the lesion is often in the clitoral or periclitoral area, and these lesions drain in both directions. Pelvic lymphadenectomy is not considered part ot the treatment at the present time, since there have been no cases reported where the pelvic lymph nodes were involved without involvement of the groin nodes. Most investigators feel that there is essentially a 100% 5-year survival rate if the lesion is confined to levels I and II of either the Clark or Breslow classification. The difference between these two classifications is not thought to be significant; however, the Breslow system is easier to interpret, since most of us are clinically oriented. The survival for most of the more advanced lesions progressively decreases, with level V lesions having a less than 25% survival rate.

Currently, most gynecological oncologists consider radical wide local excision with adequate margins or radical hemivulvectomy as the treatment of choice for levels I and II of either method of staging this disease. Patients having more than a superficially invasive melanoma should be treated with radical vulvectomy and bilateral groin lymph node dissection, even though this is probably for palliation only, especially if the groin lymph nodes are positive, since these patients uniformly succumb to their disease (5,6).

Finally, the definitive treatment of a primary malignant melanoma is some type of surgical excision. Radiation therapy has very little to offer these patients. Systemic chemotherapy has been reported, using several agents or combinations thereof; however, none are clearly better than single-agent dacarbazine (DTIC). Immunotherapy (vaccine therapy) and genetic manipulation do offer some promise, but no significant reports pertaining to these lesions of the vulva have been forthcoming and these methods of treatment are still investigational.

In summary, I believe we have made significant progress in better defining the treatment of this uncommon lesion; however, we must continue to pursue other therapeutic modalities in the hopes that some day surgical extirpation will not be required.

References

1. Bailet JW, Figge DC, Tamimi HK. Malignant melanoma of the vulva: A case report of distal recurrence in a patient with a superficially invasive primary lesion. Obstet Gynecol 1987; 70:515.
2. Podratz KC, Gaffey TA, Symmonds RE, et al. Melanoma of the vulva: An update. Gynecol Oncol 1983; 16:153.
3. Clark WH, from Bernardino EA, et al. The histogenesis and biologic behavior of primary human malignant melanoma of the skin. Cancer Res 1969; 29:705.
4. Breslow A. Thickness, cross-sectional areas and depth of invasion in the prognosis of cutaneous melanoma. Ann Surg 1970; 172:902.
5. Jaramillo BA, Ganjei P, Averette HE, et al. Malignant melanoma of the vulva. Obstet Gynecol 1985; 66:398.
6. Trimble EL, Lewis JL, Williams LL, et al. Management of vulvar melanoma. Gynecol Oncol 1992; 45:254.

13

Vulvar Cancer: Stage I

CASE

A 66-year-old woman presented to her local physician with a sore on her vulva. He took a small biopsy and referred her to a gynecological oncologist. The patient has some mild cardiac disease and takes digoxin as well as a thiazide diuretic. She is 5 ft, 4 in tall and weighs 140 lb. The physical examination shows no palpable supraclavicular nodes. The chest is clear. The heart shows a regular rate and rhythm. No suspicious inguinal nodes are palpable. On examining the vulva, a 1 cm lesion is found in the posterior third of the right labium minus; it does not appear to be more than 1 or 2 mm in gross thickness.

PHYSICIANS' RESPONSE

BRADLEY J. MONK
MICHAEL L. BERMAN

Since Way reported an improved survival using en bloc radical vulvectomy and inguinal lymphadenectomy instead of local excision in women with carcinoma of the vulva, this procedure has been the mainstay of therapy in the treatment of this disease. Over the last two decades, however, many physicians have chosen to individualize operative management and, where appropriate, to perform more limited surgery in order to reduce treatment-related morbidity. Several series of patients so treated generally have confirmed excellent cure rates with marked reduction in complications including wound infections, chronic lower extremity edema, and sexual dysfunction.

The management of vulvar cancer may be considered to include two distinct components: treatment of the primary lesion and treatment of the regional lymphatics. The primary lesion may be excised separately from or in continuity with the lymph nodes. When the vulvar excision is distinct from that of the lymph nodes, it may be a radical local excision, hemivulvectomy, subtotal vulvectomy or radical vulvectomy; however, when the primary tumor is removed in continuity with the lymph nodes, it usually is done only as a radical vulvectomy. More extensive lesions may even require exenterative surgery or a combination of two or even all three modalities of chemotherapy, radiation, and surgery.

The case presentation is of a woman with a T1 lesion (less than 2 cm in diameter). Although the criteria for an adequate local excision of such a limited cancer is not standardized, we believe that a radical vulvectomy would be excessive. This opinion is supported by the experience of the Gynecologic Oncology Group (GOG) with modified radical hemivulvectomy in the treatment of early stage I (T_1 lesions, no suspicious adenopathy) carcinoma of the vulva. Among 101 evaluable women treated with a radical local excision (defined as a depth of at least 1 cm below the lesion and a 2-cm margin of normal skin around the lesion), there were 19 (16%) recurrences and 7 (6%) deaths. Of 10 patients whose disease recurred on the vulva, 8 were salvaged by further operation. Thus, only two deaths were related to local recurrence. The remaining deaths occurred among patients whose first recurrence was in the groin. As expected, the acute and long-term morbidity as well as the hospital stay was substantially less than had been reported among patients treated according to GOG protocols, which required more radical resection, such as radical vulvectomy and bilateral inguinofemoral lymphadenectomy. Although there was a significantly greater risk of recurrence, most recurrences were local and most of these were salvaged with further surgery, so that the risk of death in the limited-surgery group was not different from that of historical controls. Such a conservative surgical approach for the primary lesion would be recommended for this patient.

Several criteria should be assessed in considering the management of regional lymph nodes. It is axiomatic that inguinofemoral lymphadenectomy should be omitted if the risk of lymph node metastasis is negligible. In order to estimate this risk, one must assess the maximal depth, tumor size, histological grade, presence or absence of vascular space invasion, and clinical nature of the groin lymph nodes. Patients with clinically suspicious nodes or those whose tumors invade the lymphovascular spaces should undergo inguinofemoral lymphadenectomy and be considered for radical vulvectomy rather than radical local excision. Indeed, the GOG data for early vulvar cancers 5 mm or less in thickness showed a 17% rate of groin node metastases when lymphovascular space invasion was absent and 65% when lymphovascular space invasion was present. Fortunately, lymphovascular space invasion is present only 5 to 10% of early lesions. The risk of nodal metastases also increases with larger lesions and tumors that are more deeply invasive, a condition which does not exist in the current case presentation.

As with lymphovascular invasion, tumor size is an important risk indicator for nodal metastasis. For example, cancers less than 1 cm in size will have approximately a 4% rate of nodal spread; however, lesions between 1 and 2 cm in size have a 13 to 15% risk. In the absence of lymphovascular space invasion, perhaps the most important predictor of nodal metastases is depth of invasion. Unfortunately, there is a lack of standardization regarding measurement of depth of invasion. In most recent publications, invasion is measured from the dermal-epidermal junction of the most superficial adjacent papillae; however, others have measured from the surface of the lesion. Using either definition, the risk of lymph node metastases approaches 0% if the depth of invasion is ≤ 1 mm. With cancers invading 1 to 2 mm, the risk of nodal metastases increases to 5 and 10%. Since the current lesion appears to be at least 1 mm in thickness, a superficial inguinal lymphadenectomy with sparing of the underlying femoral lymph nodes would be indicated. Only if nodal metastases are found among the superficial nodes, do we perform a bilateral inguinofemoral lymphadenectomy. If one or even two unilateral lymph nodes contain metastatic cancer, adjuvant irradiation might not be required; however, bilateral nodal spread or the presence of three or more nodes with metastatic cancer would warrant adjuvant radiotherapy.

References

Berman ML, Soper JT, Creasman WT, et al. Conservative surgical management of superficially invasive stage I vulvar carcinoma. Gynecol Oncol 1989; 35:352–357.
Stehman FB, Bundy BN, Dvoretsky PM, et al. Early stage I carcinoma of the vulva treated with ipsilateral superficial inguinal lymphadenectomy and modified radical hemivulvectomy: A prospective study of the Gynecologic Oncology Group. Obstet Gynecol 1992; 79:490–497.

PHYSICIAN'S RESPONSE

FRANK MAJOR

This 66-year-old woman was seen in consultation. The biopsy performed prior to referral for consultation has been returned; it is a small, Keyes-punch type of biopsy with squamous cell carcinoma, invasive to a depth of 1 mm. The patient is apparently in reasonable health status, with a history of mild congestive heart failure, which is well controlled with daily digoxin and a thiazide diuretic. The examination, as noted, shows no palpable adenopathy, and the lungs are clear. The patient shows no evidence of congestive heart failure. The examination reveals a 1-cm slightly raised lesion in the posterior third of the right labium minus. There is a small 3-mm central defect, apparently the result of the recent biopsy.

On further history, the patient denies smoking and uses alcohol only occasionally at social functions. She is fully active, retired from her secretarial position after many years. She is quite anxious concerning the pathology report showing "cancer."

I have explained to the patient that this biopsy, while it does indeed show very early invasion, may not represent the whole picture, and I feel that a more extensive biopsy would be appropriate at this time. I have discussed with the patient and arranged for a wide local excision to be carried out under intravenous sedation with local lidocaine (Xylocaine) anesthesia. This procedure will excise the 1-cm lesion completely with approximately a 5-mm margin. The depth of excision will incorporate the full thickness of the dermis without taking a substantial amount of the underlying fatty tissue. The defect will be closed with a subcuticular suture following hemostasis. We will then await the final report from the pathologist, who will have carefully marked the margins of this wide local excision.

Should there be more extensive invasion, greater than 1 mm, we would recommend to the patient that a modified radical vulvectomy with unilateral groin dissection be carried out. Preferably, this could be done under conduction anesthesia and would produce a cure rate of better than 90% for this early stage I lesion. Prior to scheduling the more extensive procedure, we would obtain a computed tomography (CT) scan to look for lymphadenopathy; also, we would again make sure that the chest x-ray shows no evidence of any lesions. Should there be no evidence of deeper invasion other than the 1-mm focus noted on the biopsy, the wide local excision would be therapeutic. The patient would be advised to have follow-up examinations, either with a good gynecologist or gynecological oncologist, at 3- to 6-month intervals for the rest of her life. She would be told that the recurrence rate runs as high as 50% over a 10-year period and would be instructed in good perineal hygiene as well as the avoidance of tobacco—but, as already noted, she is a nonsmoker. I would feel from the history given that the most likely scenario would be the second one described, namely a microinvasive carcinoma of the vulva.

References

Chu J, Tamimi HK, Ek M, Figge DC. Stage I vulvar cancer: Criteria for microinvasion. Obstet Gynecol 1982; 59:716–719.

Stehman F, Burdy B, Dvoretsky P, Creasman W. Early stage I carcinoma of the vulva treated with ipsilateral superficial inguinal lymphadenectomy and modified radical hemivulvectomy: A prospective study of the Gynecologic Oncology Group. Obstet Gynecol 1992; 79:491–497.

PHYSICIAN'S RESPONSE

DANIEL SMITH

A 66 year old woman is referred for evaluation of a vulva lesion. She notes that this lesion is sore and has been present for an unknown period of time. Pertinent previous medical history includes mild congestive heart disease. The patient takes digoxin and a diuretic. Prior gynecological/obstetric history is not available. The physical examination is unremarkable except for the genital findings. Lymph node areas in the supraclavicular and inguinal regions are not clinically suspicious. On examination of the vulva, there is a 1-cm lesion located on the posterior third of the right labium minus. The lesion appears to be no more than 1 to 2 mm in gross thickness.

Because of the small size of the lesion and its easy accessibility, excisional biopsy with a 1- to 2- cm margin of surrounding skin can be readily performed under local anesthesia. Excisional biopsy as opposed to punch or incisional biopsy is preferred to minimize sampling error and allow the pathologist to determine depth of invasion, degree of differentiation, pattern of spread, and presence or absence of lymphovascular invasion.

The differential diagnosis for such a vulvar lesion includes a wide range of conditions including trauma, infection, and neoplasia. Considering only gynecological neoplasia, possible diagnoses include a vulvar dystrophy with or without atypia, squamous cell dysplasia, Paget's disease, or invasive cancer. Management of any dystrophy and most dysplasias would be complete with local excision unless the lesions are multifocal. Were the biopsy to show Paget's disease, more extensive excision would be necessary to ensure clear margins and to determine that there is no underlying adenocarcinoma. If this patient had a Paget's lesion, a right posterior excision of the labium majus would be required. Further surgery would be indicated if an adenocarcinoma were present.

If the excisional biopsy revealed an invasive squamous cell carcinoma, further questions would include (a) the thickness of the neoplasm, (b) the depth of stromal invasion, (c) the pattern of spread, (d) the degree of differentiation, and (e) the presence of lymphatic or vascular invasion. Patients with disease 1 to 5 mm thick without vascular space invasion or spray patterns of infiltration can be successfully managed with radical hemivulvectomy and ipsilateral inguinal lymphadenectomy. The exceptionally rare patient with a positive inguinal lymph node needs more extensive therapy.

Of special interest is the fact that the patient has a lesion less than 1 mm in thickness with no lymphatic or vascular invasion. Such a patient may easily be cured simply with wide local excision. In borderline cases, the choice of hemivulvectomy and ipsilateral lymphadenectomy would seem appropriate.

In the care of this patient, standard radical surgery does not seem to be required due to the size, location, and limited thickness of the lesion. If the excision revealed either an adenocarcinoma or melanoma, the traditional approach of more radical surgery would be necessary.

References

Hacker NF, Berek JS, Lagasse LD, et al. Individualization of therapy for stage I squamous cell vulvar carcinoma. Obstet Gynecol 1984; 63:155–162.

PHYSICIAN'S RESPONSE

MALCOLM G. IDELSON

The original "small biopsy" taken by the referring physician, although probably inadequate for full decision making, should be carefully reviewed. If the pathology reveals noninvasive intraepithelial squamous neoplasia or a microinvasive squamous cell carcinoma (defined below), I would next remove the entire lesion visible with a deep, 2.0-cm-diameter punch biopsy under local anesthesia. This would most likely provide the information needed to make the best decision for treatment in this controversial area as well as affording time for reviewing and studying the fixed pathological sections and recuts if necessary.

If the lesion reveals only intraepithelial neoplasia (VIN) with clear margins, no further therapy is indicated at this time. If there are dystrophic dysplastic or nondysplastic changes present at the margins, additional wider local excisions should be done.

If the lesion, carefully considered, meets the present criteria for microinvasion, a wide and deep local excision should follow with margins of 1.0 to 2.0 cm around and deep to the original lesion. Any marginal remnant of dystrophy should be further excised or laser-vaporized. This would complete the therapy.

Microinvasion is defined as (a) a lesion less than 2.0 cm in surface size, (b) stromal invasion no deeper than 1.0 mm below the epithelial-stromal junction of the adjacent most superficial normal dermal papilla, and (c) absence of lymphovascular space invasion. Poorly differentiated lesions or spray rather than pushing patterns of invasion, particularly with areas of confluence and stromal penetration near to 1.0 mm, would change my diagnosis to stage I with frank invasion.

Stage I with the interpretation of frank invasion *in this case* would alter the recommended therapy to (a) a radical local excision with at least 2.0-cm margins and depth of dissection down to the deep or inferior fascia of the urogenital diaphragm and (b) an ipsilateral "complete" groin dissection or lymphadenectomy via a separate incision. This would include removal of the deep nodes with or without preservation of the saphenous vein. If one or more nodes were involved, the contralateral groin dissection should be done. If two or more nodes are positive, adjuvant external beam irradiation should be given to the involved inguinal areas and pelvis. If deep nodes are involved, consideration for a pelvic lymphadenectomy should be made primarily to remove gross nodal disease, followed by radiotherapy.

If the lesion as described in the posterior third of the right labium minus is closer than 2.0 cm from the posterior fourchette and lymphadenectomy is indicated, a bilateral groin dissection would be done.

Finally, careful scrutiny of the remainder of the vulva, perineum, perianal area, vagina, and cervix would complete the above recommendations.

References

Kelley JL III et al. Minimal invasion vulvar carcinoma: An indication for conservative surgical therapy. Gynecol Oncol 1992; 44:240–244.

Stehman FB et al. Early stage I carcinoma of the vulva treated with ipsilateral superficial inguinal lymphadenectomy and modified radical hemivulvectomy: A prospective study of the Gynecologic Oncology Group. Obstet Gynecol 1992; 79:490–497.

14

Vulvar Cancer: Locally Advanced Disease

CASE

A 60-year-old woman presents to your office having been referred by her local physician with a large vulvar tumor. The patient tells of having had some soreness on her bottom for the past year, but she was afraid to go to the doctor. She currently takes no medications. Prior to this recent episode, she had not seen a doctor for 20 years. She has smoked a half pack of cigarettes daily for 30 years. On examination, there are no palpable supraclavicular nodes. The chest is clear. The heart shows a regular rate and rhythm. No abdominal masses are noted, no breast masses are noted, and no suspicious inguinal nodes are palpable. On examination of the vulva, a 6-by 9-cm ulcerated vulvar lesion is found involving the anal sphincter and extending up the left labium majus to within ½ cm of the external urethral meatus. The midportion of the tumor also involves approximately 1 cm of distal vaginal wall. The patient demonstrates no swelling of the lower extremities and is experiencing no pain in them. A chest x-ray and abdominal pelvic computed tomography (CT) do not demonstrate any evidence of metastatic disease.

PHYSICIAN'S RESPONSE

ALEXANDER W. KENNEDY

The initial step in managing this patient with apparent advanced vulvar cancer is to perform a representative incisional biopsy of the patient's neoplasm. It is most likely that this will demonstrate an invasive squamous cell carcinoma. Alternatively, although much less common, malignant melanoma, basal cell carcinoma, or Paget's disease of the vulva might be encountered. These latter less common lesions would be managed significantly differently than invasive squamous cell carcinoma. For the purposes of this discussion, it will be assumed that the biopsy indicates squamous cell carcinoma.

This unfortunate woman has a locally advanced vulvar cancer and, both by clinical and radiologic examination, does not have evidence of apparent metastases. The patient should therefore be considered potentially curable and a candidate for definitive surgical therapy.

Several investigators have attempted to limit the extent of surgery for advanced vulvar cancers by employing preoperative radiation therapy, possibly in conjunction with chemotherapy radiosensitizers. While some reports indicate improved resectability of these advanced tumors, our experience has been disappointing in this regard. It is unlikely that in this patient, radiation therapy, even in conjunction with chemotherapy, would cause sufficient tumor regression to allow preservation of the anal sphincter with satisfactory function. Therefore, if exenterative surgery is to be employed, it is preferred that this be done prior to any radiation therapy. Following satisfactory medical evaluation of this patient, I would advise that she undergo a posterior exenteration in conjunction with radical vulvectomy. I would advise an en bloc resection of this patient's lesion with the above-mentioned procedures. Total abdominal hysterectomy, bilateral salpingo-oophorectomy, and resection of the posterior vaginal wall would be included. I would attempt to preserve the anterior vaginal wall for use in closure and reconstruction. At the time of the operative procedure I would carefully assess the pelvic lymph nodes for any suggestion of pathological enlargement. An end-sigmoid colostomy would be fashioned. If the surgical defect were large or the patient wished to maintain sexual function, consultation with a plastic surgeon for reconstruction using myocutaneous flaps could be considered.

The patient can anticipate a significant postoperative hospital stay and recovery. Careful pathological review of the resected specimen is necessary to ensure adequate margins of resection. I would advise the patient, following satisfactory healing of her primary procedure, to undergo bilateral inguinal lymphadenectomy. This portion of the procedure could be delayed until her primary defect had healed, so as to decrease complication and morbidity. I would also wish to be reassured, based on the pathology report of the resected tumor, that the patient could still be considered potentially curable. At the time of the bilateral inguinal dissection, superficial and deep groin lymph nodes would be removed. If involvement of these nodes were noted, adjuvant postoperative groin radiotherapy would be considered.

References

Boronow RC. Therapeutic alternative to primary exenteration for advanced vulvo-vaginal cancer. Gynecol Oncol 1973; 3:233–243.

Levin W, Goldberg G, Altaras M, et al. The use of concomitant chemotherapy and radiotherapy prior to surgery in advanced stage carcinoma of the vulva. Gynecol Oncol 1986; 25:20–25.

PHYSICIAN'S RESPONSE

GILLIAN THOMAS

The patient appears to have a classic primary carcinoma of the vulva. The lesion should be biopsied. It is likely that incisional biopsy of the lesion will reveal a grade 1 or 2 squamous cell cancer, and treatment recommendations are based on a squamous cell carcinoma (SCC) histology. I am assuming that the patient is fit to undergo radical treatment.

The vulvar carcinoma is clearly advanced by virtue of its size, its encroachment upon the anal sphincter, its proximity to the external urethral meatus, and its extension proximally into the vaginal wall. The patient's long-term prognosis is dependent not only on the probability of obtaining local control of the vulvar disease but also on whether there are involved superficial or deep inguinal nodes or pelvic lymph nodes. The considerations for managing this patient's vulvar cancer are focused on defining appropriate treatment of the primary cancer in the vulva and of the inguinal lymph nodes to obtain locoregional control of disease and provide cure while minimizing the possible attendant morbidity of therapy.

The first step is to decide on optimal management of the primary in the vulva. In the past, primary posterior exenteration and radical vulvectomy would have been recommended. However, that surgery does not provide satisfactory local control and cure rates and does mean loss of the anus and rectum, a partial vaginectomy, and removal of the distal half of the urethra. More recently, numerous clinical studies have shown that squamous cell carcinomas of the vulva are very sensitive to radiation therapy with or without adjunctive sensitizing chemotherapy. This treatment may cure small cancers and obviate the need for radical or exenterative surgery in more advanced disease [1]. In view of the lesion size and its encroachment on critical midline structures, I would recommend that the patient have the cancer in the vulva treated with radical irradiation, reserving surgery for removal of residuum after irradiation. It is unclear whether the addition of radiosensitizing chemotherapy improves control compared to radiation alone. Skin and subcutaneous morbidity limit the dose of radiation that can be delivered to the vulva. In view of the size of this lesion, I would therefore favor attempting to get increased tumor cell kill by the addition of 5-fluorouracil (5-FU) as "radiosensitizing" chemotherapy.

Prior to initiating that therapy to the vulva, appropriate management of the inguinal regions is critical. Despite the fact that there are no palpably suspicious inguinal nodes, this patient is at high risk for nodal involvement. The standard therapy is inguinal node dissection. I would recommend that bilateral superficial groin node dissections be performed, since the lesion is midline. If there is involvement of the superficial nodes, the deep inguinal nodes should also be resected. There is no indication to proceed to pelvic node resection. Groin dissection may be therapeutic but is also important for diagnostic purposes, since it will guide the recommendation for postoperative radiation therapy to the groins. A large randomized study of the Gynecologic Oncology Group (2) shows that postoperative inguinal/pelvic nodal irradiation improves survival by decreasing inguinal nodal recurrences when two or more inguinal lymph nodes are involved. Macroscopic involvement of a single lymph node or extension of disease through the capsule of the single lymph node may confer the same bad prognosis as the involvement of two or more inguinal lymph nodes. Therefore, I would recommend postoperative inguinal/pelvic nodal irradiation, either uni- or bilaterally, depending on the side(s) of involvement, for microscopic involvement of two or more inguinal lymph nodes or macroscopic or extracapsular extension in a single node.

Following the lymph node dissection, consideration should be given to the technical details of radiation therapy. If the lymph node areas are to irradiated in addition to the primary in the vulva, these fields should be treated in continuity with anterior and posterior opposed parallel pairs of fields to include the vulva inferiorly and inguinal and pelvic lymph nodes up to the level of the midsacroiliac joints. If nodal irradiation is not indicated, an anterior and posterior parallel pair of radiation fields to the vulva alone will still be required to encompass the whole vulva and vagina, since the lesion extends to involve the anterior and posterior limits of the vulva. This field should extend laterally to include 2 to 3 cm of normal tissue beyond the vulvar lesion. Cystoscopy, urethroscopy, and sigmoidoscopy may be useful to determine the proximal extent of the lesion. The vulvar lesion should be treated to a radical radiation dose. The radiation should be given in 165 to 170-cGy fractions to a total dose of approximately 66 to 68 Gy. Despite the fact that full moist desquamation of the radiation field will develop, it is critical that rest periods allowing for settling of the acute reaction be kept to a minimum in order not to significantly protract the course. Infusional 5-FU should be given on the first 5 days of treatment, and at that time two fractions per day of irradiation should be given at least 6 hr apart. The 5-FU infusion should be repeated on two subsequent occasions during radiation therapy approximately 3 weeks apart.

The probability of local control following radical irradiation and resection of the residuum would be approximately 70%. It is unlikely that surgery for any residuum will require exenteration. The patient's probability of disease-free survival is clearly dependent on the presence or absence of involvement of the inguinal nodes. If the lymph nodes are negative, her probability of survival is in the order of 70%; if the lymph glands are involved in addition to the presence of this extensive primary vulvar lesion, I would suspect that her probability of survival will fall to approximately 50%.

I would recommend that the patient be seen 4 weeks after radiation therapy to ensure that the acute cutaneous reaction has settled down. At 6 to 8 weeks post-radiation, the vulva should be assessed with respect to the presence or absence of tumor residuum. If there is tumor residuum in the vulva at this time, it would be recommended that the patient undergo wide local excision of any residuum.

References

1. Thomas GM, Dembo AJ, Bryson SCP, et al. Changing concepts in the management of vulvar cancer. Gynecol Oncol 1991; 42:9–21.
2. Homesley HD, Bundy BN, Sedlis A, Adcock L. Radiation therapy versus node resection for carcinoma of the vulva with positive groin nodes. Obstet Gynecol 1986; 68:733–740.

PHYSICIAN'S RESPONSE

ERNEST W. FRANKLIN, III

Impression

Vulvar neoplasia, probably squamous cell carcinoma with invasion.

Recommendations

Biopsies to determine the presence of invasion as well as histological grade. Select biopsies should be taken from the margin at the vaginal wall, urethra, and anus to determine the degree of involvement by invasive carcinoma at these margins. If invasive carcinoma is present, particularly in the area of apparent involvement of the anal sphincter and urethral meatus, primary surgical management would require extensive resection and could result in urinary or anal incontinence requiring diversion. Primary management with radiation therapy to the inguinal nodes and vulva would then be a preferable alternative, with subsequent surgical resection of residual disease on the vulva after completion of radiation therapy. If the margins of involvement at the external urethral meatus and anus were carcinoma in situ or only superficially invasive, primary surgical resection would be feasible.

Discussion

The clinical presentation of this patient is not unusual, with the presence of a large vulvar neoplasm and a history of 1 year's symptomatology. Previous epidemiological studies of vulvar cancer show that delay on the part of physician and patient in seeking appropriate management is common. In addition, smoking appears to be an associated factor for increasing the risk for squamous cell carcinoma of the cervix, vagina, and vulva. Thorough assessment of the vagina and cervix, including colposcopy, should be carried out because of the association of cervical neoplasia with vulvar carcinoma. Sometime 20% to 40% of patients with vulvar carcinoma will develop cervical neoplasia, either prior to, concurrently with, or subsequent to the vulvar disease.

The physical findings on examination of the patient are consistent with a large primary carcinoma of the vulva. These lesions may reach considerable size in an invasive pattern of spread over the vulva and adjacent organs without metastasis to the inguinal nodes. The risk of occult metastasis with nonpalpable inguinal nodes remains at about 10 to 15%, however. Treatment of the nodes should not be neglected in this patient. If the invasive carcinoma is well lateralized, superficial and deep inguinal lymphadenectomy will suffice, with bilateral lymphadenectomy reserved for midline or bilateral vulvar carcinoma. The resection of the primary lesion, if that is elected based on the biopsies of anus and urethra, may require rotational flap or myocutaneous flap reconstruction of the vulvar defect. The management of the inguinal nodes is to be determined by the biopsies of the vulva confirming the presence of invasive carcinoma. Were suspicious inguinal nodes present, needle biopsy would be appropriate to determine whether metastatic disease is already present within the groin nodes. If that were the case, preoperative radiation to the pelvis and groin would improve local control and long-term survival. If the biopsies confirm extension of carcinoma to the urethra and anus, primary surgery would have two limitations. The first of these would be resection sufficient to obtain clear margins of resection. While a considerable portion of the distal urethra can be resected as long as the proximal urethrovesical angle mechanisms of continence remains intact, resection of the anal sphincter can be carried out over only a limited circumference without compromising anal function. Thus, involvement of the anus and urethra will be the primary determinant of whether radiation therapy should be the chief means of treatment. If radiation therapy is to be used, the inguinal lymph nodes should be included within the radiation field rather than being scheduled for subsequent surgical resection. This would be carried out to avoid the possibility of completing radiation therapy to the vulva only to find that metastatic disease within the inguinal nodes had become clinically evident. Upon completion of radiation therapy, some small amount of residual disease might still be present on the vulva and might require resection.

Reference

Perez CA, Grigsby PW, Galakatos A, et al. Radiation therapy in management of carcinoma of the vulva with emphasis on conservation therapy. Cancer 1993; 71:3707–3716.

PHYSICIANS' RESPONSE

SERGIO PECORELLI
LUCIEN VANUYSTEL
MARIO SIDERI
FRANCO ODICINO
ANTONELLA TESSADELLI

Vulvar cancer is uncommon, representing about 1% of female genital tract malignancies. Squamous cell carcinomas account for about 90%. Invasive vulvar cancer is predominantly a postmenopausal malignancy, the mean age at diagnosis being about 65 years. The staging criteria for vulvar cancer are based on tumor size and clinical evaluation of lymph nodes status and the tumor site. Recently the staging system was changed to a surgical one that incorporates the pathological status of the regional lymph nodes, found to be one of the strongest prognostic factors. Nodal involvement is strongly related to tumor diameter, depth of invasion, and grade of differentiation. Lateral vulvar lesions tend to metastasize to superficial and deep lymph nodes of the ipsilateral groin, while median lesions can metastasize directly to the deep pelvic nodes. The modern approach to the management of patients with carcinoma of the vulva is based on individualization of treatment. No "standard operation" is applicable to every patient, and emphasis is on performing the most conservative surgery that is consistent with cure of the disease.

This is an unusual case of a wide T_3 vulvar cancer involving the urethra, the vagina, and the anal sphincter with no clinical evidence of nodal involvement or distant metastasis. Once the vulvar biopsy confirms an invasive squamous cell carcinoma, surgery is the standard treatment for this locally advanced lesion, with a survival rate for these cases ranging between 50 and 65%.

The optimal surgery for this patient should include radical vulvectomy with bilateral groin and pelvic node dissection as well as distal urethral resection followed by the reconstructive procedures of the plastic surgeon. However involvement of the anal sphincter will force the surgeon to perform a posterior exenteration.

An alternative option for such a locally advanced lesion could be a neoadjuvant treatment in order to reduce the tumor burden, thus avoiding the exenterative procedure.

The role of preoperative concurrent radiation and chemotherapy to reduce the tumor volume in locally advanced vulvar cancer has been demonstrated. Clinical complete response in up to 75% of cases has been reported, thus allowing for less extensive surgery. A 5-week course of concurrent radiation (45 Gy at 1.8 Gy per day) and chemotherapy (CDDP 100 mg/m² on day 1 plus 5-fluorouracil 800 mg/m² for 5 days), this regimen being scheduled to start on days 1 and 21 of the radiation treatment. This could serve as an alternative to a purely surgical approach for this patient. If a reduction greater than 90% of the tumor were achieved, an additional boost of radiotherapy (e.g., 9 × 1.8 Gy) plus chemotherapy could be administered for treatment consolidation. On the contrary, if the tumor were reduced to less than 90% of the initial volume, the probability of obtaining a complete remission with further chemotherapy would be too low and one should proceed with surgery. The extent of the surgical approach would be radical. The possibility of avoiding posterior exenteration by combining surgery with intersitial brachytherapy at the anal sphincter should be considered.

Since quality of life is a critical issue in this case, emphasis should be placed on the need to discuss the therapeutic options with the patient in order to clarify the risks and benefits of each treatment modality.

References

Cavanagh D, Shepherd JH. The place of pelvic exenteration in the primary management of advanced carcinoma of the vulva. Gynecol Oncol 1982; 13:318–322.

Boronow RC. Combined therapy as an alternative to exenteration for locally advanced vulvo-vaginal cancer: Rationale and results. Cancer 1982; 49:1085–1091.

Thomas G, Dembo A, De Petrillo A, et al. Concurrent radiation and chemotherapy in vulvar carcinoma. Gynecol Oncol 1989; 34:263–267.

Berek JS, Heaps JM, Fu YS, et al. Concurrent cisplatin and 5-fluorouracil chemotherapy and radiation therapy for advanced-stage squamous carcinoma of the vulva. Gynecol Oncol 1991; 42:197–201.

Russel AH, Mesic JB, Scudder SA, et al. Synchronous radiation and cytotoxic chemotherapy for locally advanced or recurrent squamous cancer of the vulva. Gynecol Oncol 1992; 47:14–20.

15

Gestational Trophoblastic Disease: Persistent Mole

CASE

A 20-year-old woman, gravida I, para O, AB1 was diagnosed approximately 6 weeks ago with a molar pregnancy. She presented initially to her local emergency room with a pulse of 160, feeling unable to catch her breath, and terribly distressed by the pounding sensation in her chest. Her temperature was 101°F and she was sweating profusely. An ultrasound revealed the presence of a uterus 16-weeks in size, highly suggestive of a molar pregnancy. A beta-hCG (human chorionic gonadotropin) at that time was 430,000 mIU/ml and a T_4 was 12 μg/dL. A suction curettage was done without incident while the patient was covered by beta blockers. Her hCG level fell rapidly over the next 3 weeks to 6000; in the fourth week postevacuation, it returned as 9200. A repeat 6 days later was 10,800 mIU/mL. Computed tomography (CT) of the chest and an abdominal pelvic CT were negative for metastatic disease.

PHYSICIANS' RESPONSE

ANDREW K. SALTZMAN
LEO B. TWIGGS

The case describes a young, primigravid patient who initially presents with a hydatidiform mole. With an estimated incidence in the United States of approximately 1/1000 pregnancies, the practicing obstetrician and family practitioner will surely encounter such patients. Malignant sequelae will develop in perhaps 20%

of women with complete hydatidiform moles, so gynecological, medical, or radiation oncologists will *not* be involved in the majority of cases. The primary care physician must have an understanding of the complications and sequelae of molar pregnancy.

The clinical characteristics listed for the patient in this case study indicate a "high-risk" patient. In this instance, the term *high risk* must be differentiated from the classic usage in patients with *metastatic* gestational trophoblastic disease (GTD), whereby *high risk* (synonymous with *poor prognosis*) connotes a patient for whom combination chemotherapy is indicated. In this setting of molar pregnancy, *high risk* can be understood in terms of both the risk for nonneoplastic complications of molar pregnancy as well as the risk for postmolar GTD (malignant sequelae). A variety of signs and symptoms that characterize the patient at risk for complications have been described (1). In our case, this patient was tachycardic, hyperthermic, and short of breath, with palpitations and an enlarged uterus; she was sweating profusely. The clinical findings are consistent with trophoblastic hyperthyroidism. While the T_4 of 12 μg/dL may be elevated depending on the particular laboratory, a free thyroxine would have been a better test to obtain. It is estimated that, although increased thyroid function is frequently found in patients with molar pregnancy, only about 10% have clinical hyperthyroidism.

At the time of suction curettage in this patient, it is important for the primary care physician to remember that she is at high risk for cardiogenic dysfunction, respiratory complications, and hematological and coagulation abnormalities (1). Beta blockade at the time of evacuation is important, so that thyroid storm does not ensue. It is equally important to obtain preevacuation arterial blood gas, chest x-ray, and hematological and coagulation profiles. This patient might well have needed pulmonary artery catheterization, ventilatory support, and/or blood product transfusion, depending on the results of further evaluation. The fact that suction curettage usually proceeds without incident for most molar pregnancies should not lull the physician into complacency.

The constellation of presenting signs and symptoms in this case is also indicative of an increased risk for postmolar trophoblastic disease; namely, a uterus of 16-weeks' size, and an hCG of over 100,000 mIU/mL. Several papers report rates of malignant sequelae as high as 40 to 50% in patients with uterine size large for date, theca lutein cysts, and high preevacuation hCG titers (2). The literature on the incidence of postmolar malignant GTD in the United States, in general, can support figures from 19 to 36%. We and others believe that *all* patients with hydatidiform mole should be followed with weekly hCG titers until these normalize. Many investigators have constructed regression curves similar to that of Morrow et al. (2); they then compare each patient's falling hCG to the standard normal curve. In this case, the patient is clearly beyond the confidence intervals by the third week postevacuation, and her titers continue to rise.

Some clinics support the notion of using prophylactic chemotherapy following evacuation of a hydatidiform mole. Others have looked retrospectively at risk factors, such as those above, in order to define a subpopulation in which prophylactic chemotherapy would be of greater benefit. Currently we do not differentiate among patients with and without risk factors, and we do not recommend prophylactic therapy. Rather, we follow all patients, whether they have complete (classic) or partial hydatidiform moles, with serial hCG titers until they normalize.

There is some question as to what the diagnostic criteria should be for postmolar GTD. While U.S. figures quote the incidence of malignant GTD as above, Bagshawe and colleagues in the United Kingdom instituted treatment in only 6% of their patients. The difference lies in the common U.S. use of the hCG regression curves for determining the need for treatment. We treat patients with rising hCG titers (three values over 2 weeks), for hCG values that maintain a plateau over three determinations and for the appearance of metastatic disease. We institute a metastatic survey once the diagnosis of postmolar GTD is made, so as to stratify the patient into the categories of nonmetastatic versus metastatic disease; then we utilize a scoring system (modified from that of the World Health Organization or a clinical system) to further separate patients with metastatic disease into good and poor prognosis groups.

This patient has nonmetastatic malignant GTD. A tissue diagnosis is not necessary to institute therapy, and we do not recommend pretreatment curettage. In this clinical scenario, the pathological diagnosis would most likely be invasive mole (formerly chorioadenoma destruens) rather than choriocarcinoma, but our treatment recommendation would not be different for either histological entity. We use single-agent chemotherapy for patients with nonmetastatic disease and would treat this patient with weekly intramuscular methotrexate. We follow weekly hCG titers and continue the weekly methotrexate for three courses past a "normal" hCG. We use pulse actinomycin-D if the patient could not tolerate methotrexate or if the methotrexate was unsuccessful. If there are findings that would place the patient into the poor-prognosis metastatic category, we use combination chemotherapy. Overall, the presented patient has virtually a 100% chance of cure with appropriate treatment. We encourage referral of such patients to a center with experience in the treatment of GTD.

References

1. Twiggs LB. Nonneoplastic complications of molar pregnancy. Clin Obstet Gynecol 1984; 27:199–210.
2. Morrow CP, Kletzky OA, DiSaia PJ, et al. Clinical and laboratory correlates of molar pregnancy and trophoblastic disease. Am J Obstet Gynecol 1977; 128:424–430.

PHYSICIANS' RESPONSE

ROSS BERKOWITZ
DON GOLDSTEIN

This patient presented with the typical picture of a high-risk complete hydatidiform mole with uterine size larger than date, an hCG level > 100,000 mIU/mL,
and evidence of hyperthyroidism. This clinical entity is associated with an increased risk of persistent gestational trophoblastic tumor (GTT) approaching 40%.

All patients with molar pregnancy should be followed with weekly quantitative hCG values following evacuation. A diagnosis of persistent GTT is made
when the hCG level plateaus for 3 or more weeks or reelevates, as in this patient.

Alternatively, persistent GTT can also occur in a patient with a falling hCG
level who exhibits radiological or clinical evidence of invasive or metastatic
disease. When a patient develops GTT following molar evacuation, she should
undergo a thorough pretreatment evaluation to determine the FIGO stage and
WHO prognostic score in order to select optimal treatment. Pretreatment evaluation should include a complete blood count (CBC); a quantitative β-hCG; tests
for hepatic, renal, and thyroid function; chest x-ray or computed tomography (CT)
scan; and pelvic ultrasound.

If we assume that there was no evidence of metastases on physical examination, this patient would be characterized as having low-risk nonmetastatic disease
[Fédération International de Gynécologie et d'Obstétrique (FIGO) stage IA;
World Health Organization (WHO) prognostic score < 7]. Many single-agent
chemotherapeutic regimens using methotrexate or actinomycin-D have been
effective in the management of nonmetastatic GTT. At our center, we would treat
the patient with methotrexate administered either IV or IM with folinic acid
rescue (Table 1). After the first course of single-agent chemotherapy, further

Table 1 Protocol #1

Drug	Dose	Route	Schedule
Methotrexate	1 mg/kg	IM	Days 1, 3, 5, 7
Leucovorin	0.1 mg/kg	IM or PO	Days 2, 4, 6, 8
		or	
Methotrexate	100 mg/m^2	IV bolus × 30 min	Day 1, then leucovorin as below
	200 mg/m^2	IV infusion over 12 hr	
Leucovorin	15 mg	IM or PO	q12hr × 4 doses (to start 24 hr after starting methotrexate bolus)

treatment would be withheld as long as the hCG level were falling progressively. A second course of chemotherapy is administered if the hCG level plateaus for more than 3 consecutive weeks, reelevates, or if the hCG level does not decline by one log within 18 days after completion of the first course. In the latter situation, the treatment protocol would be changed to a combination regimen including etoposide, methotrexate, and actinomycin-D (Table 2).

Single-agent methotrexate induces complete remission in approximately 90% of patients with stage I disease, with 80% requiring only the initial course. The risk of relapse after three normal weekly hCG levels using this regimen is approximately 1%. Resistance is more commonly seen in patients with choriocarcinoma, metastases, and with pretreatment hCG levels > 50,000 mIU/mL.

Once remission is achieved, the patient should be followed with hCG levels at monthly intervals for 12 months. She should be advised to use birth control pills or some other effective contraceptive program. After 12 months of normal hCG levels, pregnancy may be undertaken. When the patient conceives, we recommend that an ultrasound examination be performed at approximately 10 weeks to rule out another molar gestation (either complete or partial), since the patient has a tenfold increased risk for developing subsequent molar disease. Otherwise the pregnancy should be managed in routine fashion and the outcome should be the same as in the general population. After delivery, we recommend that an hCG test be obtained at the 6-week checkup to rule out postterm GTT.

An alternative to chemotherapy in patients with nonmetastatic disease is hysterectomy. This treatment is usually reserved for those patients who no longer wish to preserve reproductive function or when hemorrhage or infection due to a large, bulky, invasive mole becomes a problem in management. When a surgery is carried out, strict gonadotropin follow-up is still mandatory because of the possibility that occult metastasis might already have occurred. For this reason we feel it wise to treat patients adjunctively with single-agent chemotherapy at the time of surgery.

Table 2 Protocol #2

Drug	Dose	Route	Schedule
Etoposide	100 mg/m^2	IV infusion × 30–60 min	Days 1 and 2
Actinomycin-D	12 µg/kg	IV bolus	Days 1 and 2
Methotrexate	100 µg/m^2	IV bolus × 30 min	Day 1, then as below:
	200 mg/m^2	IV infusion over 12 hr	Day 1
Leucovorin	15 mg	IM or PO	q12hr × 4 doses to start 24 hr after starting methotrexate bolus

References

Berkowitz RS, Goldstein DG. Management of molar pregnancy and trophoblastic tumors. In: Knapp RC, Berkowitz RS, eds. Gynecologic Oncology, 2d ed. New York: McGraw-Hill, 1991:328–340.

PHYSICIAN'S RESPONSE

ERNEST KOHORN

Presentation

This 20-year-old patient presented with a hydatidiform mole associated with hyperthyroidism, diagnosed by a T_4 value of 12 μg/dL. She had tachycardia, dyspnea, pounding in the chest, profuse sweating, and a temperature of 101°F. Appropriately, the patient's uterus was evacuated with beta-blocker coverage without incident.

Comment

Clinical hyperthyroidism associated with molar pregnancies is well described but rare, though chemical hyperthyroidism is common. Pulmonary embolization of trophoblastic tissue is also associated with these symptoms (1). The diagnosis may be elusive if only chest x-ray is performed, but a low arterial oxygen tension measured with a finger oximeter is virtually diagnostic. As the patient did so well following the evacuation, it would appear that pulmonary embolization was not present in this case. The issue is important as pulmonary embolization of molar tissue is invariably associated with persistently elevated levels of hCG, requiring chemotherapy. Pulmonary metastases do not usually occur and are rare.

Further Clinical Course

Following the evacuation, the hCG value fell over 3 weeks. There was no bleeding requiring curettage. We have not found uterine exploration useful in the absence of bleeding even if hCG titers are elevated (2). Physicians following patients after hydatidiform mole must plot the weekly hCG values on semilog paper (Fig. 1) to provide a visual presentation of tumor load. At 3 weeks, the value was 6000 mIU/mL; at 4 weeks, it was 9200; and at 5 weeks, it was 10,800 mIU/mL. Examination of the graph shows that the hCG rise is decreasing and the level is beginning to plateau. At 6 weeks the hCG may begin to fall, may continue to plateau, or may continue to rise. Waiting one more week is safe because chemotherapy given to patients with postmolar trophoblastic neoplasia is 99.99%

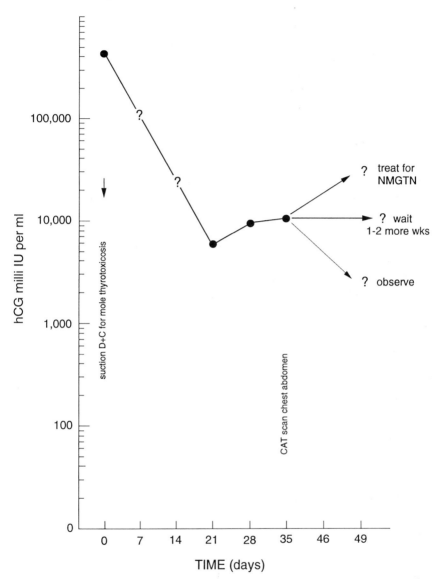

Figure 1   HCG regression curve. (See text for description.)

effective, while an inappropriate diagnosis of neoplasia would subject the patient to unnecessary chemotherapy (3). This plan mandates that the patient be followed reliably and regularly (3).

It is our recommendation to wait for one further week before deciding to initiate chemotherapy if the hCG continues to rise or to plateau and to observe the patient further if the hCG falls.

Choice of Therapy

The present choice of the Trophoblast Center at Yale is to use pulsed actinomycin-D 1.25 mg/m^2 given every 2 weeks. This is associated with minimal toxicity and only has a slightly higher primary failure rate than the 5-day course of actinomycin 12 ug/kg or methotrexate 4 mg/kg, both over 5 days. Another alternative is to give 8 days of methotrexate 1 mg/kg alternating daily with leucovorin rescue. Methotrexate 40 or 50 mg/m^2 given every week is associated with a 30% primary failure rate.

The ensuing morbidity and mortality when the occasional physician treats this disease is nine times greater than if it is treated by a trophoblast center (4).

References

Kohorn EI. Criteria toward the definition of nonmetastatic gestational trophoblastic disease after hydatidiform mole. Am J Obstet Gynecol 1982; 142:416–419.

Kohorn EI, Keating T, Blood M, et al. Gestational trophoblastic neoplasia in southern Connecticut: The experience of the Yale Trophoblast Center, 1971– 1983.

Kohorn EI. Evaluation of the criteria used to make the diagnosis of nonmetastatic gestational trophoblastic neoplasia. Gynecol Oncol 1993; 48:139–147.

Brewer JI, Eckman TR, Dolkart RE, et al. Gestational trophoblastic disease. Am J Obstet Gynecol 1971; 109:335–340.

PHYSICIAN'S RESPONSE

JOHN CURTIN

This patient has persistent gestational trophoblastic neoplasia (GTN) and will require single-agent chemotherapy, which should be initiated as soon as possible. Prior to chemotherapy, the only tests required are serum chemistry determinations of renal and hepatic function and a complete blood count (CBC). The patient has already had a normal chest CT scan and additional imaging tests are unnecessary, since the risk of metastatic disease at other sites is low. Additional surgical procedures are also unnecessary prior to starting the chemotherapy. In the past, a second uterine curettage may have been recommended; however, a recent prospective study of this technique found that the benefits of the second curettage were minimal and the risks significant (1). Since the patient is young and nulliparous, a hysterectomy is not indicated; if the patient were older and desired permanent sterilization, then hysterectomy would be a reasonable start of therapy for a patient with GTN apparently confined to the uterus. The benefits of hysterectomy are primarily related to the reduced cycles of chemotherapy necessary to achieve a complete response.

The high degree of chemosensitivity demonstrated by most patients with GTN has led to several different regimens of single-agent chemotherapy, all of which result in essentially a 100% response rate. The two most commonly used agents are methotrexate and actinomycin-D. Methotrexate regimens include weekly intramuscular injections and a regimen that combines methotrexate with leucovorin. The weekly regimen of methotrexate is preferred. The dosage schedule is methotrexate 40 mg/m^2 IM every 7 days. If there is no toxicity after the initial treatment, the dose can be escalated in 5-mg increments to a maximum of 50 mg/m^2 given on a weekly schedule.

Prior to each treatment the patient should have blood drawn for serum creatinine/blood urea nitrogen (Cr/BUN), liver function studies and a CBC. Serum beta-hCG is measured prior to each treatment and is the sole determinant of response to therapy. The patient should continue treatment for one cycle past a beta-hCG level that is less than 3.0 mIU/mL. This regimen is well tolerated, with the primary toxicity related to mucositis.

The other commonly used regimen utilizes a higher dose of methotrexate combined with leucovorin, which acts as a "rescue" antidote to the methotrexate. The dosage and administration schedule is more complex and costly, with little difference in the overall complete response rate. The other alternative single agent is actinomycin-D. This agent is given at a dose of 1.25 mg/m^2 by intravenous injection every 2 weeks. The dose-limiting toxicity of actinomycin-D is hematological and gastrointestinal. The overall complete response to this regimen was 50/55 (89%), comparing favorably with either of the methotrexate regimens. Since actinomycin-D is a desiccant, administration of this agent requires a secure intravenous access to avoid an extravasation injury. This potential problem is rare but of such consequence to prevent the more widespread use of actinomycin-D for GTN.

While they are receiving chemotherapy for GTN, I recommend that patients consider taking oral contraceptives. There are several reasons for this: first, while on chemotherapy, the patient must avoid pregnancy, since these agents are teratogenic; second, since the measure of response to therapy is serum beta-HCG, early pregnancy would confuse the clinical follow-up. In my experience when beta-hCG begins to rise during single-agent therapy for nonmetastatic GTN, more often than not this indicates that the patient has become pregnant rather than that therapy has failed.

If the patient fails the initial methotrexate therapy, she should then be treated with actinomycin-D. In the unlikely event that she fails this second round of chemotherapy, the next regimen of choice would be etoposide, methotrexate, and actinomycin-D alternating with cytoxan and oncovin (EMA-CO). Although this scenario is rare, prompt recognition of resistant GTN and treatment with an effective combination therapy such as EMA-CO will still result in salvage of most patients.

After therapy, the patient should be monitored with beta-hCG serum levels monthly for 1 year. If the patient desires another pregnancy, she is generally advised to wait for 6 to 12 months. Any rise in the serum beta-hCG should be promptly evaluated; at a minimum, the patient should have an ultrasound of the uterus. If the patient does not have an intrauterine pregnancy, the diagnosis is recurrent GTN and treatment should be initiated in an expedient fashion. If the patient is found to have an intrauterine pregnancy, she should have repeat ultrasound at 10 to 12 weeks to confirm that the pregnancy is normal; there is a 1 to 2% chance of a second molar pregnancy after treatment for GTN. Children delivered to women treated for GTN do not appear to be at increased risk of congenital anomalies. After any future pregnancies, the patient should be followed with a serum beta-hCG due to a slight risk of postpartum choriocarcinoma.

Reference

Schaerth JB, Morrow CP, Rodriguez M. Diagnostic and therapeutic curettage in gestational trophoblastic diseases. Am J Obstet Gynecol 1990; 162:1465.

PHYSICIANS' RESPONSE

CORNELIUS GRANAI
WALTER GAJEWSKI
STEPHEN FALKENBERRY

This 20-year-old woman was diagnosed with a molar pregnancy 6 weeks prior to consultation. At initial presentation, she had tachycardia, fever, and an enlarged uterus (16-week size). The beta-hCG was elevated to 430,000, and the T_4 to 12 μg/dL. An uneventful evacuation of the molar pregnancy was followed by an appropriate steady decline in the beta-hCG levels for 4 weeks. However, during the fourth and fifth week, two beta-hCG elevations occurred. At that time, a workup, including a chest CT and abdominal/pelvic CT, was negative for metastatic disease. Further, we assume that the patient had a pelvic ultrasound or CT and had the unlikely possibility of intercurrent pregnancy ruled out. The question now is how to proceed. First some contextual background.

At certain medical centers, patients considered at "high risk" for malignant sequelae after molar evacuation are recommended to receive single-agent prophylactic chemotherapy in the hope of reducing such transformation. Although prospective randomized trials have shown a significant decrease in the risk of postmolar gestational trophoblastic neoplasia (GTN) among patients treated prophylactically, the question is whom to treat. Who is "high risk"? Since the accuracy of prognostic factors is imperfect, the malignant transformation rate after hydatiform mole is only 15% overall; if transformation occurs, it is readily treated, and today most experts do not recommend prophylactic chemotherapy after a simple molar pregnancy. Moreover, the exquisite sensitivity of the beta-hCG assay as a monitoring tool allows quick identification of malignant transformation, whereupon the problem can be treated with equivalent, excellent results.

The value of "chemotherapy prophylaxis" after molar pregnancy is, however, moot in this patient, since she has already developed malignant transformation; hence this consult. Based on the current metastatic workup, this patient would be classified as having nonmetastatic gestational trophoblastic disease (GTD). When, as in this case, chest CT and abdominal/pelvic CT are negative, it is extremely unlikely that metastases will be found at other sites, such as the brain. Hence the workup can be limited.

Virtually all patients with nonmetastatic GTD are cured, most by single-agent chemotherapy. Methotrexate or dactinomycin are the individual agents used. Multiple studies support the efficacy of such single-agent therapy with non-metastatic GTN, most reporting cure rates of 98 to 100%. Although a number of different regimens employing these agents exist, we prefer weekly IM methotrexate as per the original and now proven protocol of the Gynecologic Oncology Group (GOG) (40 mg/m^2 weekly, continued until one course after normalization of the beta-hCG). This regimen was found to be not only efficacious but minimally toxic and also cost-effective. Other single-agent methotrexate regiments may have slightly higher primary cure rates, but, all things considered, the GOG format is simpler for the patient. Furthermore, if second-line "salvage" chemotherapy is needed after failure of weekly IM methotrexate, the final results are equivalent to those achieved by the more toxic primary regiments.

As an alternative to methotrexate, dactinomycin is also used as a primary single-agent treatment for nonmetastatic disease. One regimen uses 9 to 13 µg/kg per day for 5 days, recycled at 14-day intervals. Comparable remission rates have also been achieved with single intravenous dactinomycin bolus (40 µg/kg) given every 2 weeks to resolution. Although bolus/dactinomycin produces remission rates similar to weekly methotrexate, a slightly higher toxicity is encountered, making it less preferable.

Nonmetastatic GTN should be treated with one of these single-agent regiments and the beta-hCG titer carefully monitored (weekly) for response. As long as beta-hCG continues to fall, that regimen should be continued (with occasional exception) until complete beta-hCG normalization. "Remission" is then defined as negative beta-hCG for 3 consecutive weeks. If, however, rather then declining, the beta-hCG plateaus or elevates while the patient is receiving a specific treatment, that regimen is immediately discontinued and the patient is switched to an alternative single-agent therapy. Where one single-agent regimen fails, frequently another does not. Therefore the use of more aggressive combination chemotherapy (e.g., etoposide, methotrexate, and actinomycin-D alternating with cyclophosphamide and vincristine, or EMA-CO) is usually reserved for those rare patients who fail both single-agent methotrexate and dactinomycin.

Once remission of nonmalignant GTN has been achieved, recommended follow-up is monitoring of the beta-hCG each month for 1 year, during which time effective birth control should be employed, so as not to confuse surveillance with an intercurrent pregnancy. Use of oral contraceptives is safe in these patients.

In the longer view, not only is the GTD cure rate excellent, but so is the reproductive potential of women having experienced GTD. Studies have repeatedly shown a normal reproductive capacity after chemotherapy for nonmetastatic and low-risk metastatic GTD. Encouragingly, the rate of congenital malformation appears to be comparable to, not worse than, that in the general population. The risk of having a repeat molar gestation is estimated at only 1 to 2%. As a matter of prudence, it is recommended that with future pregnancies, an early ultrasound be obtained to confirm normal fetal and placental development, which is the expectation.

References

ACOG Technical Bulletin. Management of Gestational Trophoblastic Disease. No 178, March 1993.

Homesley HD, Blessing JA, Rettenmaier M, et al. Weekly intramuscular methotrexate for nonmetastatic gestational trophoblastic disease. Obstet Gynecol 1988; 72:413–418.

PHYSICIAN'S RESPONSE

BABAK EDRAKI
JOSEPH T. CHAMBERS

Thyrotoxicosis in a setting of molar pregnancy is an unusual but recognized finding. This phenomenon is due to the stimulatory effect of the hCG molecule on the TSH receptors. The hyperthyroidism rapidly resolves after evacuation of the molar pregnancy. This patient was appropriately managed with beta blockade followed by suction curettage, which remains the most efficient method of evacuation of a molar pregnancy. Microscopic evaluation of the specimen is of utmost importance, as a diagnosis of choriocarcinoma mandates prompt chemotherapy. However, if the histological diagnosis is consistent with molar gestation, observation and serial monitoring of the hCG value is recommended. This will result in 80% spontaneous regression. The majority of the malignant sequelae of molar pregnancy occur within the first 6 months after evacuation. The initial decrease in hCG levels in this patient was reassuring; however, the subsequent rise in the levels is consistent with persistent viable trophoblastic tissue. A metastatic workup was appropriately undertaken, consisting of CT scans of the chest, abdomen, and pelvis, which were normal in this patient. We can therefore assume that the viable trophoblastic tissue is most likely still limited to the uterus. The CT scan, however, has been disappointing in evaluation of the uterine cavity and myometrium. Ultrasonography with color Doppler flow studies is a more accurate means of detecting macroscopic myometrial lesions and retained molar tissue within the uterine cavity. Given the large uterine size preoperatively, it is not unreasonable to assume that the uterus contains retained molar products. If this is corroborated by the ultrasound study, a repeat suction curettage with continued careful serial monitoring of the hCG levels may be sufficient.

An alternative and less conventional option has been proposed by Kohorn (1). He has suggested that the diagnosis of malignant trophoblastic disease may be related to tumor load and therefore to the hCG level at which the plateau or slight rise occurs. Since the hCG value is proportional to the tumor load, the therapeutic intervention should be initiated more rapidly in a patient if the plateau occurs at a higher hCG level than at a lower values. In such a case, a longer period of observation and monitoring of hCG values may demonstrate continued regression. Using this model, one may opt in this case to repeat the hCG test in 1 week and undertake therapeutic measures if there is no spontaneous decline.

Single-agent chemotherapy has been the cornerstone of treatment in non-metastatic GTN (2). For the past 30 years, the two most widely used agents have been methotrexate and actinomycin-D, reflecting their efficacy and minimal side-effects profile. Therapy may be initiated with either of these drugs. If resistance to one agent occurs, the regimen should be promptly switched to the other drug. Single-agent chemotherapy with either of these two agents yields an approximately 90% remission rate. In the unlikely event of failure, the patient should be treated with a combination drug regimen consisting of etoposide, methotrexate, and actinomycin-D alternating with cyclophosphamide and vincristine (EMA-CO). It should be emphasized that therapy should be undertaken only at centers experienced in treating GTN. Chemotherapy should be continued until three normal hCG values at weekly intervals are obtained. Follow-up after successful chemotherapy consists of measurement of hCG levels at 2-week intervals for 2 months, followed by monthly evaluation for the first year. The patient is advised against pregnancy for this first year, as the hCG levels associated with a normal pregnancy may interfere with surveillance and the possible detection of a recurrence.

References

1. Kohorn EI. Evaluation of the criteria used to make the diagnosis of nonmetastatic gestational trophoblastic neoplasia. Gynecol Oncol 1993; 48:139–147.
2. Lurain JR, Elfstrand EP. Single agent methotrexate chemotherapy for the treatment of nonmetastatic gestational trophoblastic tumors. Am J Obstet Gynecol 1995; 172:574–579.

16

Apparent Stage I Endodermal Sinus Tumor in a Woman Desiring to Preserve Fertility

CASE

A 24-year-old woman presents to her gynecologist with right-sided pelvic pain. An abdominal ultrasound reveals a right ovarian mass. The patient has recently been married and desires, if at all possible, that the left ovary and the uterus should not be removed. The gynecologist, assisted by a general surgeon, takes the patient to the operating room, where a 3-by 4-cm right ovarian mass is resected. Frozen section reveals a malignancy, possibly of germ-cell origin. Only the right ovary and mass are resected. Washings for cytology are obtained but no other biopsies are taken. The remainder of the abdominal cavity and pelvis are reported to be normal. Final pathology reveals the patient to have had an endodermal sinus cell tumor. Washings are negative for cancer.

PHYSICIAN'S RESPONSE

S.D. WILLIAMS

This patient was recently found to have an ovarian endodermal sinus tumor. This tumor, while rare, does occur in young women, and this patient is at the age when many of these tumors are diagnosed. The only mildly unusual finding in this patient is the fact that the primary tumor is rather small. These tumors are very malignant, and most patients will have a very large pelvic mass at the time of diagnosis. Further studies that should be done include a chest x-ray, hCG, and alpha-fetoprotein (AFP). The chest x-ray will likely be normal, as hematogenous spread to the lungs is not common. The AFP likely will be markedly elevated. If the AFP is normal, the diagnosis of endodermal sinus tumor is essentially excluded and careful pathology review should be obtained. The hCG may or may not be elevated; if abnormal, it indicates the presence of germ-cell elements other than endodermal sinus tumor.

The major issue to be addressed in this patient is the fact that she has been incompletely staged. While there is no obvious extraovarian spread, the surgical procedure that was done apparently did not include thorough examination of the entire abdominal cavity, random biopsies, and at least gross evaluation of retroperitoneal and pelvic nodes. I believe she should have an abdominopelvic computed tomography (CT) scan, but this is certainly an imperfect staging test. While more ovarian germ-cell tumors than epithelial ovarian cancer are localized to the ovary at diagnosis, she has a very real chance of having intraperitoneal or nodal dissemination or both. One potential course of action would be to reexplore at this point with the goal of completing surgical staging. The problem with this is that endodermal sinus tumors are sometimes extraordinarily aggressive. All are treated with similar (but probably not identical) chemotherapy, which should be initiated promptly. While more precise surgical staging would give interesting prognostic information, it would not alter therapy enough to warrant doing the procedure.

I believe that the patient should be treated with four courses of chemotherapy consisting of cisplatin, etoposide, and bleomycin (regimen shown in Table 1). If one were certain that she had stage I disease, three courses of treatment would be adequate and would virtually always prevent recurrence. In patients with stage III and IV tumors, the optimum duration of treatment is less clear, but, based on experience in testicular cancer, four courses of chemotherapy would seem to be appropriate. Should she have stage I disease, her likelihood of cure is in excess of 95%. Should she in reality have advanced disease, her likelihood for cure is 60 to 80%. As she does not have elements of teratoma in her primary tumor, second-look laparotomy will not be necessary.

Acute side effects of treatment include alopecia and some nausea and vomiting, the latter much improved by the newer antiemetic agents. She may have an episode of fever and neutropenia, but these episodes are ordinarily easily managed, and I would not use granulocyte colony-stimulating factor (G-CSF) rou-

Table 1 The BEP Regimen

Cisplatin 20 mg/m2 days 1–5
Etoposide (VP-16) 100 mg/m^2 days 1–5
Bleomycin 30 U weekly IV
Three to four courses given at 21-day intervals

tinely in low-risk patients such as this. Bleomycin pulmonary fibrosis is not common but does occur. The most important method of reducing this possibility is with regular careful physical examinations of the chest, with prompt discontinuation of the drug should the patient develop rales or a lag of expansion of one hemithorax.

References

1. Gershenson DM, Morris M, Cangir A, et al. Treatment of malignant germ cell tumors of the ovary with bleomycin, etoposide, and cisplatin. J Clin Oncol 1990; 8:715–720.
2. Williams S, Blessing JA, Liao S, et al. Adjuvant therapy of ovarian germ cell tumors with cisplatin, etoposide, and bleomycin: A trial of the Gynecologic Oncology Group. J Clin Oncol 1994; 12:701–706.

PHYSICIAN'S RESPONSE

DAVID GERSHENSON

Endodermal sinus tumor of the ovary, or "yolk sac tumor," as it is now termed, is the second most common malignant ovarian germ-cell tumor. In this case, the gynecologist and general surgeon appropriately resected the right ovarian mass and submitted it for frozen section. Although no mention is made of the appearance of the contralateral ovary, we assume that it is normal, since bilateral ovarian involvement with ovarian yolk sac tumor is exceedingly rare. The principal exception to this rule is the clinical presentation of advanced-stage disease, in which there is dissemination, including metastasis of tumor from one ovary to the other. Therefore, the contralateral ovary and fallopian tube were left in situ. Preservation of fertility potential is usually possible in such patients.

Unfortunately, however, the surgeons did not perform comprehensive surgical staging. Only cytological washings were done. In my experience, the majority of patients referred to a cancer center or tertiary referral center after the surgery elsewhere have had inadequate surgical staging. The oncologist encountering such a dilemma has several options for clinical management, including reexploration with surgical staging followed by combination chemotherapy versus combination chemotherapy alone. In the United States, standard treatment for all patients with ovarian yolk sac tumor regardless of stage includes surgery and chemotherapy. In Europe, however, some groups are studying the feasibility of treating patients with stage IA yolk sac tumor with surgery alone. In my opinion, such an approach is very risky, since several reported series from the prechemotherapy era documented cure rates of less than 20% in patients treated with surgery alone for presumed stage IA yolk sac tumor. Of course, the criticism of such older studies is that the surgical staging was inadequate in many cases. Nevertheless, I believe that such an approach today is placing the patient at undue risk, since salvage with chemotherapy at the time of recurrence is very unpredictable.

Information obtained from surgical staging will provide important prognostic data and may guide therapy. Patients with advanced-stage disease have less probability of cure; more intensive chemotherapy may be indicated, both in terms of dose intensity and total cumulative dose. In fact, since I believe that all patients with ovarian yolk sac tumor, regardless of stage, should receive postoperative chemotherapy, I carefully review the pathology and obtain routine studies, including serum tumor markers, other routine blood studies, pulmonary function tests, chest x-ray, and computed tomography of the abdomen and pelvis. I would avoid restaging surgery and proceed directly to chemotherapy with the combination of bleomycin, etoposide, and cisplatin (BEP). If this patient had obvious metastatic disease, as indicated by imaging studies, I would employ more dose-intensive treatment using the same regimen (higher doses of etoposide in conjunction with growth factors). I generally treat a patient for two cycles after a negative alpha-fetoprotein has been achieved. For patients with stage I disease (and most patients with unstaged tumors, as in this patient), three or four cycles are adequate. For patients with advanced stage disease, four to six cycles are given. The key to a successful outcome is meticulous monitoring during chemotherapy and avoidance of undertreatment. Findings from randomized studies of good-prognosis testicular cancer patients suggest that (a) bleomycin is an essential component of the regimen for patients with ovarian germ-cell tumors and (b) carboplatin should not be substituted for cisplatin.

References

Gershenson DM. Update on malignant ovarian germ cells tumors. Cancer 1993; 71:1581–1590.

Gershenson DM. Management of early ovarian cancer: Germ cell and sex cord-stromal tumors. Gynecol Oncol 1994; 55:S62–S72.

PHYSICIANS' RESPONSE

MIKE F. JANICEK
BERND-UWE SEVIN

The presentation of pain associated with a pelvic mass in a young woman is typical for reported cases of endodermal sinus tumors (EST). These tumors, also known as *yolk sac tumors*, are the second most common malignant germ-cell tumors of the ovary and are now considered distinct from *embryonal carcinomas*. An EST produces elevations in serum alpha-fetoprotein (AFP) levels (> 1000 ng/mL is strongly diagnostic); histopathologically, such tumors are characterized by Schiller-Duval bodies (invaginated papillary structures with a central blood vessel).

The median age of affected patients is 19 years. Preservation of fertility through conservative surgery is considered acceptable when the tumor is grossly limited to one ovary. With currently available chemotherapy and assisted reproductive technologies, bilateral salpingo-oophorectomy and uterine preservation when both ovaries are involved is a treatment option in carefully selected patients desiring to retain childbearing potential. Clinical disease remission for at least 1 to 2 years should precede any attempts at pregnancy so as to avoid delays or potential conflicts in the treatment of any recurrent disease. Retrospective studies have shown no long-term impairment in fertility after conservative surgery followed by adjuvant chemotherapy.

The prognostic value of optimal surgical staging procedures (omentectomy/lymphadenectomy/biopsies) and aggressive cytoreduction is not known for this disease. The gynecologist must therefore rely on clinical judgment guided by the patient's wishes in determining surgical aggressiveness. There is no justification for reexploring this patient for staging purposes provided that a careful upper abdominal exploration and retroperitoneal node palpation was performed or if a postoperative CT scan confirms the absence of residual disease. Analysis of preoperative tumor markers, including AFP in this case, might have enabled better preoperative counseling of the patient and referral to the appropriate specialist.

Before the advent of multiagent chemotherapy for germ-cell tumors, there were no long-term survivors with EST. The combination of vincristine, actinomycin-D, and cyclophosphamide (VAC) was the standard regimen for germ-cell tumors of the ovary throughout the 1970s and produced excellent stage I remissions. A Gynecologic Oncology Group study, however, found that only 21% of partially resected EST remained progression-free on the VAC regimen. The introduction of platinum chemotherapy in the late 1970s and the development of combination vinblastine, bleomycin, and cisplatin (VBP) therapy produced sustained remission rates for all stages of EST; thus VBP replaced VAC. As VP-16 (etoposide) began to demonstrate activity in VBP-resistant EST, it eventually replaced vinblastine so as to reduce neurotoxicity. The currently most popular regimen for EST treatment has therefore become three to four courses of bleomycin, etoposide, and cisplatin (BEP) (1). Sustained remission rates including all stages of germ-cell tumors exceed 90% for this regimen.

Serum AFP levels are highly *specific* markers for tumor response and recurrence, and AFP levels should be followed every 1 to 3 months for at least a year following remission. Any positive AFP level must be considered as tumor recurrence. Despite two case reports of persistent disease when AFP levels and CT scans are *negative*, recent studies and opinions argue against the need for second-look laparotomy in EST (2). Follow-up with regular (every 3 months) pelvic examinations, AFP levels, and CT scan after the conclusion of therapy is sufficient in most cases. Patients with suspected residual or recurrent disease after chemotherapy may require reassessment laparotomy and consideration for investigation protocols.

References

1. Gershenson DM. Chemotherapy of ovarian germ cell tumors and sex cord stromal tumors. Semin Surg Oncol 1994; 10:290–298.
2. Gershenson DM. The obsolescence of second-look laparotomy in the management of malignant ovarian germ cell tumors. Gynecol Oncol 1994; 52:283–285.

PHYSICIAN'S RESPONSE

STEPHEN A. CANNISTRA

This 24-year-old woman has recently been diagnosed with an endodermal sinus tumor of the right ovary. A right oophorectomy was performed, and her staging revealed no gross disease in the upper abdomen and pelvis, with negative peritoneal washings. Biopsies of the omentum, paraaortic lymph nodes, and contralateral ovary were not obtained.

Endodermal sinus tumor, also known as yolk sac tumor, is the second most common malignant germ-cell neoplasm of the ovary. It is known for its ability to secrete alpha-fetoprotein (AFP), which is a useful marker of disease activity, and it is also known for its high propensity for distant recurrence, even in cases of stage I disease. Unlike dysgerminoma, which may present in a bilateral fashion and involve paraaortic lymph nodes, endodermal sinus tumor almost never occurs bilaterally and may be associated with both regional lymph node involvement and distant hematogenous metastasis to the lungs.

For these reasons, this patient should be staged postoperatively with a chest x-ray and CT scan of the abdomen and pelvis. Serum markers including AFP and beta-hCG should be performed on preoperative blood, if available, as well as postoperatively. The beta-hCG level is sometimes elevated in the rare instance of a mixed germ-cell tumor containing elements of embryonal cells or choriocarcinoma (which may not have been detected in the original specimen). Since relapse without further therapy is likely with this histology, adjuvant chemotherapy is a reasonable consideration regardless of whether disease is found outside of the ovary. Therefore, further surgical staging is not necessary for obtaining additional biopsies of the omentum and lymph nodes in this situation; it will not alter postoperative management and will delay the initiation of chemotherapy in a tumor known for its propensity for rapid growth. Also, since this tumor almost never occurs bilaterally, biopsy of the contralateral ovary is not indicated and may lead to infertility due to the development of adhesions. Baseline pulmonary function testing is required in view of the need for bleomycin chemotherapy, and a creatinine clearance should be obtained in anticipation of cisplatin administration.

Adjuvant chemotherapy with bleomycin, etoposide, and cisplatin (BEP) for three cycles administered every 3 weeks is a reasonable option for this patient, assuming normal pulmonary and renal function. Although large series evaluating the results of BEP in ovarian endodermal sinus tumor do not exist, the available literature suggests that platinum-based therapy is curative for many patients with this disease (1). The BEP regimen has now largely replaced VBP (velban, bleomycin, and cisplatin) in view of its lower incidence of neurological toxicity (2). It is important that the patient be fully informed of the toxicities of this regimen, including the small chance of bleomycin-induced pulmonary damage and etoposide-related myeloid leukemia. Although it is important to inform her of a small chance of sterility after pelvic surgery and chemotherapy, she should be told that fertility after BEP is often preserved and that healthy children have been born to mothers treated in this fashion.

The patient's pulmonary and renal function must be followed carefully during treatment. Serum markers, if elevated, usually normalize after the first cycle of therapy in patients with chemosensitive disease. If the patient has no evidence of disease at the end of treatment as assessed by examination, radiographic studies, and tumor markers, there is no need to perform a second-look laparotomy in view of the low yield of this procedure for germ-cell patients in clinical remission.

References

1. Williams S, Blessing JA, Liao SY, et al. Adjuvant therapy of ovarian germ cell tumors with cisplatin, etoposide, and bleomycin: A trial of the Gynecologic Oncology Group. J Clin Oncol 1994; 12:701–706.
2. Williams S, Birch R, Einhorn L, Irwin L, Greco A, Loehrer P. Treatment of disseminated germ cell tumors with cisplatin, bleomycin, and either vinblastine or etoposide. N Engl J Med 1987; 316:1435–1440.

PHYSICIANS' RESPONSE

THOMAS J. RUTHERFORD
SETSUKO K. CHAMBERS

Unfortunately, this young patient was not surgically staged: biopsies of the pelvic or abdominal peritoneum, retroperitoneal nodes, or omentum were not obtained. Regardless of the findings at surgery, surgical staging is important to determine the extent of disease, prognosis, and adjuvant therapy. For most patients with a nondysgerminomatous cell tumor, unilateral salpingo-oophorectomy with preservation of the contralateral ovary and uterus is appropriate. It is presumed that the left ovary appeared normal; however, if bilateral ovarian masses had been encountered and the opposite ovary contained tumor or was known to be dysgenetic, a bilateral salpingo-oophorectomy would have been indicated. The uterus could be maintained to allow donor oocyte transfer and hormonal support for an intrauterine pregnancy. As the specific diagnosis is critical and germ-cell tumors of the ovary are relatively uncommon, it is recommended that the cytology and pathology slides be reviewed by a gynecological pathologist.

This patient could be given the option of reexploration for staging purposes. If surgery is not an option, a baseline CT scan of the abdomen and pelvis to assess lymph node status and chest x-ray should be obtained. No mention was made as to whether a serum alpha-fetoprotein (AFP) level was obtained. Elevated serum AFP levels may indicate more advanced disease than was apparent at the time of surgery. For any patient with an endodermal sinus tumor, administration of adjuvant chemotherapy is the current standard of care. Studies have suggested that "second-look" laparotomy is unnecessary in patients with germ-cell tumors associated with an elevated serum AFP level at presentation.

Short-term (three to six cycles) of vincristine, actinomycin-D, and cyclophosphamide (VAC) therapy has been used for patients who have a surgical stage I germ-cell malignancy. More commonly, a bleomycin, etoposide, and cisplatin (BEP) regimen is utilized, especially in patients with endodermal sinus tumors who are unstaged. We recommend that this patient received BEP for one cycle beyond a negative AFP titer.

This patient should be followed with serial serum AFP titers and examinations. She should be counseled about not becoming pregnant for 1 year after completion of therapy. In a review of reproductive function at Yale University, 15 women with retained reproductive capacity after surgery for ovarian germ-cell tumors ultimately had successful pregnancy outcomes. Ten patients had one, four had two and one patient had three successful pregnancies following chemotherapy. There have been no congenital anomalies in the offspring of these patients. The single most common reason that pregnancy was not achieved in the remaining women was that pregnancy was not desired. Wedge biopsies of the contralateral ovary had no effect on pregnancy rates.

References

Gershenson DM. Management of early ovarian cancer: Germ cell and sex cord–stromal tumors. Gynecol Oncol 1994; 55:562–572.

Schwartz PE, Chambers SK, Chambers JT, et al. Ovarian germ cell malignancies: The Yale University experience. Gynecol Oncol 1992; 45:26–31.

PHYSICIAN'S RESPONSE

JAMES SPEYER

This young woman, who presents with an endodermal sinus tumor in one ovary, wishes to maintain fertility. These tumors, also known as yolk sac tumors, typically produce alpha-fetoprotein (AFP), which can be helpful in following these patients.

The first issue is whether it is necessary to do a total abdominal hysterectomy/bilateral salpingo-oophorectomy (TAH/BSO), as is recommended for epithelial ovarian tumors. The answer obtained from large series is that unless the contralateral ovary is obviously involved, unilateral salpingectomly and oophorectomy is sufficient surgery for women with malignant germ-cell tumors and that further surgery does not contribute to the cure rate. Careful staging procedures are recommended. The extent of surgery may, however, remain limited. Concern about anatomic barriers to fertility from subsequent scarring will still exist. Even if this were to result, pregnancy might still be achieved using transfer of fertilized donor oocytes and treatment with exogenous hormones. Some fertility experts might advocate harvesting oocytes from such a patient prior to surgery if the medical situation permits.

Regardless of the apparent surgical result, the risk that this patient will have a recurrence of disease with surgery alone is quite high. Systemic chemotherapy is therefore the recommended postoperative treatment regardless of stage. This treatment has developed analogously to the treatment of testicular cancer in men. Initial regimens of vincristine, dacarbazine (DTIC) and cytoxan have been replaced by platinum-containing regimens. First, platinum, vinblastine, and bleomycin and more recently platinum, etoposide, and bleomycin (a less toxic regimen) have been employed. The role of bleomycin in this regimen is not clear. However, given that in a patient like this three to four courses would be recommended, the inclusion of bleomycin seems prudent.

Follow-up monitoring will be physical examination, CT scan, and/or ultrasound and tumor markers. If fertility is desired, one may wish to limit the radiation exposure from CT scans, even though these are generally more accurate than ultrasound and provide more information. The AFP level should be determined monthly for two years and less frequently thereafter. With initial therapy, the AFP should decline rapidly to the normal range. One can plot the rate of fall in AFP. Knowing the half-life of $3^1/_2$ days, one can determine if the rate of decline is indicative of disease response or partial response with residual disease. Any rise in the AFP thereafter is evidence for disease recurrence. A thorough search for the site of disease should be made and second-line chemotherapy instituted.

Finally, some consideration must be given to any possible effect of the chemotherapy on future fertility and the outcome of pregnancies. Much of the long-term follow up data we have comes from women treated for Hodgkin's disease. Different drugs are used here and may have different results. The general principles are that the earlier in her reproductive years a woman receives chemotherapy, the more likely she is to maintain fertility. This is also related to the drugs received. We do not have as much long-term follow with VP-16, bleomycin, and platinum. However, pregnancies have been reported in patients who have received this therapy. Again from the Hodgkin's data and in men who received this regimen for testicular cancer, there appears to be little effect on the outcome of subsequent pregnancies. There may be a slightly higher rate of spontaneous abortion. Given the caveat that more experience is needed, especially with VP-16, there is no obvious increase in teratogenicity.

Overall, the outlook for this patient is quite good. While the number of patients in published series is limited, the probability of complete response and cure for a patient with completely resected disease treated with the above chemotherapy remains high. If we again extrapolate from testicular disease, if the patient is free of disease 2 years after treatment, her survival may be similar to that of age-matched controls.

References

Gershenson DM. Management of early ovarian cancer: Germ cell and sex cord stromal tumors. Gynecol Oncol 1994; 55:S62–S72.

Williams SD, Gershenson DM, Horowitz CJ, Scully RE. Ovarian germ cell and stromal tumors. In: Hoskins WJ, Perez CA, Young RC, eds. Principles and Practice of Gynecologic Oncology. Philadelphia: Lippincott, 1994:715–730.

Williams SO, Blessing JA, Moore DH, et al. Cisplatin, vinblastine, and bleomycin in advanced and recurrent ovarian germ-cell tumors. Ann Intern Med 1989; 111:22.

Curtin J, Rubin SC, Hoskins WJ, et al. Second-look laparotomy in endodermal sinus tumors: A report of two patients with normal levels of alpha-fetoprotein and residual tumor at reexploration. Obstet Gynecol 1989; 73:893.

Gershenson DM. Menstrual and reproductive function after treatment with combination chemotherapy for malignant ovarian germ cell tumors. J Clin Oncol 1988; 6:270.

17

Ovarian Cancer: Germ-Cell Tumor (Yolk Sac)

CASE

The patient is a 19-year-old woman, gravida O, who is 5 ft, 1 in tall and weighs 200 lb. She was experiencing some pelvic pain and her pediatrician ordered an ultrasound. A 12-cm pelvic mass was noted with both solid and cystic components. Preoperative physical exam was normal with no evidence of cul-de-sac nodularity. Blood tests were all normal except for the alpha-fetoprotein level, which was 155. A lower abdominal midline incision was made at the time of surgery and a right salpingo-oophorectomy and omentectomy performed. The tumor turned out to be a yolk sac tumor with multiple 1-cm nodules in the omentum. There was no other evidence of gross tumor. Because of the patient's size, it was decided not to do a paraaortic dissection. No tumor was grossly evident in the retroperitoneum. The patient's postoperative course was smooth and she now returns to the office 12 days postoperatively for a discussion and recommendations concerning any additional therapy and follow-up.

PHYSICIAN'S RESPONSE

MICHAEL GOLDBERG

This patient has a grossly normal left ovary and the remainder of the abdomen and retroperitoneum are also considered negative. Assuming the pathology of the omental nodules has been determined also to be a yolk sac tumor, this patient had a stage IIIB endodermal sinus tumor of the ovary. For this type of malignancy, the tumor is quite advanced, since most are found in stage I. It is unfortunate that the lymph nodes could not be sampled, since they would have provided valuable information; hopefully the decision not to perform the lymphadenectomy was made after consultation with a surgeon skilled in that procedure. Prior to being given definitive recommendations on adjuvant therapy, the patient needs to have a computed tomography (CT) scan of the abdomen, pelvis, and chest as well as a beta-hCG test to rule out the presence of choriocarcinoma, embryonal carcinoma, and polyembryoma. There is no question but that chemotherapy is indicated, and my choice at the present time would be a regimen of bleomycin, etoposide, and cisplatin. This patient should have a minimum of four and a maximum of six courses of therapy, with alpha-fetoprotein being monitored monthly and with a CT scan repeated at the termination of therapy. There is no indication for adjunctive radiation or additional immediate surgery. The question of second-look surgery following complete clinical regression of disease, in my opinion, has been resolved and there would not appear to be any value to that operation in a patient whose alpha-fetoprotein, as here, is elevated prior to the initiation of therapy. The patient should be counseled that pregnancy is possible following successful completion of chemotherapy and that, should she become pregnant, the incidence of congenital anomalies will not be elevated over that of the general population. Assuming that all gross tumor has been removed, the alpha-fetoprotein should return to normal soon after the initiation of chemotherapy. Persistence of elevated levels would be cause for an extensive search for any isolated metastatic sites, since these can be successfully attacked surgically. I would expect this patient's overall prognosis to be good, with survival in the range of 70 to 90%. In the event that a mixed germ-cell tumor was found, especially with elements of choriocarcinoma, the prognosis would be somewhat less favorable but the chemotherapy regimen would remain the same. Most mixed germ-cell tumors contain a predominance of dysgerminoma, which, if present, would respond at least as well as the endodermal sinus tumor to this regimen and therefore would not affect prognosis.

References

Williams SD, et al. Second-look laparotomy in ovarian germ cell tumors: The Gynecologic Oncology Group Experience. Gynecol Oncol 1994; 52:287–291.
Gershenson DM. Update on malignant ovarian germ cell tumors. Cancer Suppl 1993; 71(4):

PHYSICIAN'S RESPONSE

JOHN KAVANAGH

This patient has a yolk sac tumor with surgically resected extraovarian disease in the omentum. At this time, the patient has no evidence of gross tumor. She has recovered from her surgery well. The examination following her surgery shows a healing surgical incision with no evidence of infection. The pelvic examination does not reveal any abnormalities.

The first issue of concern is the pathology of the tumor. The preoperative alpha-fetoprotein titer of 155 is relatively low considering the extent of disease. Additional sections should be made to make sure this is not a mixed germ-cell tumor, particularly with a teratomatous component. The latter component, having no tumor marker, would require follow-up with radiographic imaging or even the possibility of laparoscopic restaging. Also, carcinoid should be ruled out.

The major issue is whether stage III ovarian germ-cell tumors that are surgically resected have the same prognosis and curability as stage I and II tumors. Previous studies have shown that patients with gross residual disease following surgery and advanced stages have a relatively poor prognosis with standard chemotherapy compared to patients with stage I disease. However, the observation may not be applicable in this particular case.

Considering the absence of residual disease, there remains concern over the advanced stage of disease at presentation, the reports of inferior results in male testicular tumor with the deletion of bleomycin, the correlation of the outcome in germ-cell tumors in both sexes with the volume of disease, and the lack of a large number of patients with stage III yolk sac tumors treated with abbreviated courses of chemotherapy, I recommend that the patient initiate a combination of chemotherapy with etoposide (VP-16) 100 mg/m^2 daily for 5 days, cisplatin 100 mg/m^2 on day 1, and bleomycin 15 U daily as continuous intravenous infusion for 3 days. This combination should be given every 21 days. If severe neutropenia is encountered, then granulocyte colony-stimulating factor (G-CSF) support is recommended. Cytokine support has been used in testicular tumors with no adverse effect. The total number of courses should be a minimum of four, given every 3 weeks. If the patient shows subjective intolerance, neuropathy, renal failure, or ototoxicity with cisplatin, it should be deleted and carboplatin substituted. After four courses, depending on toxicity, the patient should receive an additional four courses of carboplatin/VP-16 as a consolidation. Carboplatin should be dosed to a Calvert's formula with a target area under the curve (AUC) of 6, and the VP-16 should not be reduced but maintained at 100 mg/m^2 daily for 5 days. The G-CSF should be utilized for these chemotherapy courses. The total number of chemotherapy courses will be eight. The patient will then be followed without a surgical restaging procedure. The patient will have a monthly alpha-fetoprotein measurement for approximately 1 year, then every 2 to 3 months for the second year, and then once every 6 months for the third year. The patient should receive oral contraceptives during chemotherapy if there is no contraindication. If there is a teratomatous component, the patient should have a CT scan of the abdomen and pelvis at the completion of chemotherapy, and this should be repeated every 4 to 6 months for 2 years. Consideration should also be given to a restaging laparoscopy at the end of chemotherapy, depending on the clinical course and results of the CT scan. The patient should be advised that pregnancy, if desired, is possible and that the gestational course and offspring are the same as in normal women.

Reference

Williams SD, Gershenson DM, Horowitz CJ, Scully RE. Ovarian germ cell and stromal tumors. In: Hoskins WJ, Perez CA, Young RC, eds. Principles and Practice of Gynecologic Oncology. Philadelphia: Lippincott, 1992:715.

PHYSICIANS' RESPONSE

CLAUS TROPÉ
GUNNAR KRISTENSEN

This tumor type, originally called a mesonephroma, constitutes about 20% of ovarian germ-cell tumors. In 1965, the Danish pathologist Teilum demonstrated that the architecture of yolk sac tumors resembles that of the labyrinth placenta of the rodent, where yolk sac diverticula invade the extraembroynal mesenchyme as papillary structures with central capillaries, called Schiller-Duval bodies. Yolk sac tumors are also called endodermal sinus tumors. They contain not only extra-embryonal structures but also embryonal structures such as intestinal glands with goblet cells and a hepatoid type where the embryonal differentiation resembles liver tissue and produces alpha fetoprotein (AFP). Yolk sac tumors are the prototype of tumors producing AFP and human chorionic gonadotropin (hCG).

Macroscopically, yolk sac tumors are big, cystic, partly necrotic, yellowish, slimy, and malignant looking. They often rupture during operation. Unilateral oophorectomy is sufficient if the contralateral ovary looks normal, as these tumors occur bilaterally in only 1% of cases. Biopsy of the contralateral ovary is not recommended, as it may disturb fertility. In the report of Kurman and Norris (1), conservative fertility-sparing surgery did not jeopardize the prognosis. Yolk sac tumors spread via the peritoneal fluid and/or lymphatic dissemination, but hematogenous spread to the lungs or liver can also occasionally occur. Because of the relative frequent lymphatic spread, the retroperitoneal space should always be explored during surgery. In 60 to 70% of cases, these tumors are in stage I or II and in 25 to 30% in stage III. Stages II and IV occur rarely.

This patient had multiple omental metastases of 1 cm, which were removed during surgery. As in epithelial ovarian carcinoma, a better response to chemotherapy is seen in cases with little or no residual tumor. This patient should be offered adjuvant chemotherapy, as the tumor was in stage IIIB. In 1970, combination chemotherapy with vincristine, dactinomycin-D, and cyclophosphamide (VAC) was introduced to patients with yolk sac tumors, resulting in an increase in cure rate from 50% to about 80% in stage IA and from 0 to 50% in patients with metastatic disease. In testicular germ-cell tumors, the combination of cisplatin, vinblastine, and Bleomycin (PVB) proved successful; with this combination, cure rates of about 95% for stages I to II and about 80% for stage III ovarian yolk sac tumors was achieved. Recently, etoposide has replaced vinblastine because it involves less neurologic toxicity and has no adverse effect on survival. In a recent GOG report on radically operated patients in stages I to III, 93% were still alive after 3 years of follow-up. They received three cycles of cisplatin 20 mg/m^2 on days 1 to 5, etoposide (VP-16) 100 mg/m^2 on days 1 to 5, and bleomycin 30 U IV weekly (2).

It is important to monitor AFP and hCG during treatment to follow the response and to decide whether three cycles are enough. In case of relapse, it is important to decide whether the tumor is resistant to cisplatin or not. In case resistance to cisplatin has not been proven, cisplatin can be used in combination with vinblastine and ifosfamide (VIP). Recently, high-dose chemotherapy with stem cell rescue has been used, but the toxicity is high and no unequivocal improvement in disease-free survival has been achieved.

References

Kurman RJ, Norris HJ. Endodermal sinus tumor of the ovary: A clinical and pathological analysis of 71 cases. Cancer 1976; 38:2404–2419.

Gershenson DM. Management of early ovarian cancer: Germ cell and sex cord-stromal tumors. Gynecol Oncol 1994; 55:S62–S72.

18

Recurrent Ovarian Dysgerminoma Confined to the Pelvis

CASE

A 28-year-old woman is found on a routine pelvic examination to have a right-sided pelvic mass. At exploratory laparotomy she is found to have a stage 1 right ovarian dysgerminoma. The patient is treated conservatively with surgery only (removal of the right ovary).

The patient continues to do well, but on follow-up pelvic examination 16 months later, she is found to have a new right-sided pelvic mass. Computed tomography (CT) scan confirms the presence of this mass. No other disease is evident. The left ovary appears normal.

PHYSICIANS' RESPONSE

A. MENZIN
S. RUBIN

This case of recurrent ovarian dysgerminoma raises several important issues in the management of patients with this condition. Dysgerminomas account for about 2% of cases of ovarian cancer and nearly half of malignant germ-cell tumors. As opposed to other germ-cell tumors, approximately 10% of patients with dysgerminomas will present with gross bilateral ovarian involvement and another 10% will have occult disease in the contralateral ovary (1). It is noteworthy that dysgerminomas occur at an increased rate in women with gonadal dysgenesis, which raises the issue of the appearance of the patient's contralateral ovary. Documentation of this diagnosis is important both for this individual's management and to further her counseling.

That this patient has been considered to have stage I disease, having been documented by "conservative" surgery, raises the concern that an inadequate staging procedure was performed for suspected early disease. Thorough sampling is critical, particularly with regard to lymph nodes, given the known propensity of dysgerminomas to metastasize via the lymphatic route. Furthermore, documented extraovarian disease might have argued against the expectant management employed after this patient's initial surgery.

With regard to the consideration for reexploration in patients suspected of having recurrent dysgerminoma, guidance may be obtained from the experience with epithelial ovarian cancer. If inadequate staging was performed initially, prompt reexploration will afford the opportunity to define the extent of disease. In this particular patient with recurrent disease after 16 months, identifying an isolated, resectable focus of recurrence may allow for "optimal" disease status and perhaps an improved response to subsequent therapy. Furthermore, the subgroup of patients who may benefit from secondary cytoreduction (e.g., those with chemoresponsive tumors and those with extended disease-free intervals) may be larger than that for epithelial varieties of ovarian cancer, given the marked chemosensitivity of germ-cell tumors.

In the past, radiation therapy had been recommended for patients with dysgerminoma, based on histological and clinical similarities with the exquisitely radiosensitive testicular seminoma. The efficacy of combination chemotherapy in this disease, together with the potential preservation of fertility following chemotherapy, have relegated radiation therapy to an infrequently employed modality in patients with ovarian dysgerminoma.

Marked improvements in the survival of patients with dysgerminoma and germ-cell tumors in general relate primarily to the effectiveness of chemotherapy, particularly with agents such as bleomycin, etoposide, and cisplatin (BEP). Effective in both early and advanced disease, the BEP combination, used in brief regimens, will produce durable remissions in the vast majority of patients, obviating reassessment laparotomy as a standard (2).

It may also be of value to assess the tumor marker status of this patient. Though previously considered to be devoid of markers, dysgerminomas may secrete human chorionic gonadotropin (when the tumor contains syncytiotrophoblasts, as it does in about 5% of cases), certain LDH isoenzymes, neuron-specific enolase, and rarely CA-125. If these prove informative, serial measurement of tumor markers could aid in the follow-up of this young patient, who may want to preserve her reproductive capacity.

Our recommendation is for reexploration with excision of all visible tumor. The left ovary should be biopsied; it may be retained if it is uninvolved. Subsequent treatment should be with combination chemotherapy.

References

1. Williams SD. Ovarian germ cell tumors. In: Rubin SC, Sutton GP, eds. Ovarian Cancer. New York: McGraw Hill, 1993.
2. Gershenson DM. The obsolescence of second-look laparotomy in the management of malignant germ cell tumors (editorial). Gynecol Oncol 1994; 52:283–285.

PHYSICIANS' RESPONSE

LARRY J. COPELAND
JAMES L. NICKLIN

The patient is said to have had a stage I dysgerminoma about 16 months earlier. Did the patient undergo a complete surgical staging procedure, including aortic node sampling? It would also be of interest to read the prior operative note to obtain a feel for the surgical technique related to the right oophorectomy. Was there any intraoperative tumor disruption? If there was such disruption, a local recurrence would be less surprising. Was the right tube also removed? Did the patient have any tumor marker evaluation done at the time of the original surgery or subsequently? (Such markers would include LDH, CA-125, or beta-hCG, all of which can serve as potential markers for dysgerminoma tumors, although there is no reliably consistent marker.) Since it is possible that the prior tumor was a mixed germ-cell tumor, redrawing a complete panel of tumor markers, including an alpha-fetoprotein (AFP), would be appropriate. We assume that the patient's chest x-ray is normal and the CT scan reveals no other significant abnormalities. This patient's fertility expectations are important factors in the potential evaluation and management of this probably recurrence.

While it is possible that the current process is new and unrelated to the prior history (e.g., a fibroid), one certainly has to place recurrent dysgerminoma at the top of the list. In view of the apparently unusual nature of this suspected recurrence, a review of the prior pathology material would be appropriate. Specifically, it would be nice to rule out a possible lymphoma or mixed germ-cell tumor. Stage I dysgerminomas, if they recur, tend to recur in the aortic nodes, but it is quite possible that this patient now has a local pelvic recurrence. While tumor marker information could increase one's index of suspicion, it is necessary to confirm histologically that this mass is a recurrent dysgerminoma. While a needle biopsy or fine needle aspirate would probably confirm the diagnosis, we would lean toward surgical excision of the mass and a comprehensive surgical staging procedure. Either irradiation or chemotherapy following percutaneous confirmation have a reasonably good likelihood of eradicating a recurrence of dysgerminoma. There is little information to guide us regarding the contribution of tumor debulking for germ-cell tumors in general. However, a laparotomy would also offer the opportunity to both confirm whether this is a pure dysgerminoma or a mixed germ-cell tumor and to stage the recurrence pathologically. This staging will provide information that could potentially limit the extent of treatment, either the irradiation field or the duration of chemotherapy.

If this mass was a local recurrence and the contralateral ovary and uterus were grossly normal, there remains the potential to preserve childbearing, and these organs could be left without significantly compromising the patient's cancer treatment or the result. Even assuming that all gross tumor was removed, the patient should receive postoperative adjuvant therapy with either irradiation or chemotherapy. If her childbearing expectations are high, the radiation would not be a good choice, even though the uterus and contralateral ovary could be shielded. Of course, if the recurrence were adherent or adjacent to the uterus, one would be hesitant to shield any area at risk for microscopic metastasis. Even if future pregnancies were not a priority, we would tend to recommend chemotherapy rather than the radiation therapy unless the patient had requested removal of her uterus and contralateral adnexa, a somewhat drastic intervention for a 28-year-old. It must be kept in mind that this tumor is exquisitely sensitive to irradiation and that the doses required for either the treatment of tumor masses or for adjuvant therapy are quite low and usually not associated with serious toxicity or sequelae. In this particular patient, we would recommend the bleomycin, etoposide, and cisplatin (BEP) regimen in the standard doses for three to four cycles.

There is limited information about menstrual and childbearing function following chemotherapy for germ-cell tumors. In general, for a 28-year-old with normal menstrual function prior to chemotherapy, the likelihood of maintaining ovarian function should be in the range of 80 to 90% after four cycles of BEP. However of equal concern for this patient will be the potential for adhesive disease to complicate the fertility potential.

PHYSICIANS' RESPONSE

JIANAN GRAYBILL
MARCUS E. RANDALL

Nearly three-fourths of patients with dysgerminoma present with stage I disease. Because most of these patients are of childbearing age, preservation of fertility is an important factor in treatment selection. Conservative surgery with unilateral salpingo-oophorectomy has been the treatment of choice in these patients. The relapse rate is approximately 10 to 20%, with a high expectation of salvage.

Unlike the case in epithelial ovarian carcinoma, the principal mode of dissemination for this tumor is nodal, although transperitoneal spread can be seen. Recurrences often appear in the pelvis, as in this case, or the retroperitoneum. Published data in the prechemotherapy era document a consistently high salvage rate with radiation therapy (RT) alone or the combination of surgery and RT.

Therefore, 10-year survivals are generally 90 to 100%, whether conservative or nonconservative treatment is administered initially.

Additional workup in this patient is necessary to aid in decision making. First, serum marker studies including alpha-fetoprotein (AFP) and beta-human chorionic gonadatropin (beta-hCG) should be obtained. Elevation of AFP indicates the presence of a nondysgerminomatous element even if not detected pathologically. Elevation of beta-hCG has been noted in approximately 10% of patients with pure dysgerminoma and this can serve as a useful marker of disease status and response to treatment. Also, this patient needs pathological confirmation of recurrence, probably best obtained by CT-directed fine needle aspiration biopsy. For patients with pure dysgerminoma, there is no evidence that surgical debulking improves survival or local control.

Treatment options, assuming that this patient has pure dysgerminoma, include RT encompassing the pelvis and paraaortic chain and systemic chemotherapy. Dysgerminomas are exquisitely radiosensitive and are curable with doses limited to 2500 to 3500 cGy in 100 to 125-cGy fractions. However, this approach would render this patient menopausal and infertile. Systemic chemotherapy using active germ-cell regimens is associated with high response rates and appears to have curative potential (1). It has also the advantages of treating subclinical hematogenous or transperitoneal spread and of treating unrecognized nondysgerminomatous elements. A disadvantage of this approach is the possibility that patients not salvaged with chemotherapy might be less suitable for RT salvage, either because of compromised hematological tolerance or the emergence of radioresistant tumor clones during chemotherapy exposure.

Although chemotherapy salvage data are not as well established in large numbers of patients compared to RT salvage, the high response rates that have been reported, the efficacy of chemotherapy in the adjuvant setting, and the potential advantages given above justify an initial approach of salvage chemotherapy and close follow-up in this patient. Consolidation RT to initial sites of bulky disease following chemotherapy is controversial in chemoresponsive germ-cell tumors but should be considered, especially if this patient had a large initial tumor burden, elevated markers failed to return to normal, or there is less than a complete response to chemotherapy. Recent data suggests that positron emission tomography might provide an accurate way of evaluating patients for residual active tumor following chemotherapy.

Reference

1. Jacobs AJ, Harris M, Deppe G, et al. Treatment of recurrent and persistent germ cell tumor with cisplatin, vinblastine, and bleomycin. Obstet Gynecol 1982; 59:129–132.

PHYSICIAN'S RESPONSE

S.D. WILLIAMS

This patient almost certainly has recurrent dysgerminoma. She was appropriately observed after oophorectomy for stage I disease. About 15% of such patients will develop recurrent tumor, with nearly all such events occurring within the first 2 to 3 years after oophorectomy. It is probably reasonable to confirm the diagnosis with fine needle aspiration biopsy, but this will almost certainly be the case. Human chorionic gonadotropin (hCG) and alpha fetoprotein (AFP) levels should also be determined and they in all likelihood will be normal. However, an elevated AFP in this situation connotes the presence of germ-cell elements other than dysgerminoma, in which case the patient should be managed accordingly.

Assuming that the AFP is normal and the pathology is dysgerminoma, the patient should be treated with chemotherapy. Dysgerminoma is very responsive to radiation; in earlier years, the patient would have been treated in this fashion. However, a number of observations make the choice of radiation less desirable. They are as follows:

1. Some patients, such as this one will not remain disease-free with radiation. This number is probably 25 to 40%.
2. Radiotherapy is associated with loss of fertility in most or all patients so treated.
3. Modern chemotherapy will cure nearly all (in excess of 90%) patients with recurrent dysgerminoma.

She should be treated with bleomycin, etoposide, and cisplatin (BEP) (see Case 16). Three courses of chemotherapy is probably sufficient in this patient with a relatively small volume tumor and a favorable prognosis.

It should be noted that many patients with dysgerminoma will have a persistent mass after chemotherapy. These masses are almost invariably fibrosis and necrosis and second-look laparotomy is not necessary.

References

1. Gershenson DM, Morris M, Cangir A, et al. Treatment of malignant germ cell tumors of the ovary with bleomycin, etoposide, and cisplatin. J Clin Oncol 1990; 8:715–720.
2. Williams SD, Blessing JA, Hatch KD, Homesley HD. Chemotherapy of advanced dysgerminoma: Trials of the Gynecologic Oncology Group. J Clin Oncol 1991; 9:1950–1955.

PHYSICIAN'S RESPONSE

ALEXANDER W. KENNEDY

My initial recommendations for this patient are a careful pelvic examination and review of the CT scan to determine the feasibility of surgical resection of her recurrent tumor. I would advise obtaining the following serum tumor markers: the beta subunit of human chorionic gonadotropin (hCG), alpha-fetoprotein (AFP), lactic dehydrogenase (LDH) and CA-125. Elevated levels will be helpful to monitor response to later chemotherapy and unexpected marked elevations in AFP, CA-125, or hCG would suggest the possible presence of other germ-cell or epithelial elements in her tumor. I also recommend that her original pathology slides be reviewed by an experienced gynecological pathologist to confirm the original diagnosis as well as to exclude other germ-cell elements.

If all of the above are favorable, I would advise surgical reexploration to attempt tumor debulking as well as for thorough and accurate staging. While this is still somewhat debatable, results of prior Gynecologic Oncology Group (GOG) trials suggest that minimal residual tumor volume at the initiation of subsequent chemotherapy improves the overall response and cure rates for patients with advanced or recurrent ovarian germ-cell tumors (1). The patient's present recurrence is most likely within lymph nodes along the pelvic side wall, and adjacent lymph node groups need to be sampled. I would advise careful inspection of the left ovary but would not advise wedge biopsy except on the basis of clinical suspicion. I would advise careful inspection of all peritoneal surfaces but do not recommend random biopsies unless clinically suspicious areas are encountered.

Following postoperative recovery and pathological confirmation of recurrent pure dysgerminoma, this patient will require adjuvant chemotherapy. While encouraging results were previously obtained with radiotherapy or with the combination of vincristine, actinomycin-D, and cyclophosphamide (VAC), recent GOG experience would favor platinum-based chemotherapy in this setting (2). I would not advise radiotherapy, the previous standard treatment, since chemotherapy should be equally effective and reproductive potential possibly preserved. I would consider with the patient the possibility of Depo Lupron ovarian suppression with add-back low-dose estrogen therapy to potentially reduce the risk of chemotherapy-induced ovarian failure.

Although cisplatin, vinblastine, and bleomycin (PVB) have yielded excellent results, etoposide has now generally been substituted for vinblastine due to concerns of severe toxicity. Three courses of the PEB regimen, with the following doses, should be administered:

Cisplatin 20 mg/m^2 IV on days 1 to 5 every 3 weeks
Etoposide 100 mg/m^2 IV on days 1 to 5 every 3 weeks
Bleomycin 30 U IV weekly

During therapy, tumor markers and DLCO should be monitored in addition to weekly blood counts. At the completion of chemotherapy, the patient will need regular follow-up clinical examinations and CT scans. Second-look laparotomy would not be advised in the absence of clinical suspicion of persistent tumor or elevation of tumor markers.

References

1. Slayton RE, Park RC, Silverberg SG, et al. Vincristine, dactinomycin, and cyclophosphamide in the treatment of malignant germ cell tumors of the ovary. Cancer 1985; 56:243–248.
2. Williams SD, Blessing JA, Moore DH, et al. Cisplatin, vinblastine, and bleomycin in advanced and recurrent ovarian germ cell tumors. Ann Intern Med 1989; 111:22–27.

19

Recurrent Ovarian Germ-Cell Tumor (Endodermal Sinus Tumor) Following a Response to Chemotherapy

CASE

A 26-year-old woman is found to have stage IV (several pulmonary nodules) endodermal sinus tumor of the ovary. Following tumor debulking, she is treated with three courses of cisplatin, etoposide, and bleomycin and achieves a complete response (including normalization of markers and normal CT scan of the chest and abdomen). The patient remains symptom-free but marker studies obtained 1 year after the completion of chemotherapy reveal a beta-hCG (human chorionic gonadotropin) of 57 (confirmed on repeat studies).

PHYSICIAN'S RESPONSE

WIM TEN BOKKEL HUININK

Germ-cell tumors of the ovary mainly afflict young women and represent 20% of all tumors of the ovary. More than 90% consist of major cystic teratomas and only 5 to 8% are malignant. The entity of endodermal sinus tumor has been defined during the last decade to consist of 10 subtypes, of which some have been identified to have worse prognostic features than others. It has become clear that platinum-containing regimens, preferably with etoposide and bleomycin, lead to a better prognosis than the previously used regimen consisting of dactinomycin, vincristine, and cyclophosphamide. The treatment performed in this case has, therefore, been adequate, but instead of four cycles of chemotherapy, as would be standard in Europe, only three courses were given.

The patient has achieved a complete remission. Data are lacking as to whether other significant tumor markers of teratocarcinomas (such as beta-hCG and/or LDH) have ever been elevated in the past. It is stated that markers have become normalized. Has there ever been an elevation of hCG? Such an increase would suggest the diagnosis of recurrent tumor activity.

Endodermal sinus tumor is sometimes only part of a composite germ-cell tumor. Sometimes pathology reports overlook syncytial cells, which are well known to produce hCG and may be part of choriocarcinomatous elements of either an embryonal cell carcinoma or real choriocarcinomatous parts of the mixed germ-cell tumors.

Since it remains unknown whether other markers have previously been found to be increased in this patient, an elevation of the beta-hCG may be related to increased activity of other parts of a mixed germ-cell tumor, of which only the endodermal sinus tumor was recognized previously. The short duration of treatment may well be responsible for such a partial remission, seemingly achieved in this case.

I think that the elevation of beta-hCG to a value of 57, which is clearly elevated in this patient, seems to point to a renewed activity of a previously possibly overlooked component of a mixed germ-cell tumor of the ovary consisting of embryonal cell carcinoma or choriocarcinomatous parts.

Renewed chemotherapy after industrious staging procedures is, therefore, justified. It should consist of high-dose platinating agents such as cisplatin or carboplatin, preferably followed by further dose-increased regimens with peripheral stem cell transplantation salvage procedures. However, if a single lymph node or lung metastasis could be demonstrated, surgical excision may be worthwhile.

The differential diagnosis in this patient comprises the possibility of an inclining pregnancy (in very early-stage of development), since data on the surgical procedures are lacking. Notwithstanding the fact that treatment outcomes in teratocarcinomatous tumors of the ovary are still not as favorable as they are in tumors arising from the testis in men, the prognosis of female patients suffering from teratogenous tumors after treatment with cisplatin-based chemotherapy, even in the case of hematogenous metastases, is favorable enough that organ-sparing surgical procedures should be sought. Therefore, a surgical procedure whereby the contralateral ovary can be saved is appropriate. Other diagnostic tests to exclude pregnancy should be performed.

PHYSICIANS' RESPONSE

ROBERT A. BURGER
ALBERTO MANETTA

Most endodermal sinus tumors secrete alpha-fetoprotein (AFP), a reliable serum tumor marker used to monitor disease status during treatment and follow-up. Clearly an elevated serum AFP detected during the posttreatment follow-up is diagnostic of recurrent germ-cell tumor (GCT), even in the presence of a negative metastatic workup. Although most endodermal sinus tumors (ESTs) are pure, 70% of mixed GCTs have been reported to contain EST as one component. Furthermore, mixed GCTs contain choriocarcinoma in 20% and embryonal carcinoma in 16% of cases. The latter two lesions are noteworthy for their elaboration of beta-hCG. In the absence of an abnormal AFP, an elevated serum beta-hCG in this asymptomatic young woman with a 1-year clinical remission following treatment for stage IV disease could arise from either a gestational or nongestational source.

Obviously the possibility of a gestational source for beta-hCG production, either an early first-trimester pregnancy or, less likely, gestational trophoblastic neoplasia (GTN), could be gleaned from additional history alone. The EST is exclusively unilateral, and the uterus and contralateral adnexa are commonly preserved during initial surgical management of advanced-stage disease in women who wish to retain childbearing potential. Such fertility-conserving surgery has not been shown to compromise clinical outcome. If, based on this patient's surgical and reproductive history, a gestational source cannot be excluded, an immediate workup is indicated, since the only likely nongestational source would be a recurrent mixed GCT initially misdiagnosed as a pure EST. The latter case would reflect an incomplete initial response of a mixed lesion to primary chemotherapy, with the resultant outgrowth of a beta-hCG–secreting component.

The evaluation should begin with a repeat serum beta-hCG level obtained 48 hr from the time of the initial determination. A rapidly falling level would indicate a degenerating gestation, in which case the patient could be observed clinically with serial serum beta-hCG determinations.

A plateauing or rising beta-hCG would mandate further investigation with an approach that would permit prompt diagnosis of recurrence, limit morbidity from invasive procedures, and respect the patient's wishes either to maintain or terminate pregnancy. By 10 days following this patient's initial beta-hCG titer, one could safely exclude a gestational source for beta-hCG production. If a gestational source is indeed excluded, then review of the original pathological material should be conducted, with immunostaining for beta-hCG, in an attempt to identify either a choriocarcinoma or embryonal carcinoma component. At the same time, a metastatic workup including chest, abdominal/pelvic, and head computed tomography (CT) is indicated, with procedures performed for tissue diagnosis only when the benefit-risk ratio is highly favorable. Even with a negative slide review and metastatic survey, however, once a gestational source is excluded, the diagnosis of a recurrent, mixed GCT should be assumed and the patient treated accordingly.

Fortunately, three to four cycles of bleomycin, etoposide, and cisplatin (BEP) represent the standard postsurgical treatment not only for EST but also for mixed GCT (1). However, while GCT is exquisitely sensitive to standard combination chemotherapy, over 25% of patients with metastatic disease will progress or recur. If a diagnosis of recurrent, mixed GCT is made in this patient, she would be considered at high risk of ultimately succumbing to her disease. The role of secondary surgical resection for measurable recurrent disease, no "standard" salvage regimen exists. Therefore, this patient should first be offered entry onto a clinical trial of second-line therapy. Currently, dose-intensive platinum-containing combination chemotherapy regimens with autologous hematopoietic support are undergoing phase II testing in patients who relapse after previous platinum-based treatment (2). Given the patient's prior complete response to BEP and 1-year period of clinical remission, a suitable off-protocol recommendation would be retreatment with the standard BEP regimen. If a rapid fall in beta-hCG levels were observed, treatment would be continued for two courses beyond attainment of a biochemical remission. Therapy would be discontinued at any time a plateauing or rising beta-hCG level was documented.

References

1. Gershenson DM. Treatment of ovarian germ cell tumors and sex cord stromal tumors. Semin Surg Oncol 1994; 10:290–298.
2. Gershenson DM. Update on malignant ovarian germ cell tumors. Cancer 1993; 71:1581–1590.

PHYSICIAN'S RESPONSE

R. GERALD PRETORIUS

The case presentation does not state whether the uterus and both ovaries were removed at the time of debulking; if they were not removed, pregnancy must be excluded. Assuming that pregnancy has been excluded, I would interpret the elevation of beta-hCG as probably evidence of persistent disease. I would be more certain of this if the patient had had an elevation of hCG at the initial diagnosis. I would examine the patient and obtain titers of serum alpha-fetoprotein (AFP) and lactate dehydrogenase (LDH). I would also order computed tomography (CT) scans of the abdomen, pelvis, and chest. If these studies strongly suggested recurrent endodermal sinus tumor (e.g., if serum AFP were elevated and/or there were lesions on examination or CT scan), I would consider laparotomy with resection of the mass if it appeared that the disease was limited to one area. However, since the original presentation was with pulmonary nodules, it seems unlikely that a recurrence would be limited to one area. Following surgery or if the disease were widespread, I would treat the patient with chemotherapy (what chemotherapy is unclear).

This case study has no simple answer. I have never seen a patient with recurrent stage IV endodermal sinus tumor. These tumors are rare; I found no reports of large series of patients with recurrent endodermal sinus tumor upon which to base therapy. In this situation, I would prevail upon Dr. Peter Schwartz at Yale, one of the handful of specialists on germ-cell malignancies of the ovary, and ask him what to do. Accordingly I contacted Dr. Schwartz and obtained the following information. In the case of an advanced endodermal sinus tumor, it may have been more appropriate to use six as opposed to three cycles of chemotherapy. Most of the tumors that recur do so within the first 6 months; recurrence at 1 year is unusual. Given the unusual time of possible recurrence, it would be useful to know whether the hCG was elevated at the initial presentation and whether the patient could be pregnant. Assuming that there is evidence of recurrent endodermal sinus tumor, laparotomy with debulking is probably not going to be particularly useful; the patient should probably be treated with high-dose carboplatin plus ifosfamide with bone marrow rescue. Dr. Schwartz advised against vincristine, actinomycin-D, and cyclophosphamide (VAC); he had one anecdotal experience in which paclitaxel (Taxol) was not effective; and he had heard of cases in which intraperitoneal chemotherapy had been used with some success.

Given Dr. Schwartz's consultation, I would be even less likely to attempt cytoreductive surgery. As I do not believe that intraperitoneal chemotherapy is of any use and there was extraperitoneal disease (pulmonary nodules) initially, and as I suspect that the dose-response curve for germ-cell malignancies may be steep, I would probably treat this patient with high-dose carboplatin and ifosfamide with bone marrow rescue.

PHYSICIAN'S RESPONSE

HOWARD D. HOMESLEY

Because of the rarity of endodermal sinus tumor of the ovary, there is scant information as to management of patients who initially are highly responsive to first-line cisplatin-based chemotherapy.

Options would be to re-treat this patient with the same regimen of therapy, especially since she "responded completely" after only three courses of therapy. There is also the possibility that the patient may be responsive to other combinations of therapy such as vincristine, actinomycin-D, and cyclophosphamide

(VAC). For malignant germ-cell tumors, the possibility of treatment with radiation therapy, where appropriate, combined with cisplatin multiagent chemotherapy is an alternative.

If the patient were discovered to again have pulmonary nodules by magnetic resonance imaging (MRI) or subsequent computed tomography (CT) of the lungs, radiation therapy to the pulmonary nodules would not ordinarily be a viable treatment. If the patient proved unresponsive to chemotherapy even if the pulmonary nodules were bilateral, the recurrences might be amenable to surgical resection because of the young age.

The secretion of hCG may well be indicative of susceptibility of the tumor to chemotherapy regimens associated with successful management of gestational trophoblastic diseases. Response to therapy could be sensitively noted by hCG-level response.

Paclitaxel may be a very attractive chemotherapy agent in this situation, as activity has been noted in gestational trophoblastic disease. It is unknown if a low dose (135 mg/m^2) would be as effective as a high dose (250 mg/m^2 with growth factor support).

There is no clear-cut approach for this patient, so the above suggested regimens would be used sequentially, based upon the patient's clinical response.

PHYSICIAN'S RESPONSE

MAUREEN KILLACKEY

In order to address the issue of an elevated beta-hCG in this 26-year-old woman, status postcytoreduction and combination chemotherapy for a stage IV endodermal sinus tumor (EST) of the ovary, more clinical information is needed:

1. Were the slides reviewed and was this a pure EST, or were there mixed malignant germ-cell elements?

2. What was removed at the patient's initial surgery? Since ESTs are usually unilateral, can I assume that her uterus and other adnexa were not removed?

3. What was her pre- or perioperative beta-hCG?

(I will assume that this is a pure EST with a normal pretreatment hCG and that her uterus and one adnexa are intact.)

Endodermal/sinus tumors produce alpha-fetoprotein (AFP) and rarely have an isolated hCG elevation. It is imperative to rule out pregnancy, whether intrauterine or ectopic, and I would obtain a repeat quantitative beta-hCG. If this were elevated, a pelvic ultrasound would be in order. If a pregnancy is confirmed, appropriate follow-up would depend on its location, viability, and the patient's desire.

If pregnancy is not a possibility, I would repeat the chest and abdominal-pelvic computed tomography (CT) and possibly also do a brain CT. Careful review of these films for occult metastases or residual, chemotherapy-resistant tumor is necessary. If there is an isolated pulmonary lesion in the setting of a persistently elevated or increasing hCG, a thoracotomy to diagnose and remove the lesion should be offered to the patient. If a malignant germ-cell tumor is confirmed, I would give the patient two or three additional courses of cisplatin, etoposide, and bleomycin. Radiotherapy can also be considered after secondary cytoreduction of isolated metastases.

Unfortunately there is not a large body of literature to cite since malignant germ-cell tumors in women are rare. Much of the experience in gynecological oncology has been extrapolated from the treatment of testicular cancers.

PHYSICIAN'S RESPONSE

JOHN CURRIE

In the majority of patients with germ-cell tumors who exhibit complete responses to combination chemotherapy, the responses are durable; that some do fail, as in this case, justifies continued monitoring of tumor markers many years after apparent cure. Some clinicians, anticipating the possibility of a late relapse, follow the induction regimen with a different consolidation course of chemotherapy. Thus, although bleomycin, etoposide, and cisplatin (BEP) are clearly the agents of first choice, consolidation with vincristine, actinomycin-D, and cytoxan (VAC) might have been appropriate in this 26-year-old female with stage IV endodermal sinus tumor.

With beta-hCG elevation one year after therapy confirmed, the first task is a thorough evaluation; initial efforts should center on ruling out other causes of hCG elevation, including missed abortion, chronic ectopic pregnancy, gestational trophoblastic disease, or another gestational cause of the hCG elevation. Diagnostic curettage, vaginal ultrasound, free-fragment hCG analysis, and human placental lactogen (hPL) (to rule out placental site trophoblastic tumor) should be considered early in the patient's evaluation.

Next, assuming that the elevation is a bona fide indication of recurrent disease, assertive imaging should be undertaken to search for the site(s) of extant tumor. Computed tomography (CT) of the chest, abdomen/pelvis, and brain should be performed and compared with previous studies. A sample of cerebrospinal fluid should be obtained for hCG determination and the value obtained compared with the serum value. A higher value than expected in the cerebrospinal fluid (CSF) might indicate central nervous system metastases. Finally, labeled hCG antibody study might locate an obscure metastasis; although such studies are frequently indistinct and subsequent testing may be clouded because of host immunological response to the test, location of a single focus of recurrent disease that might be amenable to surgical extirpation makes an exhaustive search worthwhile. Because retroperitoneal or nodal recurrences are common with endodermal sinus tumor, magnetic resonance imaging (MRI) might help delineate such locus; the utility of this modality would be limited if there were no comparison images.

If a solitary nodule of recurrent disease is responsible for the relapse, surgical therapy to remove this focus is indicated. Following removal, if markers fall to normal levels, no further therapy would be indicated, although markers should be followed closely and chemotherapy instigated immediately if values rise.

Persistent disease following surgery, multiple sites of recurrent disease found on tumor survey, or failure to demonstrate the exact location of the source of marker elevation mandates systemic chemotherapy. Choice of agents is the next problem for the clinician to consider.

Retreatment with BEP is a logical choice because of the previous dramatic response, assuming careful evaluation of toxicity to the original regimen was negative and historical information did not suggest undue toxic consequences from the original BEP treatment. However, even if repeat BEP therapy induced remission, I would favor three to six additional courses of VAC in this patient to ensure sustained control.

An alternative approach would be to initiate VAC therapy as the initial salvage regimen for six to nine courses at standard dosages. If remission were induced rapidly, no further treatment would be necessary after the planned duration of chemotherapy. If response, as judged by the rapidity of fall of the marker, were more methodical and obtuse, further therapy should be instigated.

Failure to induce remission with either BEP or VAC would suggest highly resistant disease, and the next choice of chemotherapy would be empiric. Ifosfamide, methotrexate, dacarbazine, vinblastine, doxorubicin, and hexamethamelamine—alone or in combination—should be considered. Paclitaxel (Taxol) may show activity against these tumors, but extensive data are lacking.

The initial response to chemotherapy would suggest that continued persistence of treatment should induce permanent remission.

20

Ovarian Cancer: Germ-Cell Tumors (Teratoma, Grade 2)

CASE

A 24-year-old woman, gravida O, was on her honeymoon and on oral contraceptives when she developed severe right-lower-quadrant pain. She underwent an exploratory laparotomy with a right salpingo-oophorectomy (RSO) for the removal of a 12-cm right-ovarian mass adherent to the pelvic wall. The surgeon commented at the time that he was worried it could be malignant, but a pathologist was not available for frozen section. Surgery was done through a Pfannenstiel incision. The surgeon did not notice any other suspicious areas in the pelvis or abdomen. Postoperatively the patient did well and she is otherwise in good health. The final pathology identified the tumor as a grade 2 malignant teratoma.

PHYSICIAN'S RESPONSE

S.D. WILLIAMS

This patient poses some very difficult management problems. She no doubt does indeed have a malignant teratoma and clearly has been incompletely staged. Additional studies that should be done include a chest x-ray and abdominal computed tomography (CT) scan. The chest x-ray will likely be normal. Unless clearly abnormal, the CT scan is not a particularly effective way to evaluate the peritoneal cavity and retroperitoneal nodes. Measurement of human chorionic gonadotropin (hCG) and alpha-fetoprotein (AFP) should also be done, but these results will probably not affect initial therapy.

Because of the uncertainties in the staging of this patient, it is tempting to recommend a surgical staging procedure prior to initiation of chemotherapy. I would not argue strongly against this. However, I believe that the best approach to this patient is to begin chemotherapy with bleomycin, etoposide, and cisplatin (BEP). As discussed below, this patient should have another surgical procedure, but I believe it would best be done after chemotherapy rather than before. If a surgical staging procedure were done and were negative, she would receive adjuvant therapy with BEP. If it were positive, she also would receive chemotherapy, possibly followed by a second-look laparotomy. Immature teratomas can sometimes be very aggressive. It seems best to begin therapy as quickly as possible.

Should the patient truly have disease localized to the ovary (which is likely), then three courses of chemotherapy would be adequate and her likelihood of cure high. If, on the other hand, she had more advanced tumor, the optimum duration of therapy is not clear, but patients are usually given four courses. If her tolerance of chemotherapy were good, I would give her four courses. On the other hand, if she tolerated treatment poorly, I would give here only three courses.

At the completion of therapy, I would recommend second-look laparotomy with thorough surgical staging and resection of any significant residual masses. A recent review of the Gynecologic Oncology Group (GOG) experience with second-look laparotomy suggests that the patients who potentially benefit from surgery are those who have teratoma elements in their primary tumor and who are initially incompletely resected. As this patient certainly might fall in this category, I would recommend such surgery. Again, one could argue to do the second surgical procedure before chemotherapy. If residual tumor were present, it could perhaps be resected, thus placing this patient in a favorable prognostic group. Further, patients with no residual tumor clearly would need only three courses of chemotherapy. However, I would proceed immediately to chemotherapy and recommend surgery at the completion of treatment.

The likelihood of cure of this patient is difficult to predict because of the uncertainties of stage. However, if she is free of tumor at initiation of chemotherapy (which is most likely), she almost certainly will survive. If, on the other hand, she has residual tumor, then her likelihood of survival will be less but still between 60 and 80%.

The reproductive effects of treatment are discussed in Case 16. I would hold considerable optimism that this patient would resume menses after treatment and retain fertility.

Reference

Williams SD, Blessing JA, DiSaia PJ, et al. Second-look laparotomy in ovarian germ cell tumors: The Gynecologic Oncology Group experience. Gynecol Oncol 1994; 52:287–291.

PHYSICIAN'S RESPONSE

MURRAY JOSEPH CASEY

The aggressive application of multiple antineoplastic drug regimens has proven highly effective in managing patients with completely resected malignant teratomas and in those with minimal residual subclinical disease. But cytotoxic chemotherapy is significantly less effective in cases of bulky residual measurable tumors. Among the first effective regimens used in the treatment of malignant ovarian germ-cell tumors was a combination of vincristine, actinomycin-D, and cyclophosphamide (VAC), which was successful in controlling 72% of completely resected disease and 45% of minimal residual disease, but this regimen controlled disease in just 18% of patients who were left with bulky tumor following primary surgery. In all, 68% of patients who were left with residual tumors failed treatment with VAC compared with a failure rate of 28% in patients whose tumors were completely resected.

Subsequently, cisplatin-containing regimens have proven more effective against malignant ovarian germ-cell tumors. A regimen of vinblastine, bleomycin, and cisplatin (VBP) controlled 65% of subclinical malignant ovarian germ-cell tumors and 34% of measurable residual tumors. Disease-free survival was reported for 66% of patients with less than 2-cm residual germ cell tumors treated with VBP and in 42% of patients with larger residual tumors. The proven responsiveness of similar testicular germ-cell tumors to etoposide led to the substitution of this drug for vinblastine into the regimen of bleomycin, etoposide, and cisplatin (BEP), which is less toxic than VBP and at least as effective, achieving control in 96% of completely resected malignant ovarian germ-cell tumors.

Therefore, it is incumbent upon the consultant to take reasonable steps to assure that all identifiable tumor has been primarily resected. Except for the 10 to 15% bilaterality of dysgerminomas, bilateral ovarian involvement by germ-cell tumors is rare, although 5 to 10% may be associated with benign dermoid cysts. So the most ominous features of the present case are the relatively large size of the resected tumor and its adherence to the pelvic side wall. Scanning methods, such as computed tomography (CT) and magnetic resonance imaging (MRI), may be helpful in delineating residual tumor if it exists, and expert lymphangiography may demonstrate suspicious defects and enlargement of pelvic or paraaortic nodes. In pure malignant ovarian teratomas, serum alpha-fetoprotein (AFP) may be detectable and beta-human chorionic gonadotrophin (beta-hCG) levels may be elevated if mixed elements of dysgerminoma, embryonal carcinoma, polyembryoma, or choriocarcinoma are present. Elevations in serum CA-125 and neuron-specific enolase levels have been reported with malignant teratomas. Baseline determinations of these markers should be obtained. Ultimately, laparoscopy should be undertaken for thorough exploration of the pelvic and abdominal peritoneal cavity, all serosal surfaces, and the undersurface of the diaphragm, with special attention to the previous tumor bed in the right pelvis and any questionable sites found by the preoperative scanning studies. Multiple and generous biopsies should be taken from the right pelvic peritoneum and all other suspicious sites. Then video-endoscopic retroperitoneal exploration should be performed with selective tissue biopsies and excision of all suspicious and enlarged pelvic and paraaortic nodes. If tumor is identified by scanning studies or if serum tumor markers are significantly elevated or residual malignant teratoma is found at laparoscopy, exploratory laparotomy through a vertical incision is warranted to permit maximum tumor debulking and formal staging procedures. The effectiveness of resecting large retroperitoneal nodes has not been proven but seems advisable in view of the improved results with chemotherapy in the absence of measurable tumor.

Delays in the institution of antineoplastic chemotherapy for germ-cell tumors of the testes and ovaries have correlated with poor outcomes. Therefore, the preferred BEP regimen of cisplatin 20 mg/m^2 and etoposide 100 mg/m^2 on days 1 to 5 at 21-day intervals and bleomycin 30 U weekly should be undertaken immediately following negative laparoscopy or within a week of laparotomy and debulking surgery, as soon as significant risk of infection has passed. Excellent hydration and diuresis should be employed to avoid cisplatin nephrotoxicity; modern antiemetics with or without corticosteroids will help reduce nausea during administration.

Baseline tumor markers and scanning studies should be obtained, and extended physical examinations and tumor marker determinations should be repeated just prior to each expected 21-day cycle of chemotherapy. Particular attention should be paid to fever, which may herald severe granulocytopenia, and fine pulmonary rales or decreased breath sounds may be early sings of bleomycin-induced pulmonary fibrosis. In the face of severe toxicity, chemotherapy doses should be modified or agents should even be eliminated as appropriate to permit prompt resumption of planned courses, thus avoiding deleterious delays in the 21-day schedule.

Four courses of BEP are planned, but surgical intervention should be entertained in the instance of refractory or recurrent disease, since salvage therapy with selective surgical resection of isolated tumor and alternative chemotherapy regimens have been successful in some cases of testicular and ovarian germ-cell tumors. Responses to both platinum-resistant and platinum-sensitive recurrent germ-cell tumors have been reported. For the former, regimens that include cisplatin with ifosfamide and etoposide or vinblastine have been effective; for the latter group, high-dose carboplatin with etoposide supported by autologous bone marrow transplant have successfully salvaged 20 to 34% of patients.

Though the issue is somewhat controversial, there seems to be little to recommend routine second-look laparotomies for the management of malignant ovarian teratomas in the absence of demonstrable disease by physical examination, scanning studies, or rising tumor markers. Malignant ovarian teratomas tend to be highly chemoresponsive and should have excellent prognosis if primarily debulked and adequately managed with the suggested BEP regimen.

Reference

Gershenson DM. Update on malignant ovarian germ cell tumors. Cancer 1993; 71:1581–1590.

PHYSICIANS' RESPONSE

THOMAS V. SEDLACEK
MAX A. CLARK

In the patient in question several factors must be taken into consideration. First the patient was not staged properly; peritoneal washings and biopsies were not obtained and lymphadenectomy was not performed. Also, the adhesions to the pelvic side wall were not biopsied. However, since the surgery was done through a Pfannenstiel incision, it is doubtful that the patient could have been staged properly.

In a patient who desires fertility, a unilateral salpingo-oophorectomy should be performed in stage I disease. For patients who no longer desire fertility, a total abdominal hysterectomy and bilateral salpingo-oophorectomy may be performed. However, no clear survival benefit is associated with hysterectomy. Prognosis is determined by the grade and stage of the primary tumor. Tumors are graded based on the degree of immaturity and the amount of neuroepithelial tissue present. Prognosis and survival depend ultimately on the tumor grade. Norris et al. have demonstrated that in stage I, patients with grade 1 tumor experienced an 85% survival rate. Patients with stage I grade 2 tumors and stage I grade 3 tumors experienced 55 and 33% survivals respectively with unilateral salpingo-oophorectomy (1). For patients with metastatic tumors (stages II and III), all grade 0 patients survived while less than 50% survived with grade 1 and 2 tumors. Treatment therefore depends on the tumor grade.

The approach to the patient should begin with a review of the histology specimen, taking one block of tissue for each centimeter of tumor followed by a full explanation to the patient concerning immature teratomas. If the patient's grade 2 status is confirmed, then the patient may undergo proper staging either via a laparotomy or with laparoscopy. More prudent is to simply treat the patient with chemotherapy because the tumor is grade 2. Stage is not that important at this juncture, especially with the report of the general surgeon that no gross tumor implants were noted.

However, many authors feel that tumor adherence constitutes stage III disease. Since no gross metastatic lesions were noted, there is no benefit to re-exploration for cytoreduction. Therefore we would prefer to treat the patient with three cycles of chemotherapy. Her disease should be monitored with serum tumor markers, hCG, AFP, and LDH.

The most frequently used chemotherapy regimen since 1970 has been a combination of vincristine, actinomycin-D, and cyclophosphamide (VAC). In 1985, the Gynecologic Oncology Group (GOG) reported a relapse-free survival rate of 75% with VAC. Newer approaches use a platinum-containing regimen for primary or salvage treatment. Patients who have failed therapy with VAC have been salvaged with the use of bleomycin, etoposide, and cisplatin (BEP). In a trial of 166 patients, using platinum and etoposide with and without bleomycin as primary treatment in patients with germ-cell tumors of the testes, the disease-free survival was 84% with the BEP regimen and 69% with the EP regimen (2). Thus, bleomycin is an integral part of the newer treatment regimens. Both fatal and nonfatal pulmonary fibrosis is associated with bleomycin treatment; however, if careful monitoring is used, this is usually not a problem. In general, pulmonary fibrosis is dose-related or occurs in patients who have previously had chest radiation, although it can also occur even without predisposing factors. Therefore, BEP should *not* be used as adjunctive treatment.

The patient should have three cycles of treatment and should continue to use birth control pills during the chemotherapy and probably for a year or two thereafter. If a reproductive-age patient has been treated with chemotherapy and waits 2 years following therapy before becoming pregnant, the rate of congenital anomalies is no greater than in a nontreated population. Since the immature teratoma does not produce a marker unless it contains elements of other germ-cell tumors and since this patient was not properly staged with her first operation, she should have an assessment laparotomy (second look) 1 month following completion of chemotherapy. If the patient is tumor-free, no further therapy is indicated. If persistent tumor is noted, she can then be switched to an alternate chemotherapy regimen (VAC, VPB). Almost all patients such as the one presented will be tumor-free.

Patients have successfully become pregnant 1 year after completion of VAC chemotherapy and they have even been treated successfully during the second and third trimesters with chemotherapy (1). Successful pregnancies have been reported following chemotherapy and conservative surgery for a stage III immature teratoma of the ovary (2). Since the recurrence rate for immature teratomas is low, the patient's prognosis is quite good, especially if the laparotomy following chemotherapy is negative.

Recommendations

1. Three courses of VAC chemotherapy.
2. Restage with MRI or CT scan and tumor markers 1 month following

completion of chemotherapy; perform laparotomy/laparoscopy if no clinical evidence of tumor is noted.

3. Second-line chemotherapy if laparotomy/laparoscopy is positive.
4. Continue contraceptives for 2 years following completion of chemotherapy.

References

1. Norris HJ, Zirkin HJ, Benson WL. Immature (malignant) teratoma of the ovary: A clinical and pathologic study of 58 cases. Canao 1976; 37 (5):2359.
2. Lachrer PJ, Elsono P, Johnson PH, et al. A randomized trial of cisplatin plus etoposide with and without bleomycin in favorable prognosis disseminated germ cell tumors: An ECOG study. Proc Am Soc Clin Oncol 1991; 10:540.

PHYSICIAN'S RESPONSE

THOMAS MONTAG

I would recommend obtaining computed tomography (CT) of the abdomen and pelvis postoperatively. In addition, several tumor markers should be obtained as soon after initial surgery as possible. These should include alpha-fetoprotein (AFP), lactate dehydrogenase (LDH), CA-125, and CA-19-9. Should the CT scan show bulky metastatic disease, strong consideration must be given to attempting cytoreductive surgery (debulking) prior to initiating chemotherapy (1). Studies have shown that fewer patients with completely resected disease fail chemotherapy as compared with patients with incompletely resected disease treated with the same chemotherapy (1). In addition, a higher percentage of patients with bulky residual disease fail chemotherapy as compared with patients with minimal residual disease (1).

If the CT scan does not show bulky disease, chemotherapy should be initiated as soon after surgery as possible. The combination of bleomycin, etoposide, and cisplatin (BEP) is the regimen of choice (2). This consists of bleomycin 30 units IV weekly, etoposide 100 mg/m^2 IV on days 1 to 5, and cisplatin 20 mg/m^2 IV on days 1 to 5 repeated at 21-day intervals (1). In a recent Gynecologic Oncology Group study, 96% of patients with completely resected stage I, II, or III ovarian germ-cell tumors remained continuously disease-free after three cycles of BEP (2). If any of the tumor markers are elevated, the duration of chemotherapy may be based on serial measurements of the elevated marker(s).

Following a minimum of three courses of BEP or the return of the elevated tumor marker to the normal range, a "second look" exploratory laparotomy is recommended through a vertical midline incision (2). Ascites, if present, or peritoneal washings should be submitted for cytological evaluation. Careful inspection and palpation of the entire peritoneal cavity should be performed. Any suspicious areas should be biopsied or excised. The site where the right ovarian mass was adherent to the pelvic side wall should be biopsied. If no suspicious areas are noted, standard surgical staging should be performed, including multiple biopsies of the pelvic and abdominal peritoneum, omentectomy, and pelvic and paraaortic lymph node sampling.

Should there be persistent immature teratoma at the time of surgery, additional cycles of BEP may be indicated. Alternatively, the combination of vincristine, dactinomycin, and cyclophosphamide (VAC) may be given as salvage therapy.

I would recommend continuation of the oral contraceptives while the patient receives chemotherapy, since suppression of ovarian function may theoretically minimize any potential deleterious effects on the remaining ovary.

References

1. Williams SD, Gershenson DM, Horowitz CJ, Scully RG. Ovarian germ cell and stromal tumors. In: Hoskins WJ, Perez CA, Young RC, eds. Principles and Practice of Gynecologic Oncology. Philadelphia: Lippincott 1992:715–730.
2. Gershenson DM. Management of early ovarian cancer: Germ cell and sex cord tumors. Gynecol Oncol 1994; 55:S62.

PHYSICIANS' RESPONSE

WATSON WATRING
NEIL SEMRAD

Patients with germ-cell tumors of the ovary often present as this patient did. Due to these tumors' rapid growth, it is not uncommon for a dysgerminoma, endodermal sinus tumor, or immature teratoma to present with an "acute abdomen." It was quite astute for the surgeon in this case to be "worried it could be malignant."

Even with a pathologist unavailable, it might have better served the patient had the surgeon done staging procedures. This is preferably accomplished via a vertical incision; however, if aesthetics is an issue a Maylard or Churney may be considered. In any case, all that being behind us now, what to do?

Initially markers should be obtained. These would have been more ideally obtained prior to surgery. However, they should be obtained at this time to see if they are elevated. Markers should include AFP, beta-hCG, carcinoembryonic antigen (CEA), and LDH.

In the past, patients with grade 2 disease of immature teratoma were generally given chemotherapy. Once acceptable treatment for this patient, then, would be four courses of BEP chemotherapy. No second look is needed.

Recently, Bonazzi and coworkers (1) questioned the necessity of chemotherapy in early-stage (I or II) and grade 2 immature teratoma patients. 14 of 32 patients in this category remained free of disease without chemotherapy. It should be noted that these patients "underwent follow-up laparoscopies at regular intervals." It is unknown if follow-up laparoscopies would convey greater morbidity/mortality than chemotherapy.

Clearly, in this patient, if chemotherapy is to be withheld, a complete surgical staging is necessary. If she is found to be stage I or II, then the data would seem to indicate that, with close follow-up, a good outcome can be obtained. If she is found to have more advanced disease, chemotherapy is indicated, as above.

Reference

1. Bonazzi, et al. Pure ovarian immature teratoma, a unique and curable disease: 10 Years' experience of 32 prospectively treated patients. Obstet Gynecol 1994; 84:598–604.

21

Elevated CA-125 in a Premenopausal Woman with No Known Cancer

CASE

A 35-year-old woman, gravida III, para III, had some right-lower-quadrant pain and was seen by her local gynecologist. He thought he could feel some fullness on the right side, so an ultrasound was done and a CA-125 was ordered. The CA-125 came back as 128 U and ultrasound showed a 4-cm cystic right ovary. She was referred to a gynecological oncologist who asked that the CA-125 be repeated prior to the consultation. At the time of the consultation, the pelvic exam was normal, the patient was asymptomatic, and a repeat pelvic ultrasound was normal. A repeat CA-125 came back as 78 U. The patient is obviously quite anxious about this blood test since she has been doing some reading since her initial visit to her local doctor.

PHYSICIAN'S RESPONSE

VICKI SELTZER

It is essential to do a thorough clinical evaluation of this patient prior to incorporating consideration of the CA-125 level. Begin by obtaining a complete history including all past medical history, gynecological history, family history, social history, and review of systems. Elicit a very thorough history regarding the patient's recent episode of right-lower-quadrant pain. A complete physical examination (including pelvic and rectovaginal examinations) should be performed. Then, a complete differential diagnosis regarding the etiology of the patient's previous pain should be determined. This would include such problems as salpingo-oophoritis, functional ovarian cyst, endometriosis, and so on.

Next, the differential diagnosis of an elevated CA-125 should be considered. In addition to ovarian cancer, CA-125 has been found to be elevated in a variety of benign gynecological disorders (e.g., endometriosis, pelvic inflammatory disease, uterine fibroids), physiological conditions (including pregnancy and menstruation), nongynecological malignancies (e.g., breast, colorectal, lung, and pancreas), and benign nongynecological disorders (including liver disease and heart failure). In addition, it is more common in a premenopausal than in a postmenopausal woman to have an elevated CA-125 level with no specific etiology ever found.

After having evaluated the patient's clinical circumstances, the known etiologies of an elevated CA-125 level, and the likely differential diagnosis, a determination can be made regarding what, if any, further clinical investigation would be appropriate. Does the patient require further evaluation for liver disease? for pelvic infection? Appropriate blood studies should be obtained. If a specific disease process is identified, obviously it should be treated accordingly.

What about the clinical circumstance in which the entire evaluation is negative, the family history is negative, and the presumptive diagnosis is that the patient had a functional ovarian cyst which resolved. Does a CA-125 of 128 with a repeat of 78 warrant an invasive evaluation? I personally would not perform a laparoscopy in this circumstance but would obtain a serial CA-125 in 2 or 3 months. If the values continued to fall, I would be reassured, since certainly if the patient had cancer one would expect the CA-125 to continue to rise. On the other hand, if the CA-125 did rise, I would favor more aggressive diagnostic studies, including laparoscopy.

Reference

Jacobs I. Genetic, biochemical, and multimodal approaches to screening for ovarian cancer. Gynecol Oncol 1994; 55:S22–S27.

PHYSICIAN'S RESPONSE

DANIEL SMITH

This patient was referred to me for consultation because of an elevated CA-125 blood test. On examination today, she had no symptoms, a normal pelvic exam, and a normal pelvic ultrasound examination. She was quite anxious and asked to discuss the meaning of the results and her risks of having ovarian cancer.

Following the examination, I sat with the patient to review the information.

She seemed relieved that the results, including the ultrasound, were normal. She was encouraged but not entirely reassured by the declining CA-125 test.

I explained that there were many benign, noncancerous conditions that might account for her recent medical history and test results. The CA-125 test is a measure of the body's response to a specific stimulus, usually a tumor-associated antigen. Although the test was developed to assay for the presence of ovarian cancer, other malignant and benign conditions can cause an elevation of the CA-125 test. Typically, many stimuli that cause peritoneal irritation can result in an elevated test. Possible benign causes of her test elevation might include pelvic inflammatory disease, endometriosis, ovarian cysts, leiomyomata uteri, diverticulitis, and mild appendicitis or mesenteric adenitis.

As to the risk of malignancy in this patient, it is relevant to obtain a complete family history of malignancy. In a rare instance, such a pedigree may disclose a significant clustering of relatives with ovarian, breast, colon, and/or uterine cancer. The presence of one or more first-degree relatives or several second-degree relatives with such malignancies may indicate that the patient herself is at increased risk for similar cancers and indicate further testing in any case.

However, with a negative family history, the patient appears to have a resolving problem. Nevertheless, the CA-125 blood test is still elevated. At this time, several options are possible and should be discussed with the patient. These options include (a) accepting the falling blood test as an indication of a totally resolving problem, (b) further radiological testing at this time, (c) surgical investigation such as laparoscopy to ascertain the process causing the recent course, or (d) future scheduled testing and examination. Of these choices, I recommend the last. In this case, I would reexamine the woman in 3 months and repeat the CA-125 blood test at that time. Should the test be normal, the patient could be remanded to her local gynecologist. Should the test remain elevated, increase in value, or there is a positive finding on pelvic examination, further testing would be indicated. In the face of pelvic pain or discomfort, a positive CA-125 blood test, and negative ultrasound or other imaging studies, diagnostic laparoscopy may well prove useful to identify endometriosis or chronic pelvic infection. The finding of ovarian cancer in such a situation would be rare.

In the end, the patient should be reassured that she has a resolving, benign process. Further testing and examination will be performed to assure us both that this is so. However, should she have any further symptomatology, such as abdominal discomfort, change in appetite, or alteration of bowel habits, an immediate reevaluation would be necessary. Ultimately she may need either additional imaging studies or even laparoscopy/laparotomy. However, the elevation of the CA-125 test in her case appears to result from a process that is quickly resolving.

Reference

Chem D-X, Schwartz PE, Li X, Yan Z. Evaluation of CA125 levels in differentiating malignant from benign tumors in patients with pelvic masses. Obstet Gynecol 1988: 72:23–27.

PHYSICIAN'S RESPONSE

JOHN CURTIN

The sequence of events in this case illustrates a common misuse of serum CA-125 levels. The patient had no indication for drawing a serum CA-125 in the first place; however, now the clinicians are left to explain to an anxious patient that serum CA-125 can be elevated in a number of normal physiological and benign conditions. Unfortunately the negative workup done to date does not exclude the possibility that the patient may be at some risk. My recommendation is that since the ultrasound of the ovaries is normal, there is no indication for additional studies at this time with the possible exception of a screening bilateral mammography.

CA-125 is a high-molecular-weight glycoprotein antigen; OC-125 is the monoclonal antibody which is specific for the antigen CA-125. CA-125 is produced by a variety of normal and neoplastic cells derived from coelomic epithelium. The primary clinical use of serum CA-125 levels is in the management of women with adenocarcinoma of the ovary. Bast and colleagues developed the blood test and first reported on its clinical utility in 1983; in women with ovarian cancer, the CA-125 levels were elevated in 80% patients. Subsequent publication have further defined the clinical utility of serum CA-125 determinations. For the patient with a possible ovarian neoplasm, an elevated CA-125 is associated with a high likelihood of malignancy, especially among postmenopausal women. For women with ovarian cancer, serum CA-125 levels reflect disease status and response to therapy.

The role of serum CA-125 determinations in the screening for ovarian cancer was recently reviewed by Ian Jacobs as part of the NIH Consensus Conference on Ovarian Cancer. Among premenopausal women, 5.7% will have an elevated serum CA-125. Many benign and physiological conditions can result in an elevated CA-125, including menstruation, uterine fibroids, endometriosis, pregnancy, and pelvic inflammatory disease. Less commonly, hepatic disorders or inflammation of the pleura or peritoneum also result in elevated levels of CA-125. Jacobs says that screening studies utilizing serum CA-125 as an initial test must be combined with pelvic ultrasound as a secondary test for those women with elevated levels. This combination of serum CA-125 and pelvic ultrasound had a specificity of 99% in detecting ovarian cancer. Given that this patient has had a pelvic ultrasound which is normal, no further studies are indicated at this time.

The patient should be followed at regular intervals of 6 to 12 months. There is some concern from the analysis of serum banks that, in some patients, elevated serum CA-125 levels may precede the clinical detection of ovarian cancer by 1 to 2 years. In one study of nearly 40,000 serum samples obtained from healthy women, patients who developed ovarian cancer after the serum samples were obtained were analyzed. Fifty-nine women had serum obtained more than 5 years before their clinical diagnosis of ovarian cancer. Fourteen of these serum specimens (25%) were found to have an elevated serum CA-125 level when analyzed retrospectively. Given this knowledge, I do believe that at this time we can completely reassure women who are found to have an elevated serum CA-125 level. If the level continues to be elevated in the future, I would recommend yearly pelvic ultrasound. Surgical evaluation (i.e., laparoscopy) would be indicated only if an abnormality were discovered on pelvic ultrasound.

References

Bast RC, Klug TL, St John E, et al. A radioimmunoassay using a monocloncal antibody to monitor the course of epithelial ovarian cancer. N Engl J Med 1983; 309:169–171.
Jacobs I. Genetic, biochemical, and multimodal approaches to screening for ovarian cancer. Gynecol Oncol 1994; 55:S22–S27.

PHYSICIANS' RESPONSE

LYNDA ROMAN
FRANCO MUGGIA

In premenopausal women, elevation of CA-125 must be interpreted with great caution. In fact, screening for ovarian cancer by CA-125 determinations has not been deemed cost-effective, because the percentage of false-positives is several-fold higher than the rare incident cases that are detected (1–4). These false-positives nearly all represent benign gynecological conditions or are unexplained, contrasting with the situation in postmenopausal women subjected to screening, where a substantial number of false-positives represent incidental detection of epithelial malignancies of nongynecological origin.

Having commented in general on "incidental" CA-125 elevations, we turn to consider the possible causes for the abnormalities detected in this particular patient. Given the clinical setting, the most likely explanation for both the signs and symptoms *and* the CA-125 is a benign process, that of a hemorrhagic corpus luteum. The CA-125, in fact, shows a decrease on a repeat determination performed presumably within a couple of weeks. Serial determinations of CA-125 are being explored as a way of enhancing the predictive value of this marker in screening large populations (3). However, such a maneuver will prove unlikely to generate early detection of ovarian cancer or to be cost-effective.

Since the CA-125 remains abnormal in this patient, a repeat determination in 4 to 6 weeks is warranted and should prove sufficient to rule out any serious process as long as it is not increasing. Should it increase, one could consider laparoscopy if the patient desires; however, the yield is very low. If an ultrasound had again revealed a nonsuspicious cyst, this laparoscopy would be best postponed until after a 3-month period of oral contraceptives had been administered so as to eliminate the chance of visualizing benign cysts. The overwhelming probability remains that one is dealing with a benign process.

One might argue about the wisdom of having obtained a CA-125 in this setting in the first place.

References

1. Helzlsouer KJ, Bush TL, Alberg AJ, et al. Prospective study of serum CA-125 levels as markers of ovarian cancer. JAMA 1993; 269:1123–1126.
2. Zurawski VR, Sjovall K, Schoenfield DA, et al. Prospective evaluation of serum Ca 125 levels in a normal population: Phase I. The specificities of single and serial determinations in testing for ovarian cancer. Gynecol Oncol 1990; 36:299–305.
3. Zurawski VR, Broderick SF, Pickens P, et al. Serum CA 125 levels in a group of nonhospitalized women: Relevance for the early detection of ovarian cancer. Obstet Gynecol 1987; 69:606.
4. Einhorn N, Sjovall K, Knapp RC, et al. Prospective evaluation of serum CA 125 levels for early detection of ovarian cancer. Obstet Gynecol 1992; 80:14–18.

PHYSICIAN'S RESPONSE

JOHN WEED

A simple ovarian cyst in an asymptomatic 35-year-old patient is most likely to be "functional" (follicular) or a corpus luteum. The associated elevation of CA-125 causes the dilemma. In reviewing the patient's history, one would concentrate on factors that would clarify the significance of the CA-125 levels. Were menstrual cycles truly regular in cycle, duration, and flow? What is the current means of contraception , if any? Is there a family history of reproductive/endocrine or other malignancy? Has there been dysmenorrhea or dyspareunia? The sonograms, if available, should be reviewed to comment on septation, complexity of cyst, and pulsatility. Are there any other historical factors present such as smoking, liver disease, inflammatory bowel disease, and so on, that may be associated with elevation in CA-125?

Upon confirming a normal pelvic examination with the palpation of normal adnexal structures and cul-de-sac, I would recommend cautious observation with the patient on adequate contraception. The CA-125 and pelvic examination should be repeated on a 3-month cycle until both are normal or further evaluation is undertaken. Should the CA-125 remain elevated over a 6-month period, one would be more aggressive in diagnosis. Diagnostic laparoscopy would be appropriate to see the right ovary and adnexal structures and to secure a tissue diagnosis in the case of endometriosis.

In the event that the patient is not reassured by the recommendation for cautious observation, one may be justified in proceeding with diagnostic laparoscopy. Any further surgical intervention should await a careful review of the visual and histological finding with the patient and additional discussion regarding the therapeutic options.

22

Elevated CA-125 in a Postmenopausal Woman

CASE

A 61-year-old woman presents to her local physician with a chief complaint of intermittent mild lower abdominal discomfort of several months' duration.

She has a history of diverticulosis and has been treated in the past for peptic ulcer disease. Past medical history is also remarkable for an uncomplicated inferior wall myocardial infarction 2 years ago. The patient has seen her gynecologist approximately every 2 years and has not been told of any abnormalities. She has two sisters, one of whom developed breast cancer at age 64.

Physical examination performed by her local physician reveals mild diffuse middle and lower abdominal tenderness to deep palpation. The remainder of the physical examination is reported to be unremarkable, including both the breast and pelvic examinations.

Laboratory examination reveals mild anemia (hemoglobin 10.2 g/dL). Liver and renal function studies are normal.

A CA-125 test returns 1 week after the current visit at a value of 123. She is sent to you for a second opinion.

PHYSICIANS' RESPONSE

THOMAS J. RUTHERFORD
SETSUKO K. CHAMBERS
PETER E. SCHWARTZ

This patient with a history of diverticulosis and lower abdominal pain needs to undergo evaluation of the gastrointestinal tract. A barium enema and/or colonoscopy would be a reasonable first approach. Diverticulitis would be our primary suspicion in view of her past history and the elevated CA-125. Colon cancer needs to be ruled out, since it can cause elevations in CA-125. We do not know from the given history whether she has experienced rectal bleeding. During the physical examination, the stools should be checked for guaiac positivity. If traces of blood are present, colon cancer could account not only for the increased CA-125 but also for her mild anemia. One would also have to exclude recurrent peptic ulcer disease or gastric cancer as a cause of her anemia and consider an upper GI series. We have presumed that the remaining indices of her complete blood count are normal and that there is no evidence of an infectious process. However, we do not know the status of her purified protein derivative (PPD) test or previous exposure to tuberculosis. Pelvic tuberculosis can cause abdominal pain as well as an elevation in the CA-125; however, it is a rare entity.

Other nongynecological malignant causes of an increased CA-125 are lung, pancreatic, and breast cancer. We do not know this patient's tobacco history or whether she has been exposed to asbestos. A chest x-ray might be considered if the patient has been exposed to tobacco, either by primary or secondary exposure. Pancreatic cancer is listed only for completeness. Since her abdominal discomfort has persisted for several months with normal liver function tests and no signs of pancreatic carcinoma, this possibility is remote. A mammogram should be obtained to rule out occult breast cancer because of her age and family history. Levels of CA-125 may also be elevated when breast cancer is present.

There are several gynecological malignancies that can cause elevations in CA-125. These include endometrial, endocervical, and ovarian carcinoma. Obviously, if she has vaginal bleeding, an endometrial biopsy should be performed to rule out endometrial carcinoma. We have presumed that a Pap smear was performed and found to be normal, therefore making an endocervical etiology unlikely.

Her pelvic examination did not identify an adnexal mass; however, her ovaries should not be palpable, since she is postmenopausal. If they were palpable, the use of a pelvic sonogram would be justified to help rule out an ovarian malignancy. If the sonogram demonstrated no evidence of malignancy, the CA-125 level should be repeated within a 3-month interval. In a retrospective study, those women 50 years of age or older whose CA-125 levels were 95 U/mL or more or whose levels had doubled over the course of a year appeared to be at a substantial risk for malignant disease.

In this patient, in consideration of her past history and presentation as well as the elevation of the CA-125, recurrent diverticular disease is the most likely etiology. If this proves to be the case and the diverticulitis is successfully treated, one may see a decline in the CA-125.

References

Einhorn N, Sjovall K, Knapp RC, et al. Prospective evaluation of serum CA 125 levels for early detection of ovarian cancer. Obstet Gynecol 1992; 80:14–18.

Malkasian GD, Knapp RC, Lavin PT, et al. Preoperative evaluation of serum CA 125 levels in premenopausal and postmenopausal patients with pelvic masses: Discrimination of benign from malignant disease. 1988; 159:341–346.

PHYSICIANS' RESPONSE

GEORGE A. OMURA
RONALD D. ALVAREZ

Further evaluation is clearly indicated in this case. Assuming that the repeat history and physical examination is as previously described, the CA-125 should be repeated. We will assume that the repeat value is similar. Such an elevation is nondiagnostic but very suggestive of ovarian cancer in a postmenopausal woman. False-positive elevations can occur with several conditions, including pancreatitis, liver disease, and other cancers such as breast, lung, pancreatic, and colon cancers. Diverticulitis is a possible cause. Additional tumor markers could be checked but are not likely to resolve the problem.

The anemia should be characterized. If it is hypochromic and microcytic and the patient's iron saturation is very low, gastrointestinal blood loss, perhaps from the patient's ulcer or diverticulosis, is a likely cause. Bowel cancer is possible. If the anemia is normocytic and her reticulocyte count is normal or low, the anemia of chronic disease is probable. Several types of cancer have been associated with this type of anemia, which does not, however, imply marrow invasion. In contrast, myelocytes and/or nucleated red cells on the peripheral blood smear might be a clue to marrow involvement, albeit ovarian and gastrointestinal tract cancers seldom grow in the marrow.

A chest x-ray will probably be normal but conceivably could yield a surprise such as a lung cancer, pleural effusion, or metastatic deposits; we assume that it will be unremarkable.

The serum amylase should be checked; we assume that it will be normal.

The colon should be evaluated for evidence of inflammatory disease or colon cancer, at least with a barium enema and sigmoidoscopy, and the stool checked for occult blood. Assuming that these studies are not helpful, computed tomography (CT) of the abdomen and pelvis should be done.

If the scan shows a small adnexal mass with no evidence of ascites or carcinomatosis and no pancreatic or liver lesions, and provided that the colon workup is normal, laparoscopy could be used for diagnosis. If ovarian cancer is confirmed or if there are more hints of advanced-stage cancer, a laparotomy should be done instead. If ovarian carcinoma is confirmed at frozen section, peritoneal washings, a hysterectomy, bilateral salpingo-oophorectomy, omentectomy, inspection of the entire peritoneal cavity, and, if possible, resection of all remaining gross disease should be carried out. If there is no obvious residual disease, multiple peritoneal biopsies, biopsy, or scraping of the right diaphragm and pelvic and periaortic node sampling should be done to complete the staging.

Assuming that ovarian carcinoma (not a borderline tumor) is confirmed, we would then offer protocol therapy appropriate to the stage and histological grade. In the absence of a protocol, if the patient had, for example, Stage IIIA ovarian carcinoma, six courses of cisplatin and paclitaxel (75 mg/m^2 and 135 mg/m^2 respectively every 3 weeks) should be considered.

If the abdominal CT and other noninvasive studies noted above were unrevealing, mammograms should be done, but they would probably be negative. A chest CT might reveal a small, potentially resectable lung cancer. If the problem is actually extraovarian peritoneal carcinomatosis or a very small ovarian carcinoma, 1 or 2 months of observation would not be unreasonable, but the patient will most likely come to laparoscopy in the near future, especially is she continues to be symptomatic and/or the CA-125 rises further. In the meantime, her diverticular disease could be treated with a high-fiber diet, stool softener, and so on for the remote possibility that the diverticulosis is responsible for her findings; in that case, we would expect the CA-125 to decline.

PHYSICIAN'S RESPONSE

BARRIE ANDERSON

This presumably postmenopausal woman has nonspecific intermittent lower abdominal symptoms of several months duration. Her past history of diverticulosis and peptic ulcer disease treatment mandate concern for intestinal dysfunction, including diverticulitis and "irritable bowel." Cystitis, either bacterial or inflammatory, secondary to estrogen deprivation, must also be considered. The hemoglobin of 10.2 g/dL also leads one to think of chronic blood loss, which can be associated with chronic inflammatory conditions of the stomach and intestine or with malignancy of the stomach or particularly the right side of the colon. Such individuals may also report weight loss.

Consideration must also be given to malignancy arising and/or metastatic to the uterine adnexa. While tenderness is not typical of malignancy in this area, an enlarging mass bound by pelvic adhesions could become tender on pressure.

Although no mass is described, a small mass in this area may not be detectable in a moderately obese patient. Cancers that commonly metastasize to the adnexa include breast and bowel. Breast cancer can metastasize widely in the absence of a palpable mass in the breast or even with regression of the primary breast cancer.

The elevation of the CA-125 to 123 is a nonspecific but significant finding. While the CA-125 has been studied primarily in women with ovarian cancer, it can also be elevated in other cancers or in any condition in which there is inflammation of the peritoneum.

Recommendations for workup at this time would include a mammogram, transvaginal pelvic ultrasound, colonoscopy, and consideration of gastric endoscopy. Initial management for inflammatory conditions of the bowel should be instituted, with appropriate dietary and stool-softening measures. If all tests are negative and symptomatic improvement occurs, follow-up CA-125 can be taken to determine whether this has returned to normal. If any of the tests are positive, investigation should continue in the direction they indicate.

PHYSICIAN'S RESPONSE

BONNIE S. REICHMAN

A 61-year-old female presents with the complaint of intermittent lower abdominal discomfort and clinical findings of mild diffuse middle and lower abdominal tenderness to deep palpation without palpable adnexal mass and/or ascites, elevated CA-125, and mild anemia. In this postmenopausal woman, consideration of possible etiologies include gastrointestinal and gynecological sites. A detailed history regarding the nature of the abdominal pain, exacerbating or relieving factors, change in stool habits or stool, evidence for gastrointestinal blood loss, changes in weight and appetite, abdominal girth, nausea and/or vomiting, fever, urinary symptoms, and any vaginal complaints such as discharge or bleeding would aid in a more accurate determination of the underlying disease process. Objective signs of ovarian carcinoma are frequently nonspecific and may consist of vague abdominal complaints, pelvic mass, ascites, omental cake, pleural effusion, supraclavicular lymphadenopathy, and "doughy abdomen." Further evaluation should include a bimanual rectovaginal pelvic examination with testing for fecal occult blood, repeat CA-125, and CT scan of the abdomen and pelvis. Pelvic sonogram should be done if the CT scan of the abdomen and pelvis is unremarkable. Barium enema and/or colonoscopy should be done in patients in whom carcinomatosis is suspected in the absence of a pelvic mass to detect a primary gastrointestinal malignancy. If fecal occult blood is present, colonoscopy should be performed. Bilateral mammography would be helpful to rule out metastatic breast cancer. The differential diagnosis includes ovarian carcinoma, endometrial or fallopian tube cancers, colorectal carcinoma, metastatic carcinoma to gynecological organs and/or bowel, nonneoplastic gastrointestinal disorders including diverticulitis, diverticular abcess, pancreatitis, peritonitis, and so on.

The CA-125 is elevated in more than 80% of patients with epithelial ovarian cancer, but only 1% of apparently healthy women have elevated levels. This marker, detected in tissue, is derived from mullerian ducts and coelomic epithelium and neoplasms derived from these tissues. Thus, CA-125 may be elevated in adenocarcinoma of the fallopian tube, endometrium, and the cervix as well as several nongynecological malignancies, including carcinoma of the pancreas, lungs, breast, and colon. Typically, the highest CA-125 levels are seen in patients with epithelial ovarian cancer. Lower levels may be seen in patients with nongynecological malignancies or with early-stage gynecological cancer. In a postmenopausal patient with a CA-125 greater than 95 and a pelvic mass, the elevated CA-125 has a predictive value of ovarian carcinoma of 96%. This should prompt referral to individuals who can perform appropriate staging laparotomy and cytoreduction. In this patient, the moderately elevated CA-125, in the absence of a pelvic mass and/or ascites does not clearly indicate an ovarian cancer. In addition, CA-125 may be elevated in nonmalignant gynecological and nongynecological conditions, such as endometriosis, pelvic inflammatory disease, adenomyosis, leiomyomas, pregnancy both normal and ectopic, menses, pancreatitis, cirrhosis, and peritonitis. In this postmenopausal patient, a thorough search to rule out carcinoma of the ovary is indicated, whereas if this were a premenopausal patient, endometriosis would be the leading diagnosis. Of note, a normal CA-125 level would not rule out the diagnosis of an ovarian or other gynecological malignancy. The CA-125 does not have sufficient specificity to be used as a general screening test for ovarian carcinoma. It may be useful in screening high-risk populations (i.e., hereditary ovarian cancer) when used in combination with other screening tools such as transvaginal pelvic sonography.

Further evaluation of this patient should include chest radiographs, bilateral mammography, and workup of anemia. A normal breast examination does not rule out breast cancer and an unremarkable pelvic examination does not rule out gynecological malignancy. All patients who are suspected of having ovarian cancer should have a thorough examination of the breasts and bilateral mammography, since the ovaries are a frequent site of breast cancer metastases. Patients with ovarian cancer are at increased risk for the development of breast cancer. This patient's age is her greatest risk factor for developing breast cancer, and it is not significantly increased by one first-degree relative with postmenopausal breast cancer.

23

Metastatic Carcinoma, Pelvic Mass with History of Colon Cancer

CASE

A 51-year-old woman underwent a rectosigmoid resection with low colorectal anastomosis secondary to a Duke's C adenocarcinoma of the colon 2 years ago. She has not been followed since her colon surgery. Her mother died recently of carcinoma of the ovary, and this prompted the patient to come in for a gynecological examination. On examination there was a 3- to 4-cm nodular pelvic mass fixed to the vaginal apex in the middle of the cul-de-sac. The level of carcinoembryonic antigen was 2.5 and abdominal pelvic computed tomography (CT) showed a suggestion of a perihepatic nodule. The patient had no bowel or bladder symptoms, no change in her appetite, no weight loss.

PHYSICIAN'S RESPONSE

J. YON

This 51-year-old woman has not been followed since her surgery for a Duke's C carcinoma of the colon 2 years prior to this consult. Her mother recently died of ovarian cancer. One again, given the fact that the patient is 51 and that the survival of patients who ultimately die of ovarian cancer is less than 5 years, one could assume that her mother was over 50 when she was diagnosed; therefore, I think we can exclude the young, primary patient from the family history. We do not know very much about this patient's colon cancer (i.e., whether she was given adjunctive treatment). We also do not know anything about her gynecological history, but the protocol notes that there is a nodular pelvic mass at the vaginal apex, suggesting that the patient does not have a uterus. If the patient had a hysterectomy in the past, it would be of significant to know whether her ovaries had been removed.

Be that as it may, her CEA is 2.5, which is within the range of normal. An abdominal pelvic CT scan suggests a perihepatic mass and the patient is asymptomatic. In her examination, this patient needs to have her chest evaluated, and this might be done with a plain film or possibly even a chest CT. If that is negative for metastatic disease, then one could consider fine needle aspiration of the mass at the apex of the vagina, although it is quite likely that this would show only adenocarcinoma and it would not tell us its origin. The CA-125 level would probably not be helpful. Therefore, once the above tests had been done, one should prepare the patient for laparotomy. At the time of laparotomy, the pelvic mass can be excised. If it is colon cancer, excision of isolated pelvic metastases can confer a significant disease-free survival. The same can be said for the perihepatic nodule if it is the only area involved. If the patient has other evidence of carcinomatosis from colon cancer, then her prognosis, unfortunately, is grim.

If the patient should prove to have ovarian cancer, then a straightforward, aggressive debulking operation should be performed for that disease and she should then be treated with currently recommended cytotoxic chemotherapy for front-line therapy in advanced ovarian cancer.

A question might be raised regarding the role of laparoscopy in this patient which might allow a diagnosis to be made, with better histology than a transvaginal needle biopsy, but unless the patient proved to have extensive carcinomatosis that was felt to be unresectable, she might well need a laparotomy anyway. However, one could consider a laparoscopy with a laparotomy at the same sitting if carcinomatosis was not found.

PHYSICIAN'S RESPONSE

JOHN MIKUTA

The history does not state whether the patient is menopausal or whether she still has her uterus. The finding of the pelvic mass in a patient with a prior adenocarcinoma of the colon would make one suspicious of a metastatic lesion to the ovary (Krukenberg tumor). I would advise the patient to have the following evaluations: A chest x-ray or chest CT, colonoscopy, CA-125, and better definition of the perihepatic nodule including needle biopsy. If no further problems can be defined in the colon and if the perihepatic nodule is found to be benign or some other lesion, then the patient definitely should have an exploratory laparotomy, preferably through a standard incision, to deal with the lesion in the pelvis and the area around the liver and to provide for a thorough exploration of both intraperitoneal and extraperitoneal areas, with tumor debulking and biopsies as indicated.

If the lesion is a primary carcinoma of the ovary on frozen section, a staging procedure should be carried out, removing the uterus and both tubes and ovaries if they are still present and carrying out omentectomy with multiple peritoneal biopsies, pelvic washings, and lymph node sampling of the pelvic, common iliac, and paraaortic nodes. If the lesion is a carcinoma of the colon metastatic to the ovary or to other portions of the abdominal cavity, then appropriate debulking should also be carried out. In both instances, the decisions for postoperative chemotherapy or radiation would have to be made based on the location, extent, and type of disease.

If this patient is fortunate enough to have benign lesion, her management would be based on her menarchal status and her desire to preserve her pelvic organs. I would be inclined to counsel her that in view of her own colon cancer history and her mother's ovarian cancer history, her risks of developing endometrial and breast cancer are elevated; therefore, I think removal of any residual pelvic organs is advisable.

PHYSICIAN'S RESPONSE

A. ROBERT KAGAN

Although, in the past, removal of the ovaries was "automatic" in patients who underwent either an abdominal perineal or low anterior resection, presently there is no uniform agreement among gynecological oncologists or general surgeons as to whether to take or leave the ovaries in patients. A list of the major differential diagnoses for this patient are as follows:

1. "Anastomotic" recurrence of the colorectal cancer.
2. Metastatic colonic cancer to the ovary.
3. Cancer of the ovary.
4. The hepatic nodule may represent a metastasis from cancer of the ovary or the colorectum.

The workup should include sigmoidoscopy to look for a local recurrence, chest roentgenogram, liver function tests, and CT, especially for the presence of ascites. An attempt should be made to document the malignancy of the hepatic nodule, perhaps by endoscopy, if the nodule is equal to or larger than 1.5 to 2 cm. It is important to find the etiology of this hepatic nodule. Approximately 15% of patients can be saved if colonic cancer is metastatic to the anastomotic site, but the outcome is zero if the colon cancer is found metastatic to the ovaries. The

CEA is often normal with only a local recurrence. A fine needle aspiration specimen may be too small to settle the diagnostic issues.

I would prefer not to irradiate a pelvis that has been resected, since fixed loops of bowel are invariably present. The possibility that the hepatic nodule may be a false-positive finding for colonic metastasis may suggest that this patient has a new ovarian primary, not a colonic metastasis to the ovary. Exploratory laparotomy may be the only way to sort this out. Importantly, some patients with stage I, II, and IIIA ovarian cancer may be cured by surgery, and it would be a shame to assume this patient had intraabdominal metastasis from cancer of the colon when she indeed had a curable cancer of the ovary. The satisfactory diagnosis *and* management of similar patients in my experience occur only *after* an open operative procedure.

PHYSICIAN'S RESPONSE

KENNETH D. WEBSTER

It is unfortunate that this patient was not followed more closely after surgery for her colon cancer. Patients are usually seen at 3-month intervals for 2 years, at 6-month intervals for 3 years, and annually thereafter.

It would be informative to know if there was lymph node involvement in the original resection. We must assume that the ovaries appeared normal at the time of bowel resection 2 years earlier but the ovaries should be removed in all perimenopausal and postmenopausal patients with bowel cancer to prevent subsequent ovarian cancer and remove occult ovarian metastases.

The CEA levels are useful in monitoring postoperative patients whose serum CEA level was elevated preoperatively, but this information is also not available. In Duke's stage C carcinoma of the colon, the 5-year survival is about 40%, and about 85% of all recurrences are evident within 3-years after primary surgery. Therefore the palpable pelvic mass suggests recurrent colon cancer.

A histological diagnosis of the pelvic tumor could be made by transvaginal needle biopsy, but I recommend that the patient be explored and the surgeon be prepared to resect recurrent disease both in the pelvis and elsewhere. A CT of the chest and colonoscopy should be included in the preoperative evaluation.

PHYSICIAN'S RESPONSE

MARK D. ADELSON

This is a patient with a prior adenocarcinoma and a newly diagnosed pelvic mass; is it a recurrence or a new a primary ovarian cancer? Did the patient have her ovaries/tubes/uterus removed at the time of the colon surgery? In the absence of personal, reproductive, or family risk factors for cancer, I recommend prophylactic removal of the ovaries to avoid ovarian cancer for patients with colon cancer who are 40 years of age or older. The incidence of metastasis to the ovaries with colon cancer otherwise thought to be resectable for cure is 8% in postmenopausal women and 20% in premenopausal women. This strengthens the argument to remove the ovaries routinely for patients being treated for colon cancer who have completed their childbearing. A patient with colon cancer has a higher relative risk for adenocarcinomas of the breast, ovary, and endometrium. This patient has an increased risk for cancer of the ovary because of her cancer and because of her mother's cancer. The level of that risk would depend on the age at diagnosis and histology of her mother's disease. If there are any other adenocarcinomas in the family, this further increases the risk. If the patient has any other reproductive risks, such as no prior pregnancies and never having taken birth control pills, then that would also increase her risk. A Duke's C adenocarcinoma of the colon is accompanied by a survival of 30% (> 4 nodes positive) to 60% (1 to 4 positive), so this patient could have recurrent colon cancer. Was a CEA or CA-19-9 obtained prior to the colon surgery? If either of these were elevated, I would expect that they would be elevated again with recurrence. If they were negative before, negative values now would not rule out recurrence. The CA-125 would also be helpful, since it is elevated in 64% of primary ovarian cancers and should be normal with nonmetastatic mucinous colon carcinoma. The presence of ovarian or peritoneal metastasis could elevate the CA-125 in the absence of a primary cancer of the ovary. The patient should have a pelvic sonogram, since it is more sensitive than a CT scan in identifying the location and characteristics of the ovaries. One could then determine whether the ovaries, if still present, appear normal and whether this tumor was separate from the ovaries.

Is her health good? Is she obese? Does she have diabetes, heart disease, or hypertension, which might increase the risk of surgery? If this mass is palpable vaginally, then a needle aspiration or core biopsy could be done to compare the histology with that from the colon cancer. If the histology is identical, then it would be unlikely for this to be a primary ovarian cancer. Since cytoreduction does not generally play a role in colon cancer treatment, one could spare this patient further surgery.

If these examinations do not document malignancy or reveal the presence of malignancy without determination of the primary site, then the patient should have operative laparoscopy. At laparoscopy I would evaluate the abdomino-peritoneal contents and determine the status of her ovaries. I could resect the pelvic nodule and inspect the hepatic lesion, depending on its location. If I could determine that this was not primary ovarian (or peritoneal) cancer, her surgery could end at this point. An endometrial biopsy/dilation and curettage (D&C)

should be done to rule out an endometrial primary (less likely). If this seemed to be a primary ovarian cancer, it could be resected with or without use of the CUSA Lap (the laparoscopic extension to the Cavitron) (1). If the patient had extensive or retroperitoneal disease, exploratory laparotomy to complete her staging and tumor reduction might be required.

Reference

1. Adelson MD. Cytoreduction of diaphragmatic metastases using Cavitron Ultrasonic Surgical Aspirator. Gynecol Oncol 1991; 41:220–222.

24

Metastatic Carcinoma

CASE

For the past 3 months a 52-year-old woman has had a chief complaint of back pain and "heartburn." She says that this discomfort has affected her appetite and she has gone from approximately 150 to 130 lb in those 3 months. She relates that she feels quite tired all the time but has no other symptoms. Bowel and bladder function, she says, are normal. The patient works as a secretary at a university. Physical exam shows no palpable supraclavicular nodes. The chest is clear. No abdominal masses are noted. There is no abdominal swelling. No suspicious inguinal nodes are palpable. No vulvar or vaginal lesions are present. The cervix is smooth and without lesions. On bimanual vaginal and rectovaginal examination, one can feel bilateral 6-cm pelvic masses. The cul-de-sac is without nodularity. Stool is trace-positive on test for occult blood. Laboratory: hemoglobin 10.6; electrolytes, liver, and renal function tests within normal limits. CA-125 is 250. Chest x-ray is normal.

PHYSICIANS' RESPONSE

GINI FLEMING
STEVEN WAGGONER

The presenting symptoms of ovarian carcinoma are vague and nonspecific. There are, however, a number of features in this patient's history that raise the question of whether she has a nonovarian cancer which has metastasized to the ovaries. A decision must be made as to what testing for another primary source should be performed and under what circumstances a laparotomy would not be indicated.

186

As many as 10% of patients undergoing surgery for presumed ovarian malignancy have been reported to have an extragenital primary cancer, usually in the breast or gastrointestinal tract. Metastatic ovarian tumors are frequently bilateral. An elevated CA-125 is, unfortunately, not at all specific for ovarian cancer; a variety of malignancies will present with elevated CA-125 levels, particularly pancreatic and hepatocellular cancers. This woman's striking weight loss and complaint of back pain in the absence of bowel dysfunction or evidence of abdominal carcinomatosis on physical exam are certainly consistent with a pancreatic tumor. In addition, although colonoscopy or barium enema are not part of our routine preoperative evaluation of women with ovarian cancer, a colon exam *is* indicated for a postmenopausal woman with a heme-positive stool.

This woman should have a computed tomography (CT) scan of her abdomen and pelvis and a barium enema or colonoscopy. If these studies fail to explain this patient's heme-positive stool and other symptoms, we would perform an upper GI endoscopy. If there appears to be an obvious pancreatic or gallbladder primary tumor, we would attempt to obtain tissue by the least invasive means, possibly through CT-guided needle aspiration. This patient's pelvic masses are not causing her any symptoms, and we would not operate just to remove them. However, if a colonic primary tumor is found and there appears to be no other evidence of carcinomatosis or metastatic disease, bilateral salpingo-oophorectomy at the time of resection of the colonic tumor should be considered. Resection of isolated ovarian metastases from colon cancer may, like resection of isolated liver metastases, yield prolonged survival (although a unilateral ovarian metastasis has a better prognosis than bilateral ovarian metastases).

If significant doubt about the source of the primary tumor remains after the diagnostic studies mentioned above (for example, if a possible pancreatic mass plus other intraabdominal disease is suggested on CT scan), we would proceed with a formal exploratory laparotomy; ovarian cancer is the only curable tumor this woman is likely to have, and she should be treated as having a primary ovarian cancer unless the contrary is proven. The same principle applies when the source of tumor remains in doubt after surgery, if, for example, histological examination reveals a poorly differentiated carcinoma that may have arisen from either the pancreas or the ovary. We would treat such a patient with a platinum-based chemotherapy regimen while monitoring her response carefully.

References

Brooks SE. Preoperative evaluation of patients with suspected ovarian cancer. Gynecol Oncol 1994; 55:S80–S90.

Mazur MT, Hsueh S, Gersell DJ. Metastases to the female genital tract: Analysis of 325 cases. Cancer 1984; 53:1978–1984.

PHYSICIAN'S RESPONSE

JOHN MALFETANO

This 52-year-old woman presents with anemia, weight loss, vague gastrointestinal (GI) symptoms of heartburn, bilateral adnexal masses, stools positive for blood, and an elevated CA-125. The immediate concern is of a malignancy, most likely of ovarian or gastrointestinal origin. The patient should undergo a diagnostic workup to include a GI evaluation with a barium enema followed by an upper GI series and small bowel follow-through to evaluate the heme positive stools and heartburn. Subsequently, she should be placed on a mechanical bowel prep in anticipation of surgery.

Unfortunately, it is infrequent that the exact nature of pelvic masses found in this way is known definitively before surgery. If the GI examinations show a primary GI carcinoma, then ovarian metastasis is certainly a possibility (Krukenberg tumor). If the evaluation is negative, then primary ovarian carcinoma should be a concern. In a 10-year retrospective review of 861 women of all ages with a postoperative diagnosis of ovarian neoplasm independent of size by Koonings et al. (1), teratomas were the number one ovarian neoplasm seen in 44% of the cases. The overall risk of the ovarian neoplasm being malignant was only 13% in premenopausal women but rose drastically to 45% in postmenopausal women. The elevated CA-125 is of particular concern, since an elevated CA-125 in women over the age of 50 is associated with malignancy in 80% of these cases.

Preoperatively, the patient and her family should be informed of the possible diagnosis and that she will undergo exploration with total abdominal hysterectomy and bilateral salpingo-oophorectomy. At surgery, a thorough exploration of the abdominal cavity will be performed with peritoneal washings. The total abdominal hysterectomy and bilateral salpingo-oophorectomy will be done with frozen section as needed. If the ovarian neoplasms are benign, the procedure will be terminated. However, if an ovarian malignancy is diagnosed, surgical staging and tumor-reductive surgery will be performed. In the case of a metastatic lesion to the ovaries diagnosed by frozen section, the large intestine is the most common site of metastasis in 40 to 50% of patients. Intraoperative general surgical consultation will be available if necessary. Postoperative management will be determined by the surgical and pathological information obtained.

Reference

1. Koonings PP, Campbell K, Mishell DR, Grimes DA. Relative frequency of primary ovarian neoplasms: A 10-year review. Obstet Gynecol 1981; 74:921–926.

PHYSICIAN'S RESPONSE

PETER ROSE

This patient has significant weight loss (13% of her weight), guaiac-positive stools, a pelvic mass, and an elevated CA-125. In view of these findings, it is essential to exclude a metastatic tumor to the ovary. Metastatic tumors make up 6 to 8% of malignant ovarian tumors, with the most common primary sites being the colon, breast, stomach, and pancreas. The patient's national heritage would be important, since stomach cancer is the most common origin of metastatic ovarian tumors for Oriental patients, while colon and breast cancer are the most common primary sites in the United States and western Europe. Yazigi et al. recently reported 29 patients with metastatic ovarian tumors (1). The most common symptom was abdominal pain. Interestingly, as in this patient, 63% of patients with a gastrointestinal primary cancer had normal bowel function. Primary tumor sites included the colon (52%), breast (17%), pancreas (10%), stomach (1%), appendix (3%), and lung (3%). The patient's symptoms of heartburn and back pain are suggestive of an upper abdominal primary. She should undergo an abdominal CT scan with 5-mm cuts of the pancreas; if this study is negative, gastroscopy should come next. If both of these studies are negative, colonoscopy should follow. If all of these studies are negative, a careful surgical history should be obtained, specifically with respect to a prior history of appendectomy. Although they are uncommon, appendiceal tumors frequently metastasize to the ovaries. Further consideration of an ovarian primary should be given, since the patient's symptoms do not exclude the possibility of an ovarian cancer with nodal and abdominal metastases. Further nutritional evaluation will be necessary before abdominal exploration. A serum albumin should be obtained. If the serum albumin is below 2.5 mg/dL and the patient has a weight loss of more than 10%, the operative morbidity is increased. In this case preoperative parenteral nutrition should be given for 7 to 10 days (2). Intraoperatively, following an adequate incision, a careful exploration of the abdominal organs including the pancreas needs to be performed. If the frozen section is nondiagnostic for a primary ovarian cancer or suggests a metastatic ovarian tumor and the primary tumor site is not evident, an appendectomy should be performed, since cases of appendiceal cancer have been missed with a normal-appearing appendix.

References

1. Yazigi R, Sandstad J. Ovarian involvement in extragenital cancer. Gynecol Oncol 1989; 34:84–87.
2. Baker JP, Detsky AS, Wesson DE. Nutritional assessment: A comparison of clinical judgement and objective measurements. N Engl J Med 1982; 306:969.

PHYSICIAN'S RESPONSE

LEO LAGASSE

Since the data presented suggest the possibility of an ovarian cancer, surgical exploration is required. Differential diagnosis includes benign ovarian tumors, tumor of low malignant potential, epithelial ovarian cancer, or possibly cancer from another site metastatic to the ovary. Preoperatively, a CT scan of abdomen and pelvis is often obtained and may be helpful, but accurate staging requires intraoperative evaluation. Posteroanterior and lateral chest x-rays and complete bowel preparation are carried out prior to surgery. The goal of the operation is complete removal of all visible tumor. All available studies show that patients with minimal residual tumor at the beginning of chemotherapy have longer median survival than those with large residual. Nevertheless, controversy remains in the minds of some surgeons regarding the value of cytoreductive surgery. Until clear evidence to the contrary is present, gynecological oncologists should employ all reasonable surgical means to remove or destroy all visible tumor.

All patients have a midline vertical incision extending above the umbilicus. Abdominal contents are evaluated initially and an estimate of tumor burden made. It is helpful to recall that there are five areas in the abdomen requiring surgical attention: (a) pelvis, (b) intestine, (c) lymph nodes, (d) omentum–gastrosplenic ligament, and (e) diaphragm. After examining these five areas, the surgeon should attempt to anticipate which surgical maneuvers will be required to achieve minimal residual disease status. It is usually best to direct surgery to the most difficult area first, and often this is the upper abdomen. After assessment, disease in each of these areas can be managed by resection or destruction by electrocautery or by the Argon Bem Coagulator (ABC). The Cavitron UltraSonic Aspirator (CUSA) can assist in the resection of tumors otherwise nonresectable and is especially useful when combined with the ABC, which can destroy any tumor remaining after use of the CUSA and stop any bleeding at the base of the tumor.

Operative procedures required in all patients with ovarian cancer include cytologic peritoneal washings, salpingo-oophorectomy, omentectomy, and appendectomy. For apparent early-stage disease, bilateral pelvic and paraaortic lymphadenectomy, multiple random peritoneal biopsies should be added. In late-stage disease, the procedure should include excision of all possible tumor masses and involved cul-de-sac peritoneum. Routine dissection of lymph nodes in late-stage patients is controversial unless nodes are grossly enlarged. Though intestinal resection has been as controversial, the procedure is valuable if the result leaves the patient with optimal disease status or prevents obstruction. The most common intestinal segments requiring removal are the rectosigmoid and distal ileum. Though there are still patients referred to gynecological oncologist who have been managed with only exploratory laparotomy, tumor biopsy, and colostomy, studies confirm that the experienced surgical team can achieve optimal status in more than 70% of these same patients, with only about 6% requiring colostomy.

Since recurrence on the diaphragm is so common, greater effort is needed to surgically eradicate tumor implants that are commonly found there and at the junction of the liver and diaphragm. Operations involving the diaphragm are facilitated by the simple technique of dividing the falciform ligament and ligamentum teres for liver mobilization. Lesions can then be cauterized or resected or the peritoneum of the diaphragm can be peeled off if heavily studded with tumor.

Significant postoperative morbidity in those undergoing extensive cytoreduction with complete tumor removal is seen in one-quarter to one-third of patients and is usually manageable. Mortality in this group is about 3 to 5% but was paradoxically higher in patients left with larger postoperative tumor residual (1). Cytoreductive surgery requires an experienced, committed surgical team and an appropriately equipped operating room. The importance of this initial surgical effort needs continued and further emphasis even among gynecological oncologists.

Reference

1. Heintz APM, et al. Obstet Gynecol 1986; 67:783–788.

PHYSICIAN'S RESPONSE

JAVIER MAGRINA

The outstanding findings on this patient are weight loss (1.6 lb/week over the past 3 months), anemia, bilateral pelvic masses, positive test for occult blood, increased CA-125, back pain, and heartburn.

The presence of anemia and positive guiac test should always suggest GI malignancy or ovarian carcinoma with GI involvement. Because of the anemia, trace positive occult blood, heartburn, decreased appetite, weight loss, and bilateral pelvic masses, the most likely diagnosis is gastric carcinoma with ovarian metastases. Other diagnostic considerations are colon carcinoma with ovarian metastases or primary ovarian carcinoma with colon involvement.

Preoperatively, I would request an endoscopic evaluation of the upper GI tract. This will pick up approximately 99% of gastric carcinomas. If this is negative, I would request radiological evaluation of the upper GI tract. If both are negative, a colonoscopy would be indicated to rule out colon cancer or colon involvement by ovarian carcinoma. Additionally, I would request a complete blood count, chemistry group, urinalysis, and serum CEA levels.

The management will depend on the findings of the above examinations. If a gastric carcinoma is found, surgical exploration with resection should be considered concomitantly with resection of the ovarian metastases. A similar approach would be undertaken should this be a primary colon cancer with ovarian metastases or an ovarian cancer with colon involvement.

If the preoperative endoscopic evaluations of the upper gastrointestinal tract and colon are negative, surgical exploration with resection of the bilateral pelvic masses, frozen section, staging, and/or debulking would then be indicated.

25

Primary Peritoneal Mesothelioma

CASE

A 47-year-old woman presents with abdominal bloating of 2 months' duration. On physical examination, she is found to have ascites but no definite intraabdominal masses. Pelvic examination fails to reveal any specific abnormal findings. On laparoscopic evaluation, the patient is found to have a thin sheath of tumor on the peritoneal lining, with a large omental tumorous cake. A biopsy is taken, which reveals primary peritoneal mesothelioma.

PHYSICIANS' RESPONSE

GUNTER DEPPE
VINAY MALVIYA

Recommendation

This 47-year-old woman should undergo a laparotomy with an attempt to remove large omental tumorous cake. Newer surgical techniques—including the ultrasonic surgical aspirator, the argon beam coagulator, and surgical lasers—may facilitate this cytoreductive procedure with acceptable morbidity. If only minimal tumor remains following the surgical debulking, the patient should receive cisplatin-based intraperitoneal chemotherapy. If surgical debulking cannot be accomplished, the patient should be treated with systemic combination chemotherapy consisting of cisplatin and doxorubicin.

Discussion

The diagnosis of primary malignant peritoneal mesothelioma is difficult because it is a rare disorder with an annual incidence of only 2.2 cases per million in the United States. The common presenting symptoms are nonspecific abdominal pain, weight loss, and abdominal distention. Examination reveals ascites in 90% and an abdominal mass in 16% of the patients. The epidemiology has shown a male predominance. In the majority of patients there is a history of exposure of the patient or close relatives to asbestos, or the patient has lived in close proximity to areas of intense asbestos usage. The diagnosis may be confirmed with histochemical (negative periodic acid–Schiff staining, presence of a colloidal iron-positive substance removed after hyaluronidase and sialic acid digestion) and immunohistochemical methods (weak staining for carcinoembryonic antigen and positive staining for cytokeratin and vimentin). High serum levels of CA-125 and tumor tissue immunohistochemically positive for CA-125 have been reported in some patients.

The mean reported survival for patients with malignant peritoneal mesothelioma is less than 12 months. Surgery, chemotherapy, and radiation therapy alone or in combination have been described in the literature. The role of surgery is often limited due to the advanced stage of the disease, which does not permit curative resection or optimal debulking. Thus, in most instances, only palliative procedures bypassing obstructing lesions can be performed.

Radiation therapy has usually been administered in combination with in-

Table 1 Intraperitoneal Chemotherapy Alone or Combined with Other Modalities for Malignant Peritoneal Mesothelioma

Drug	No. of Patients	Combined	Response
Cisplatin	22	—	11
Cisplatin Doxorubicin	2	—	1
Cisplatin Doxorubicin	3	Radiotherapy	3
Cisplatin Doxorubicin	3	Radiotherapy Surgery	3
Cisplatin Doxorubicin	2	Radiotherapy Surgery Systemic chemotherapy	2
Cisplatin Doxorubicin	9	Radiotherapy	7

Source: Adapted from Ref. 2.

traperitoneal instillation of various agents [radioactive phosphorus (P_{32}), gold, chemotherapeutic drugs] or together with systemic chemotherapy. Occasionally patients have survived more than 10 years.

Multiple chemotherapeutic regimens have been described; they have had limited success. A few long-term survivors have been reported (1). Doxorubicin alone or in combination with other agents appears to be moderately effective. Intraperitoneal cisplatin has been administered alone or in combination with mitomycin-C or doxorubicin. Several patients have been treated with intraperitoneal chemotherapy combined with other treatment modalities (surgery, radiation, and systemic chemotherapy). A combined response rate of 50% has been reported in a total of 70 patients. The data were collected from retrospective studies and isolated case reports. Cisplatin-based intraperitoneal chemotherapy appears to be the best available treatment for malignant peritoneal mesothelioma at present (2).

References

1. Asensio JA, Goldblatt P, Thomford NR. Primary malignant peritoneal mesothelioma. Arch Surg 1990; 125:1477–1481.
2. Vlasveld LT, Gallee MPW, Rodenhuis S, Taal BG. Intraperitoneal chemotherapy for malignant peritoneal mesothelioma. Eur J Cancer 1991; 27:732–734.

PHYSICIANS' RESPONSE

ELLEN M. HARTENBACH
LINDA F. CARSON

Proliferations of the pelvic and peritoneal mesothelial cells lacking mullerian differentiation include cystic mesothelioma, well-differentiated papillary mesothelioma, and diffuse malignant mesothelioma. Cystic mesotheliomas are benign multiloculated inclusion cysts associated with prior surgery, endometriosis, or pelvic inflammatory disease. Well-differentiated papillary mesotheliomas are rare tumors that are characterized by a benign clinical course and have been associated with prolonged survival despite bulky disease. Diffuse malignant mesothelioma is the most common type of mesothelioma and is associated with a diffuse growth pattern located in the pleural or peritoneal cavity. Malignant mesotheliomas occur in both sexes and are epidemiologically associated with asbestos exposure.

Malignant mesotheliomas are classically biphasic tumors with both epithelioid and sarcomatoid foci. Epithelioid tumors can be confused with epithelial adenocarcinoma of the ovary or carcinoma arising from mullerian duct remnants involving the peritoneum. In women, malignant peritoneal mesotheliomas are uncommon; the majority of malignant papillary tumors arising from the peritoneum are examples of extraovarian serous adenocarcinomas.

In the case described here, the clinical course and findings at laparoscopy are consistent with the diagnosis of malignant peritoneal mesothelioma. However, definitive diagnosis requires adequate tissue sampling for immunohistochemical staining and electron microscopy. A laparotomy with hysterectomy, bilateral salpingo-oophorectomy, omentectomy, and tumor debulking is recommended. Laparotomy will both provide additional specimen for definitive diagnosis and the opportunity for cytoreductive surgery. Outside pathological review is also recommended if any uncertainty exists. Extraovarian serous adenocarcinomas are managed in a similar fashion to primary epithelial ovarian adenocarcinomas, where optimal surgical debulking improves survival. Minimal information on aggressive surgical approaches to malignant peritoneal mesotheliomas is available. Antman et al. (1) reported significantly better survival in a small group of patients treated after aggressive surgical debulking with a combination of intraperitoneal cisplatin and doxorubicin (Adriamycin) and whole abdominal radiotherapy (WAR) when compared with surgically inoperable cases treated with chemotherapy. In addition, aggressive surgical management of pleural mesotheliomas with extrapleural pneumonectomy has been show to improve survival.

Assuming the definitive diagnosis in this case is malignant peritoneal mesothelioma, adjuvant therapy is recommended for this highly aggressive malignancy. An attempt to enroll this patient in a cooperative group trial should be made. Cancer and Leukemia Group B (CALGB) began a mesothelioma program in 1984. Outside of a trial setting, if optimal cytoreduction is achieved, then a combination of intravenous or intraperitoneal cisplatin and Adriamycin with WAR is recommended. If bulky residual disease remains, intravenous chemotherapy would be recommended. Minimal information and few randomized trials are available to support a given treatment regimen. Radiation therapy appears to be active against mesothelioma, with a few reported survivors. However, it has not been carefully studied and its role remains unclear. Results of chemotherapy trials for patients with pleural or peritoneal malignant mesotheliomas have also been disappointing, with overall response rates of 11% (2). Phase II trials have demonstrated responses to agents including cisplatin, mitomycin, adriamycin, carboplatin, and ifosfamide. Current interest is focused on the identification of more efficacious chemotherapy agents and exploring the use of combined-modality approaches with radiotherapy and intravenous or intraperitoneal chemotherapy.

References

1. Antman KH, Osteen RT, Klegar KL, et al. Early peritoneal mesothelioma: A treatable malignancy. Lancet 1985; 2:977–982.
2. Vogelzang NJ. Malignant mesothelioma: Diagnostic and management strategies for 1992. Semin Oncol 1992; 19:64–71.

PHYSICIANS' RESPONSE

JOHN L. LOVECCHIO
DAVID GAL
ANN ANDERSON

This 47-year-old woman who presented with a 2-month history of abdominal bloating is now status post–diagnostic laparoscopy with peritoneal biopsy. Operative findings revealed diffuse miliary intraabdominal nodules as well as an omentum completely replaced by tumor. Examination of the biopsy revealed a primary malignant peritoneal mesothelioma. A consultation is requested regarding further diagnostic and therapeutic disposition.

This clinical manifestation is rather typical of peritoneal mesothelioma, advanced carcinoma of the ovary, and primary peritoneal carcinoma. The findings of abdominal bloating secondary to intraabdominal ascites and of scattered nodular masses involving both visceral and parietal peritoneal surfaces are common to each. These diseases usually remain confined to the abdominal cavity for extended intervals of time and metastasis to distant sites is uncommon. Death is usually attributed to complications arising from inanition and cachexia.

Given these clinical similarities, it is vitally important to distinguish between each entity on the basis of additional criteria. It is accepted that the microscopic pattern of malignant peritoneal mesothelioma is quite variable and that it may manifest histological features that can make it difficult to discriminate from a poorly differentiated carcinoma. The presence of mucopolysaccharides, positive immunocytochemical reactions for cytokeratins, and vimentin as well as demonstration of tonofilaments on electron microscopy will allow one to analytically distinguish malignant peritoneal mesotheioma from the others.

Historically, a diagnosis of malignant peritoneal mesothelioma is associated with a universally poor prognosis. Most patients will expire within 2 years of diagnosis from disease-related complications. Treatment protocols for this disorder are presently evolving and parallel to some degree those for ovarian cancer. Therapeutic trials have been conducted incorporating surgical cytoreduction, systemic cytotoxic and intraperitoneally administered chemotherapeutic agents, intraperitoneal radiocolloid therapy, and local external beam teletherapy, alone or in various combinations.

Recent literature appears to support an aggressive interdisciplinary approach to affect overall long-term prognosis (1). This consists of surgically debulking the disease to minimally macroscopic dimensions followed by intraperitoneal cytotoxic chemotherapy (2) and whole-abdominal radiation therapy using an open-field technique. Given these data, it would appear prudent to advocate that this patient be surgically explored with the intent to decrease the disease maximally though cytoreduction. Although without scientific basis, such an approach may offer this patient a reasonable chance at achieving a durable disease-free interval.

References

1. Lederman GS, Recht A, Herman T, et al. Long term survival in peritoneal mesothelioma: The role of radiotherapy and combined modality treatment. Cancer 1987; 59:1882–1886.
2. Pfeifle CE, Howell SB, Markman M. Intracavitary cisplatin chemotherapy for mesothelioma. Cancer Treat Rep 1985; 69:205–207.

26

Primary Peritoneal Carcinoma

CASE

A 66-year-old woman presents to her local internist with a chief complaint of weight loss and abdominal bloating of 5 months' duration. The internist thinks the patient has ovarian cancer and refers her to you. On pelvic exam, the ovaries do not appear to be enlarged, although you feel what appears to be a large omental cake and ascites. On laparotomy, the patient has ascites and bulky intraabdominal disease. Optimal cytoreduction can be performed. Intraoperative evaluation reveals the stomach, pancreas, and colon to be normal. Pathological review reveals poorly differentiated adenocarcinoma. There is involvement of the surface of the ovaries with tumor, but the pathologist is uncertain if the tumor originated in this organ.

PHYSICIAN'S RESPONSE

R.F. OZOLS

Intraabdominal carcinomatosis frequently results from the spread of epithelial ovarian cancer. However, peritoneal carcinomatosis which cannot easily be distinguished from other sites, most frequently epithelial ovarian, can result from metastatic disease from the gastrointestinal (GI) tract or breast cancer. In addition, peritoneal carcinomatosis may be the presenting manifestation of an adenocarcinoma of unknown primary. Furthermore, a distinct clinicopathologic syndrome of peritoneal carcinomatosis of müllerian origin has been described.

The first step in the management of this patient would be to carefully evaluate the histology. The classic primary peritoneal carcinoma developing in

199

the presence of normal ovaries or with ovaries only superficially involved has the microscopic appearance of a papillary serous cystadenocarcinoma. While there is some controversy regarding its natural history compared to that of ovarian serous papillary carcinoma, it does appear that the most important prognostic factors are the same as in epithelial ovarian cancer: namely, the volume of residual disease and the grade of the tumor. The treatment for such papillary serous cystadenocarcinomas of the ovary is identical to that for epithelial ovarian cancers and consists of cytoreductive surgery followed by combination chemotherapy. Consequently, I would strongly recommend the use of paclitaxel plus a platinum compound.

If the tumor appears to be a poorly differentiated adenocarcinoma without ovarian involvement, the tissue of origin becomes more difficult to establish. As noted, metastatic disease from the gastrointestinal tract is a strong possibility. The presence of mucin-containing adenocarcinoma cells would favor the possibility of a GI primary. Frequently patients with peritoneal carcinomatosis undergo a radiological and endoscopic evaluation of the GI tract to search for an occult primary. Most of the time these efforts are not successful in identifying any primary site. Serum carcinoembryonic antigen (CEA) and CA-125 levels are also frequently not helpful in establishing the site of disease, as both of these tumor markers can be elevated, one can be elevated, or neither can be significantly elevated.

Chemotherapy for adenocarcinoma of unknown origin is not as effective as for ovarian cancer. Because it is often impossible to be absolutely certain of the site of origin of peritoneal tumors, one can use the old standard of "treat what is treatable." If the tumor is of müllerian origin, the likelihood of a response to chemotherapy is substantial and can be associated with a prolonged remission. Consequently a course of paclitaxel plus a platinum compound should be administered.

In this particular case the patient underwent cytoreductive surgery and, from the extent of disease found at surgery, there is little doubt that microscopic disease was left behind. The pathologist is uncertain whether the tumor originated in the ovary. If the ovary had been involved, then the diagnosis of a poorly differentiated adenocarcinoma of the ovary would be established and be followed by chemotherapy with paclitaxel and platinum. Similar to the reasoning described above for a patient with poorly differentiated tumor of unknown origin, the possibility that this is a primary peritoneal tumor of müllerian origin would be the motivating factor for selecting paclitaxel plus a platinum-based regimen in this particular patient as well. I would not recommend further studies of the GI tract. I would obtain serum CEA and CA-125 primarily for their potential benefit in following a response to chemotherapy but not as an aid in establishing the diagnosis, and I would begin treatment with paclitaxel and a platinum-based compound. I would re-evaluate after two cycles, but determining response may be difficult. Most importantly, if the patient was established to have disease progression, then alternative treatment would be instituted. Consequently, a pretreatment computed tomography (CT) scan of the abdomen may provide background on which to assess whether there is disease progression after two cycles of treatment. If there is no clear-cut evidence of disease progression, I would continue with a full six cycles of paclitaxel plus a platinum-based compound. At that point, I would recommend follow-up until disease progression.

References

Fowler JM, Nieberg RK, Schooler TA, Berek JS. Peritoneal adenocarcinoma (serous) of müllerian type: A subgroup of women presenting with peritoneal carcinomatosis. Int J Gynecol Cancer 1994; 4:43–51.
Mulhollan TJ, Silva EG, Tornos C, et al. Ovarian involvement by serous surface papillary carcinoma. Int J Gynecol Pathol 1994; 13:120–126.

PHYSICIAN'S RESPONSE

RICHARD BARAKAT

This 66-year-old patient underwent an exploratory laparotomy for a presumed ovarian carcinoma. Optimal cytoreduction was accomplished. However, the final pathology revealed only surface involvement of the ovaries with the primary tumor site being uncertain.

Since multiple cancers can present in a manner similar to this, it is extremely important that a detailed search for the primary site be performed. Intraoperatively, the patient was noted to have a normal stomach, pancreas, and colon. Did the patient have a recent breast exam and mammogram performed, as breast cancer can also present in this manner? Other potential sites of origin include the gastrointestinal tract. A full evaluation of both the upper and lower digestive system is warranted, including an upper endoscopy and colonoscopy. A baseline abdominal/pelvic CT scan would also be useful to rule out any other possible primary sites. In addition, a CA-125 level should be obtained, as this, if elevated, may prove to be a useful tumor marker.

If a detailed survey for the primary tumor site does not reveal the origin of the patient's disease, one may be dealing with a primary papillary carcinoma of the peritoneal surface. Patients with this disease entity present in a manner that is very similar to classic ovarian cancer, with symptoms including abdominal pain/bloating, weight loss, and dyspepsia. These symptoms typically persist for several months before they prompt the patient to seek medical attention. Preoperative CA-125 levels are usually elevated.

At the time of surgical exploration, these patients will be found to have extensive carcinomatosis involving peritoneal and visceral surfaces as well as the omentum. The ovaries are usually small (< 4 cm) in diameter and are either free of tumor or will show serosal studding. There is some evidence that patients with a primary peritoneal adenocarcinoma may have a shorter disease-free survival than those with primary ovarian cancer, possibly due to a greater difficulty in achieving optimal cytoreduction (1). Overall survival, however, appears to be similar to that for classic epithelial ovarian cancer.

This patient was able to undergo optimal cytoreduction. At this point, she is a candidate for cytotoxic chemotherapy. Patients with primary peritoneal carcinoma are usually treated in a similar manner to patients with epithelial ovarian cancer. Standard therapy for this patient would therefore be considered to be combination intravenous chemotherapy with platinum and paclitaxel (Taxol). This is usually given for a total of five or six cycles. The level serum CA-125 tumor markers should be established prior to each cycle of chemotherapy to assess response.

At the end of her treatment course, if the patient is clinically free of disease based on physical examination, CT scan of the abdomen and pelvis, and CA-125 level, she may be a candidate for surgical reevaluation. The purpose of this procedure would be to document the presence of persistent disease and possibly place an intraperitoneal catheter. Patients such as this who have responded to front-line platinum-based chemotherapy and have small-volume (< 5 mm) disease at second-look surgery have a 30 to 40% chance of having a complete response to intraperitoneal chemotherapy.

Reference

1. Killackey MA, Davis AR. Papillary serous carcinoma of the peritoneal surface: Matched-case comparison with papillary serous ovarian carcinoma. Gynecol Oncol 1993; 51:171–174.

PHYSICIAN'S RESPONSE

EDDIE REED

True primary peritoneal carcinoma in a middle-aged woman is a diagnosis wherein treatment should be approached as if the patient carried the diagnosis of cancer of the ovary. However, establishing the diagnosis of primary peritoneal carcinoma should be approached with reasonable rigor. Ancillary tests that might assist include a chest x-ray, breast exam, CA-125, and CEA.

At surgery, the ovaries were not enlarged in this patient, although the surfaces of the ovaries were involved with tumor. A markedly elevated CA-125 (in excess of 1000 U, for example), would strongly suggest that the ovary may be the source of this tumor, although the size of the ovary is normal. If the CA-125 were normal but there was a markedly elevated CEA, this could suggest that a more thorough search for a bowel origin for this tumor might be in order. Whereas simple, readily available tests should be seriously considered if they would assist in evaluating the differential diagnosis, this consultant would not suggest a lengthy, costly search to rule out unlikely possibilities. Of major importance is an examination of the breasts, with the possible inclusion of mammography; and, of course, posteroanterior and lateral chest x-rays to rule out a lung mass. Lung cancer or breast cancer metastatic to the abdomen should be considered when the primary source of intraabdominal adenocarcinoma is not obvious. Endometrial carcinoma should also be considered, although this is unlikely as well.

Once the diagnosis of primary peritoneal carcinoma is made, treatment should be with either of three regimens: cisplatin-cyclophosphamide, carboplatin-cyclophosphamide, or cisplatin-paclitaxel. In women, primary peritoneal carcinoma is frequently responsive to this type of systemic chemotherapy. The prognosis is generally similar to that of cancer of the ovary of similar stage and grade. Second-look surgery should be considered after about six cycles of therapy, particularly if the findings would affect the physician's decision with respect to subsequent intraperitoneal or intravenous chemotherapy. This consultant believes that second-look surgery should be done, with a plan for debulking of possible residual disease and/or intraperitoneal chemotherapy.

References

1. Strand CM, Grosh WW, Baxter J, et al. Peritoneal carcinomatosis of unknown primary site in women. Ann Intern Med 1989; 111:213–217.
2. Ransom DT, Patel SR, Keenay GL, et al. Papillary serous carcinoma of the peritoneum: A review of 33 cases treated with cisplatin-based chemotherapy. Cancer 1990; 66:1091–1094.
3. Chen KT, Flam MS. Peritoneal papillary serous carcinoma with long-term survival. Cancer 1986; 58:1371–1373.

PHYSICIAN'S RESPONSE

MAUREEN KILLACKEY

Several studies have addressed the clinical entity of "papillary serous adenocarcinoma of the peritoneal surface (PSPS)" or "normal-sized ovary–carcinoma syndrome" (1,2). The etiology of this clinical entity is unclear, but two theories have been proposed. The first suggests that it arises from malignant degeneration of nests of ovarian tissue remnants left in the pathway of embryonic gonadal migration; the second is that an unidentified stimulus causes malignant transformation of the peritoneal mesothelium. In approximately 10 to 15% of exploratory laparotomies for presumptive ovarian cancer, there is extensive abdominal carcinomatosis with papillary serous tumor, but the gross examination of the ovaries shows minimal surface involvement. Stage-, grade-, and age-matched patients show similar clinical presentations, initial CA-125 levels, time from symptom onset to surgery, amount of ascites at surgery, and overall survival. However, more limited cytoreduction and a shorter disease-free interval differentiates PSPS from primary ovarian cancer. These papers report an initial favorable response to platinum-based combination chemotherapy as demonstrated by the early decrease in CA-125 levels and control of ascites, and there are cases where response to paclitaxel has been described.

In view of the optimal cytoreduction, I would recommend treating this patient with a combination of carboplatin or cisplatin and paclitaxel. Careful monitoring of her response to therapy with serial CA-125 levels, pelvic examinations and CT scans is also advised. Second-line treatment regimens utilizing etoposide, ifosfamide/mesna, and hexamethylmelamine have also shown some efficacy.

References

Fromm G, Gershenson D, Silva E. Papillary serous carcinoma of the peritoneum. Obstet Gynecol 1990; 75:89–95.

Killackey MA, Davis AR. Papillary serous carcinoma of the peritoneal surface: Matched case comparison with papillary serous ovarian carcinoma. Gynecol Oncol 1993; 51:171–74.

27

Ovarian Cancer, Epithelial Tumor with Multiple Previous Therapies

CASE

A 56-year-old woman was diagnosed 2 years ago with a stage III poorly differentiated endometrioid carcinoma of the ovary. She was initially treated with cytoxan/platinum chemotherapy. On completion of six courses of 75 mg/m^2 of platinum I.V. and 1000 mg/m^2 of Cytoxan, she had a negative computed tomography (CT) scan and a negative CA-125. It should be noted that her initial CA-125 was 1100; on completion of three courses of chemotherapy, it was 62; and it declined to 28 after four courses. After six courses of chemotherapy, it was less than 7. A decision was made not to do a second look, and 6 months after completion of the patient's initial course of treatment, a CA-125 was reported as 123 and the patient was experiencing some left-upper-quadrant pain. An abdominal pelvic CT scan showed some focal 1-cm densities just medial to the spleen as well as some perihepatic fluid and some fluid in the cul-de-sac. Surgical exploration revealed diffuse nodularity (1 cm). Histological exam showed high-grade endometrioid carcinoma. Postoperatively, the patient received six courses of paclitaxel (Taxol). Thereafter CA-125s returned to normal and she became symptom-free. Unfortunately, within 4 months on stopping the Taxol, the patient began to have some feelings of abdominal gas and bloating and her CA-125, which had fallen to 10, was reported out as 45 and then, 1 month, later, at 78. The patient at that time felt she did not want any additional cytotoxic chemotherapy, so she was placed on megestrol (Megace) and tamoxifen. She received 160 mg/day of megestrol and 30 mg per day of tamoxifen. She was maintained on this regimen for approximately 4 to 6 months, during which her CA-125s remained stable. Over the next 3 to 4 months, the CA-125s gradually increased and the patient began experiencing severe back pain, requiring oxycodone/acetaminophen and then morphine (MS Contin). She had lost a considerable amount of weight but still appeared to be reasonably strong and was able to eat. An abdominal pelvic CT scan revealed three 4-cm paraaortic masses from 3 cm above to 4 cm below the renal vessels. The back pain appeared to be localized to this area. It should be noted that the bony skeleton was normal.

The patient is very desirous of additional therapy and has come to your office seeking your opinion.

PHYSICIANS' RESPONSE

CORNELIUS GRANAI
WALTER GAJEWSKI
STEPHEN FALKENBERRY

This patient demonstrates the relentless biological history of most advanced epithelial ovarian cancers (EOC), which, although modified by today's treatment, eventually progress. Over 2 years she received thoughtful, appropriate, beneficial treatment; nevertheless, she now confronts recurrent/progressive disease. Understandably she wishes for more and better therapeutic options. At this late date, however, there are no clear medical choices. Thus, now more than ever, the patient's philosophy establishes the course. To make the best decision possible, a fuller medical (and philosophical) understanding of epithelial ovarian cancer in general, in the context of this specific case, may help.

From the history it is unclear whether the malignancy, "stage III" (not otherwise defined according to the Fédération Internationale de Gynécologie et d'Obstétrique, or FIGO), was optimally debulked. Regardless, at initial surgery, an advanced EOC of endometrioid histology was found. This particular cell type portends a better prognosis. Unfortunately, the favorable histology was offset by the lesion's grade, poorly differentiated.

Appropriate combination chemotherapy for the time, (Cytoxan and cisplatin), was begun. An excellent response ensued: the clinical examination was normal and the CA-125 fell dramatically in only three cycles; it was normal after six. Generally the rate of CA-125 decline is predictive of outcome, rapid decline being good. Contrary to this expectation, however, the disease-free interval was brief. Typical of disease progression, the patient began to experience vague gastrointestinal symptoms and an elevating CA-125. These development virtually flag recurrence—here, within 6 months of completing platinum-based chemotherapy—suggesting that residual cells are cisplatin-resistant.

Starkly confronted by disease progression, a somewhat controversial medical decision was made—to investigate the rising CA-125 by a second surgery. Not unexpectably, despite an "unremarkable" preop clinical exam and radiographic studies, diffuse, unresectable nodularity (i.e., gross cancer) was encountered at laparotomy. Disease distribution such as this does not permit meaningful resection. Consequently, although "optimal secondary debulking," which, like primary debulking, is thought advantageous, is rarely relevant since, as this case demonstrates, it is usually unachievable.

Anticipating platinum resistance, single-agent paclitaxel (Taxol) was used as a second-line chemotherapy. Again, an excellent clinical and chemical response followed, but it was short-lived. Within 4 months came renewed symptoms and a reelevating CA-125. Then, having exhausted the two best agents again EOC (cisplatin and paclitaxel), a less aggressive, but less toxic strategy was adopted. Specifically, tamoxifen and megestrol, both oral agents with some reported activity against epithelial ovarian cancer, were employed and yielded a stable CA-125 for the 6 months immediately preceding this consult. Evidence of further disease progression now exists, including a CT showing several periaortic nodules.

Despite everything, the patient wishes additional therapy. From the outset but particularly upon recurrence, the difficult realities of EOC must be understood by the patient and her family, so that they can select strategies realistically. The hard fact is that few meaningful anticancer therapies remain for the patient. Certainly her decision is not easy. But, by understanding the nuances of EOC (compared to the nonanalogous public stereotypes about the behavior and treatment of breast or other common malignancies) and with the reassurance that her cancer had been treated appropriately, there may be some consolation in knowing that what could be done was done. What then is left? To answer this question it is sometimes helpful to simplify to just two options: observation and more treatment.

First we consider observation (i.e., supportive/comfort care). Having failed two previous chemotherapies, some patients, families, and physicians would consider this the best option. Supporting medical rationale would indicate that the likelihood of achieving a meaningful, durable response to further chemotherapy is small, especially after the precipitous failure of platinum and paclitaxel. Why, then, endure possible drug/treatment side effects if the probability of benefit is remote or nonexistent? Why indeed, if the patient is feeling reasonably well or, at the other extreme, is doing very poorly? This judgment about quality of life is deeply personal.

The alternative, of course, is more treatment—in this case fourth-line treatment. In discussing treatment per se, it is clarifying to begin generically and consider each possibility: surgery, radiation, and chemotherapy. Though valuable in other (generic) oncological situations, surgery and radiation have no role in this case of advanced EOC. Even the second surgery, done much earlier in the disease process, was not therapeutically constructive. Thus, the chance of achieving optimal cytoreduction now is more remote still. Lacking a generally effective fourth-line chemotherapy furthers the argument against surgery, with its inherent morbidities. One theoretical advantage surgery does have is in obtaining malignant tissue for chemosensitivity testing. The practical (patient) value of this technology is controversial, however. Sensitivity testing may help select chemotherapy agents not otherwise expected to have antineoplastic activity. Alternatively, sensitivity testing can help avoid chemotherapies to which resistance has already developed. On balance, however, in this case surgery does not seem an intervention worth the attendant morbidity.

Radiation is another important cancer treatment, but it has little role in the management of EOC. Tumoricidal radiation doses are not tolerable when administered to a widespread field, as would be required here and with EOC in general. Compromised radiation doses are without overall therapeutic value.

Therefore, if (fourth-line) treatment is to be pursued, systemic therapy is the only possibility, limited though it may be. Accordingly, the patient may be eligible for a national or institutional chemotherapy protocol (e.g., bone marrow transplant). If perchance she is neither eligible or not interested in such a protocol, there are still a few chemotherapies that have shown response rates (e.g., 15 to 30%), usually of short duration (e.g., months). Such agents include ifosfamide, doxorubicin (Adriamycin), VP-16, and hexamethylmelamine. The latter two have the potential advantage of being oral. An occasional long-term response (several years) has been reported, though this is the exception. Drug side effects do occur.

In summary then, as it comes to be for most women late in the course of EOC, few good therapeutic alternatives remain for this patient. Though she has benefited from today's treatment, now her prognosis is poor. As she proceeds, regardless of the interventional strategy she elects, thoughtful, maximal physical and emotional support will be called for to help with the inevitable symptoms (e.g., GI dysfunction, obstruction, ascites) and the difficult days she faces. Philosophically, as physicians involved in these circumstances, our greatest practical care to such patients and their families may be in this line.

Reference

1. NIH Consensus Conference. Ovarian cancer: screening, treatment, and follow-up. JAMA 1995; 273:

PHYSICIAN'S RESPONSE

DAVID MOORE

The vast majority of epithelial ovarian cancers that are cured will be cured with first-line therapy. Consequently, all women first diagnosed with ovarian cancer—

coexisting medical conditions permitting—should undergo maximal attempted tumor cytoreduction and multiagent chemotherapy. Salvage therapies for ovarian cancers that persist or recur following cisplatin based chemotherapy have been generally disappointing. The available medical information pertinent to this case largely consists of uncontrolled descriptive studies. There are no randomized, comparative studies from which to derive a recommendation of one treatment over another.

First and foremost must come the recognition that this patient is incurable with conventional therapy. If she is willing and eligible for an investigational study, I would consider the investigational therapy to be "standard treatment" and strongly recommend that she enroll as a study subject. Regardless, any treatment must be considered as palliative in nature with the admonition to "do no harm" being the overriding principle.

The case history does not detail prior operations. If the patient has not undergone numerous operative procedures or has no other high-risk factors for bowel toxicity, I would recommend that she see a radiation oncologist in consideration for palliative radiation therapy. Radiologically evident disease is geographically limited, minimizing the risk for complications and maximizing the likelihood for effective palliation of her pain.

If radiation therapy is not feasible and she is willing to reconsider cytotoxic drug therapy, I would recommend carboplatin chemotherapy. The response to initial platinum-based therapy was excellent and, considering the long time interval since exposure, the tumor plausibly is still platinum-sensitive. Carboplatin can be given on an outpatient basis and, aside from myelosuppression, has a better toxicity profile than does cisplatin. Other chemotherapy options would include altretamine, ifosfamide, or oral etoposide. The brief disease-free interval between paclitaxel treatment and clinical recurrence suggests that the patient's ovarian cancer may be refractory to retreatment with paclitaxel.

Although operative intervention is a consideration, I would not attempt surgical resection of this patient's aortic nodal disease. The palliative benefits of surgery over less invasive approaches do not outweigh the expense and morbidity of a major operation. It is quite likely that more widespread disease is present than is evident on computed tomography. Furthermore, any benefit of surgery becomes tenuous if the residual cancer proves to be drug-resistant.

References

Christian MC, Trimble EL. Salvage chemotherapy for epithelial ovarian carcinoma. Gynecol Oncol 1994; 55:143S–150S.

Corn BW, Lanciano RM, Boente M, et al. Recurrent ovarian cancer: Effective radiotherapeutic palliation after chemotherapy failure. Cancer 1994; 74:2979–2983.

Moore DH, Valea F, Crumpler LS, Fowler WC. Hexamethylmelamine/altretamine as second-line therapy for epithelial ovarian carcinoma. Gynecol Oncol 1993; 51:109–112.

Sutton G. Ifosfamide and mesna in epithelial ovarian carcinoma. Gynecol Oncol 1993; 51:104–108.

PHYSICIAN'S RESPONSE

BARRIE ANDERSON

The course of this patient has been ominous from the start. Although we do not know if she was optimally debulked at the time of her original surgery, with individual tumor nodules reduced to less than 1 cm in diameter, her response to significant doses of platinum and cytoxan chemotherapy reveal a prolonged decrease in CA-125 levels. Such a flat course has been associated with poor prognosis (1). A normal CA-125 in postmenopausal cancer patients whose uterus, tubes and ovaries have been removed, is less than 20 (2). This level was not reached until after six cycles of chemotherapy. Signs and symptoms of recurrent disease were confirmed on CT scan by 6 months after completion of chemotherapy treatment. Recurrence within 6 months of treatment is generally interpreted as resistance to the drugs used. The patient's secondary response to paclitaxel (Taxol) chemotherapy was encouraging but consistent with lesser effectiveness of subsequent cycles of chemotherapy. Her disease clinically recurred again within 6 months. Hormonal therapy is a reasonable choice at this point, as stabilization of disease can sometimes be seen. In addition, megestrol (Megace) can be an appetite stimulant and give a sense of well-being.

The patient's current status, with enlarged paraaortic lymph nodes producing pain, is difficult to manage. Consideration should be given to surgical excision if possible, followed by either radiation or chemotherapy. This patient would be a possible candidate for experimental protocols, as there is no well-defined third-line treatment for ovarian cancer. Debulking could also be accomplished by chemotherapy, with subsequent radiation for longer term control. Cyclosporine has also been added to platinum to overcome resistance and can lead to secondary responses in some patients.

Whatever treatment is chosen, strongest consideration should be given to entering the patient on a prospective protocol and should be directed at symptom control to enhance the quality of life of this individual.

References

1. Buller RE, Berman ML, Bloss JD, et al. Serum CA125 regression in epithelial ovarian cancer: A correlation with reassessment findings and survival. Gynecol Oncol 1992; 47:87–92.

2. Alagoz T, Buller RE, Berman M, et al. What is a normal CA125 level? Gynecol Oncol 1993; 52:423–428.

PHYSICIAN'S RESPONSE

BONNIE S. REICHMAN

Endometrioid cancers account for less than 10% of all epithelial ovarian tumors and most are malignant. They range from borderline to poorly differentiated. The poorly differentiated endometrioid carcinomas are difficult to differentiate from poorly differentiated serous tumors of the ovary. However, when endometrioid tumors are well differentiated, the prognosis may be more favorable than that for serous tumors. The endometrioid ovarian cancers are often seen in concert with endometriosis and synchronous tumors of the endometrium. Chemotherapy for endometrioid carcinoma of the ovary is similar to treatment of other ovarian epithelial tumors. Appropriate surgical evaluation with optimal debulking should be attempted, if possible, followed by chemotherapy. This patient was appropriately treated with primary chemotherapy with cyclophosphamide and cisplatin, which were administered at appropriate doses. The details of initial surgery should be obtained.

The serum CA-125, if elevated, is a useful marker of response to chemotherapy. It has been determined that the rate of decline of CA-125 is an important prognostic indicator of chemotherapy sensitivity. It has been demonstrated that patients with elevated CA-125 after completion of chemotherapy have persistent disease. However, of patients with a normal CA-125 after completion of chemotherapy, approximately 50% will have residual disease at second-look laparotomy. Elevation of CA-125 (> 35 U/mL) at the time of second-look laparotomy predicts recurrence of disease with 96% accuracy.

The role of second-look laparotomy remains controversial due to the lack of evidence that it improves overall survival. Although it is the most sensitive means of diagnosing persistent disease for patients who appear to be clinically free of disease, 30 to 50% of patients who have a negative second-look laparotomy will eventually recur. The long-term benefit of secondary cytoreduction at second-look laparotomy remains controversial. This may be beneficial for a small subset of patients. In April 1994, the NIH Consensus Development Conference on the treatment of ovarian cancer determined that "Second-look laparotomy should be done only for patients on clinical trials or for those patients in whom the surgery will affect clinical decision making and clinical course. It should not be employed as routine care of all patients (1).

After the initial short response to platinum-based chemotherapy, the elevation in CA-125 to > 100, in concert with the CT scan findings and symptoms, confirmed the presence of recurrent disease. Pathological confirmation, if needed, could have been obtained with radiologically guided biopsy or laparoscopy rather than laparotomy. In the absence of participation in a clinical trial and the absence of need for symptomatic relief of bowel obstruction, the role of repeat laparotomy in this poor-prognosis patient remains unclear.

This platinum-resistant patient received appropriate second-line treatment with paclitaxel with normalization of CA-125 and resolution of symptoms. Unfortunately, the duration of response was brief. Objective responses to the taxanes, paclitaxel and taxotere, are in the range of 30% in the setting of platin-refractory disease (2). Prior to the taxanes, there was no effective second-line treatment in this setting. The optimal dose, schedule, and combinations for these agents have not been determined. Further treatment in the setting of both platin and taxane resistance is palliative at best. Salvage treatments such as hormonal manipulation, ifosfamide, doxorubicin, mitomycin-C, hexamethamelamine, and 5-fluorouracil, administered as single agents or in combination, do not have significant long-term term benefit. Palliative radiation therapy for pain control due to retroperitoneal adenopathy could be considered. Participation in Phase I investigational protocol should be encouraged.

References

1. National Institutes of Health Consensus Development Conference Statement. Ovarian Cancer: screening, treatment, and follow-up. Gynecol Oncol 1994; 55(suppl):4–14.
2. Trimble EL, Arbuck SG, McGuire WP. Options for primary chemotherapy of epithelial ovarian cancer: Taxanes. Gynecol Oncol 1994; 55(suppl):114–121.

PHYSICIAN'S RESPONSE

MALCOLM G. IDELSON

The salient features of this case for myself, the patient, and her family are as follows:

1. The patient is relatively young (age 56), has lost considerable weight, but still appears to be "reasonably strong" and is able to eat.
2. She has significant back pain, paraaortic tumor masses, and is very desirous of further therapy at this time.
3. The patient has had quite a good response (although short lived) to both platinum-cytoxan and paclitaxel. Time to recurrence of symptoms following cessation of chemotherapy was 6 months and 4 months respectively. Hormonal manipulation also achieved stability for awhile.

With this summary further clarified if necessary, I would realistically emphasize that, in view of multiple relapses, curative therapy would be remote and any salvage therapy must be considered palliative, with a temporary response rate no higher than 15 to 20%. Issues regarding quality of life remaining, the possible risks and hardships of resuming active therapy at this stage as well as psychological support, pain control, and the ongoing, ever-present aid and comfort provided by myself and my staff would be discussed.

Having covered all this ground and with the patient's continued interest in therapy, a program of chemoradiation followed by chemotherapy alone would be employed. Radiation oncology consultation would be sought in order to deliver 4000 to 4500 cGy of external beam therapy to the paraaortic area of gross involvement with tumor. Techniques with lateral, oblique, or rotational fields to protect the spinal cord would be utilized. Concomitant chemotherapy, cisplatin and paclitaxel, would also be utilized, with attention to dose, schedule, and supportive measures if necessary (granulocyte colony-stimulating factor, erythropoietin, platelet or blood transfusion) in order to complete the radiotherapy without protraction. Once the radiation was completed, chemotherapy would continue if response and tolerance were documented. After several postradiation cycles of chemotherapy, the cisplatin would be dropped out and paclitaxel continued until signs of progression of disease or toxicity. Alternative plans at this point or even before (while stable on paclitaxel) might include the use of hexamethylmelamine or other agents with occasional responses seen (fluorouracil with biomodulators including methotrexate, leucovorin and hydroxyurea, ifosfamide, etoposide).

Finally and in addition, one of the choices that can be offered anywhere along the way would be investigational protocols such as topoisomerase inhibitors, reducing drug resistance, and/or decreasing drug toxicity as well as other avenues of research.

In short, this case is relatively hopeless, but occasionally surprising palliation can be achieved for significant periods of time.

References

1. NIH Consensus Conference. Ovarian cancer screening, treatment, and follow-up. JAMA 1995; 273:491–496.
2. Corn BW, et al. Recurrent ovarian cancer: Effective radiotherapeutic palliation after chemotherapy failure. Cancer 1994, 74:2979–2983.
3. Schink JC, et al. Altretamine (Hexalen): An effective salvage chemotherapy after paclitaxel (Taxol) in women with recurrent platinum resistant ovarian cancer. Poster presentation and 1994 ASCO meeting, University of Wisconsin.

PHYSICIANS' RESPONSE

WATSON G. WATRING
NEAL SEMRAD

Unfortunately, this patient's scenario is a most common one for stage III epithelial ovarian carcinoma. The only way she might be more typical is if she developed intermittent symptoms of small bowel obstruction/dysfunction. We have been using carboplatin with paclitaxel (Taxol) up front for some years now, but it is too soon to know if there will be improved survival.

Even with preliminary data, however, it is clear that this clinical course will be repeated in patients with ovarian carcinoma for some time. The still ineffectual screening tests, representing a first baby step, reflect our knowledge that to prevent stage III ovarian carcinoma would be preferable to treating it. To date, the majority of women present with advanced stage disease and treatment is less than ideal.

While our future expectations for possible screening tests and/or better "bullets" remains, this typical patient with ovarian carcinoma has some potentially helpful options remaining.

First, the patient should have additional medication to help control her pain. We have used the antidepressants and antipsychotics (major tranquilizers) with good success. These medications seem to potentiate the narcotic, and the sedative side effects often bring welcome rest for the first 1 or 2 weeks of use.

There is no curative second- or third-line drug in ovarian carcinoma. It is unlikely that good palliation could be obtained, and most agents would, of course, reduce her quality of life. Before hospice referral or concurrently, consideration should be given to palliative radiation therapy. We have on occasion seen some striking responses.

Corn and coworkers (1), in a more quantitative fashion, reviewed 33 patients treated with radiation therapy at 47 separate sites and reported an 83% success rate in terms of pain relief. Likewise, Davidson et al. (2) found that limited-field therapy could prolong symptom-free survival.

It should be noted and, of course, discussed with the patient, that there is a potential for harm as well. One small bowel obstruction and a 14% grade 3 toxicity in the studies mentioned above were noted.

References

1. Corn, et al: Recurrent ovarian cancer: Effective radiotherapeutic palliation after chemotherapy failure. Cancer 1994; 74:2979–2983.
2. Davidson, et al. Limited field radiotherapy as salvage treatment of localized persistent or recurrent epithelial ovarian cancer. Gynecol Oncol 1993; 51:349–354.

28

Intraabdominal Cancer: Advanced Disease at Presentation

CASE

A 68-year-old woman with a 2-month history of abdominal bloating arrives in your office. She tells of feeling "gassy" all of the time and rapidly becomes full when eating. She notes that her appetite is good. The patient says she has increased pelvic pressure, with frequent urination. Her bowel movements are difficult for her and, on close questioning, she reports that her stools are much thinner than normal. The patient also reports that her feet have been swelling for the past month, making it difficult for her to put on her shoes.

Family Hx	Gravida II, para II
	Mother and father died age 68 of "heart attacks"
	One brother age 65 two years s/p coronary artery bypass surgery
Past Hx	Pt. is currently on a daily thiazide for hypertension
	Cholecystectomy done 8 years ago
Physical Exam	Generally thin appearing except abdomen, looks ill
	One small, firm, 8-mm left supraclavicular node
	Chest is clear with decreased sounds at the right base
	Heart with irregularly irregular rhythm
	Abdomen distended with a firm mass palpable across the upper abdomen
	Pelvic exam reveals normal-appearing cervix with firm nodularity in both the vesicovaginal as well as the rectovaginal septum. The cul-de-sac is fixed with leatherlike tissue involving both uterosacrals

Laboratory   CA-125 = 1125
                    Hb = 9.8
                    Na = 132, K = 3.6
                    Alk phos = 28
                    Albumin = 2.9, total protein 5.8
                    Remainder of CBC and SMA-16 is WNL
X-rays   Chest with small right pleural effusion
                    CT scan with tumor in omentum, cul-de-sac, involvement of
                        P/A nodes, SB mesentary and peritoneum. Ascites is also
                        present.

PHYSICIAN'S RESPONSE

C.R. HARRISON

This individual presents with a significant intraabdominal tumor burden, early satiety, small-caliber stools, anemia, probable atrial fibrillation, and evidence of malnutrition. An evaluation of her gastrointestinal (GI) tract should be performed to include the stomach and colon. Primary tumors of the GI tract will be diagnosed in approximately 36,000 women this year. If this patient has only extrinsic compression of her stomach plus small and large bowel, the likelihood that she has ovarian cancer is very high. The significantly elevated CA-125 supports that possibility. Cytology of the ascitic fluid, pleural fluid, or supraclavicular node would confirm metastatic disease and may confirm a carcinoma consistent with an ovarian primary.

In patients who are surgical candidates, an exploration, attempt at debulking, and institution of platinum-based chemotherapy would be common practice. Approximately 75% of women with epithelial ovarian cancer have advanced-stage disease noted at the time of diagnosis. There is considerable published clinical experience demonstrating that residual, not initial tumor burden directly correlates with survival. Patients who are explored and optimally debulked have a longer disease-free interval and median survival than those with unresected, large-volume disease. Griffiths et al. (1,2) reported on the survival of 102 patients, noting median survival of 18 months for residual over 1.5 cm, 29 months for less than 0.5 cm, and 39 months if there was no gross residual.

Some patients have a significant risk of operative morbidity and mortality at presentation yet may be able to undergo a debulking procedure safely at a later time. This woman has a strong family history of ischemic heart disease, a personal history of hypertension, and presents in apparent atrial fibrillation. Thyroid function tests, blood gases, and a cardial evaluation to include an electrocardiogram (ECG), echocardiography, and assessment for ischemic disease is indicated.

Her perioperative risk of significant cardiac complications is as high as 33%. With atrial fibrillation, she has an increased risk of stroke, reduced by anticoagulation if there is no clear contraindication. Cardioversion may improve overall cardiac function; however, it should be delayed until she has been anticoagulated for several weeks. Her dependent leg edema is likely due to intraabdominal carcinomatosis; however, it may also be reflective of a thrombus in the iliofemoral venous systems. An evaluation to rule out disseminated vascular thrombosis (DVT) would be appropriate. Finally, her nutritional status is comprised, the risk of anergy high, and her potential surgical morbidity and mortality increased. Institution of enteral tube feeding, if tolerated, or parenteral feeding will be an important element of her overall care.

In light of her poor surgical risk and the need for extended medical intervention, it would be reasonable to complete an evaluation quickly and begin chemotherapy, should she elect to pursue therapy. Three cycles of cyclophosphamide and a platinum analog given every 3 to 4 weeks would permit sufficient time to evaluate and stabilize her and to determine if her tumor was chemotherapy sensitive. If her ascites resolved, nutritional status normalized, and no disease progression was evident, she should be reassessed and offered surgical exploration. There is 50 to 75% chance that she could be optimally debulked to less than 1 cm. Curtin et al. (3) reported that in patients with stage IV disease, those patients who are optimally debulked have a median survival of 40 months, versus 18 months in patients with larger residual disease.

With such a potential response, it is reasonable to suggest that the patient's care team include those who routinely take care of ovarian cancer patients, so as to facilitate delicate balance of art, science, experience, and compassion as efforts are directed toward restoration of function, comfort, and cure if possible for this patient.

References

1. Griffiths CT. Surgical Resection of Tumor Bulk in the Primary Treatment of Ovarian Carcinoma: Symposium on Ovarian Carcinoma, NCI Monogr 1975; 101.
2. Griffiths CT, Parker LM, Fuller AF Jr. Role of cytoreductive surgical treatment in the management of advanced ovarian carcinoma. Cancer Treat Rep 1979; 63:235.
3. Curtin J, Malik R, Venkatraman E, et al. Surgical debulking of patients with stage IV ovarian cancer: Impact on survival. Abstr Soc Gynecol Oncol, annual meeting, 1995.
4. Schwartz PE, Chambers JT, Makuch R. Neoadjuvant chemotherapy for advanced ovarian cancer. Gynecol Oncol 1994; 53:33–37.
5. Hoskins WJ, McGuire WP, Brady MF, et al. The effect of diameter of largest residual disease on survival after primary cytoreductive surgery in patients with suboptimal residual epithelial ovarian carcinoma. Am J Obstet Gynecol 1994; 170:974–980.

PHYSICIAN'S RESPONSE

JAMES ROBERTS

This woman's history and physical are extremely suggestive of an advanced ovarian cancer. She has abdominal bloating, changes in bowel function, an upper abdominal mass suggestive of an omental mass, extensive pelvic tumor, and an elevated CA-125. However, there are several other factors to consider. She notes that she "rapidly becomes full when eating." Her stools are much thinner. She appears thin and her albumin is low, suggesting poor nutritional status. In addition, she is anemic. All of these factors point to a possible gastrointestinal tumor. In order to evaluate this possibility, one should obtain a carcinoembryonic antigen (CEA) level and order a barium enema to look for a colon cancer as well as an upper GI series to detect a stomach or small bowel cancer now presenting as a Krukenberg tumor. Both of these cancers would be more likely to present with the extensive lymph node involvement seen in this woman. If these studies return showing a gastrointestinal primary, consultation with a surgical oncologist should be obtained.

If these studies show only extrinsic tumor, it can be assumed that this woman has an ovarian cancer. She should be subjected to a bowel prep because of the likelihood of extensive tumor involvement of the transverse and sigmoid colon. This should minimize the need for a colostomy. At the same time, she should be informed preoperatively that a colostomy may still be necessary. No other preoperative studies or preparations are necessary, though a fine needle aspiration of the firm left supraclavicular node would be of interest. If this were to return showing an adenocarcinoma, this information could be used in the preoperative counseling.

The surgical dissection planned should include a total abdominal hysterectomy, bilateral salpingo-oophorectomy, omentectomy, pelvic/paraaortic lymphadenectomy, and maximal tumor resection. This approach, which is appropriate for both stages III and IV, will provide good data for staging as well as begin the therapy for this woman. The goal of this resection is to remove enough tumor that the largest remaining single tumor mass will be less than 2 cm. This will place her in the optimally resected group. This subset of patients shows a superior response rate to chemotherapy. A measure of the degree of resection can be obtained by drawing a CA-125 on the third postoperative day. At this time, the maximal degree in CA-125 decrease will be reached before it begins to elevate as a result of surgically induced peritoneal inflammation.

When the patient recovers her bowel function (usually 4 to 5 days postoperatively), she can be started on chemotherapy. The regimen now in use includes cisplatin 75 mg/m^2 and paclitaxel 175 mg/m^2, which is administered intravenously every 3 weeks. Starting chemotherapy this soon after surgery is not associated with any increase in postoperative complications, and it can eliminate one hospital admission for chemotherapy.

As she undergoes chemotherapy, the patient's disease status can be followed with regular pelvic examination and CA-125 measurements. It has been found that if the CA-125 level has not returned to normal (< 35) by the start of the fourth course, it is unlikely that a complete response will be obtained. Therefore, it may be reasonable to consider a change in the chemotherapy regimen if the CA-125 level is > 35. If the level is < 35, one should complete a total of six courses of cisplatin and paclitaxel. At the completion of this therapy, one should consider a second-look laparoscopy to access the status of disease.

PHYSICIAN'S RESPONSE

SCOTT JENNINGS

This case history describes many of the symptoms and findings of the unfortunate patient who presents with advanced epithelial ovarian cancer, although this obviously requires histopathologic confirmation. Historically it may be useful to explore the patient's prior use of oral contraceptives, hormone replacement therapy, and/or tubal ligation, although none of the above would alter prognosis or therapy at this point. A few of her symptoms related to bowel function suggest the possibility of either bowel encroachment or primary bowel disease, which would be easily documented by colonoscopy or at least by sampling for occult fecal blood.

Physical examination suggests there may be both local and distant disease from the pelvic tumor. Laparotomy will be the most expeditious method of assessing the character of the patient's abdominal disease, but it may be prudent to proceed with an evaluation for extraabdominal metastases prior to laparotomy. The right-sided effusion on chest radiograph certainly indicates the probability of metastasis at this site, and this should be confirmed cytologically. If the effusion is cytologically negative, attention may be turned to biopsy of the left supra-clavicular node. If a surgical specialist will not be available to biopsy her enlarged paraaortic lymph nodes, this could be performed percutaneously under radio-graphic direction; but it seems more expeditious to have the laparotomy con-ducted by surgeons facile in the methods for staging of this probably ovarian cancer. Cardiac examination suggests the need to address optimization of her medical status if laparotomy is pursued.

If the disease is confirmed to be ovarian cancer, metastases identified in either the pleural space or the distant node will designate her disease as Fédération Internationale de Gynécologie et d'Obstétrique (FIGO) stage IV, which is signif-icant prognostically. Large studies rarely note more than 8% of patients with stage IV disease to survive 5 years, and there are a few reports of 10-year survival. Even given this pessimistic prognosis, however, there are at least three roles for surgery. The first is for biopsy confirmation of the patient's disease. This can be performed by less invasive methods of biopsy such as CT-directed biopsy or by laparoscopy, but most surgical oncologists will utilize laparotomy for both safety and the additional information derived from visual inspection of the intraperitoneal contents. Little success has been credited in the past to laparoscopic staging followed by neoadjuvant chemotherapy, but innovative small trials utilizing this approach are now in progress.

The other two roles for surgical exploration in this patient are somewhat more controversial, given the poor prognosis of stage IV disease, but aggressive surgical debulking may offer both survival and quality-of-life advantages. Survival advantages may accrue to patients following debulking by several mechanisms, most importantly by decreasing tumor burden (often by as much as 90%) and possibly by decreasing the fraction of tumor cells in inactive or dormant (G_0) cellular phases that are less responsive to cytotoxic therapy. Most investigators, including those of a recent review from Memorial Sloan Kettering Hospital, suggest a clear survival advantage even for patients with stage IV disease who can be optimally cytoreduced surgically. In this study, presented only in abstract form at this time, over 40% of patients with stage IV ovarian cancer could be left with residual disease less than 2 cm, and the median survival for these patients was 40 months, versus the 18-month median survival of those with residual disease greater than 2 cm. If this aggressive approach to laparotomy is pursed, it seems reasonable to utilize the given preoperative studies in an attempt to demonstrate how likely the success of surgical debulking may be. The success rate of primary cytoreductive surgery for metastatic ovarian cancer has ranged from 24 to 66%, with an overall mean estimated by Hoskins in 1989 to be 33%. The likelihood of optimal surgical debulking may appear to be somewhat less than usual given the reported CT findings of mesenteric disease as well as aortic adenopathy, but aggressive surgical effort can quite frequently see impressive results even in these settings.

Even if a survival advantage can be measured only in months, cytoreductive surgery may play a significant role in palliation of symptoms and improvement in the quality of life, as demonstrated in early studies by Blythe. The putative mechanisms of this advantage include improved gastrointestinal function, decreased fluid retention due to ascites, and lessened pain due to tumor impingement upon other abdominal organs.

An additional possibility for this patient that should be entertained is that of interval cytoreduction using the approach of "chemosurgical debulking", i.e., a combination of aggressive chemotherapy followed by interval surgical cytoreduction to further chemotherapy, depending on tumor response. In a small series, complete pathological responses were doubled by this type of approach over that of primary surgical debulking followed by chemotherapy. The exact role of interval cytoreduction procedures, particularly for patients with stage IV ovarian carcinoma, remains to be elucidated.

Chemotherapy choices for stage IV disease have classically centered on combination chemotherapy, including cisplatin and cyclophosphamide with or without doxorubicin. Recent studies suggest that a combination of cisplatin and paclitaxel may be somewhat more efficacious, but maturation of these data awaits more time and more experience with these unique patients with stage IV ovarian cancer.

References

Blythe JG, Wahl TP. Debulking surgery: Does it increase the quality of survival? Gynecol Oncol 1982; 14:396–408.

Ng, LW, Rubin SC, Hoskins WJ, et al. Aggressive chemosurgical debulking in patients with advanced ovarian cancer. Gynecol Oncol 1990; 38:358–363.

Curtin J, Malik R, Denkatraman E, et al. Surgical debulking of patients with stage IV ovarian cancer: Impact on survival. Abstr Soc Gynecol Oncol annual meeting, February 22, 1995, abstr 18.

29

Ovarian Cancer, Epithelial (Stage IA, Clear Cell)

CASE

A 31-year-old woman, gravida I, para I, with a 2-year-old child came to her gynecologist complaining of some pain in her left lower quadrant. Physical examination and pelvic ultrasound confirmed the presence of a 7-cm solid and cystic left adnexal mass. CA-125 was 28. During subsequent surgery, through a lower abdominal midline incision, the patient underwent a left salpingo-oophorectomy, left pelvic and left paraaortic lymph node dissection, cul-de-sac biopsies, bilateral biopsies of the lateral gutters, and rubbings of the diaphragm. Omental biopsies as well as peritoneal washings were performed. The final diagnosis was a stage 1A clear-cell carcinoma. The patients postoperative course was smooth. The patient's hemoglobin postoperatively was 14.1. Her electrolyte, liver function tests, and renal function tests were within normal limits.

PHYSICIANS' RESPONSE

CLAUS TROPÉ
GUNNAR KRISTENSEN

Early stages make up about one-third of all ovarian cancer (OC) cases. The overall 5-year survival in stage I is about 81%. Ovarian cancer spreads via peritoneal fluids, lymphatics, and occasionally the bloodstream. It has been shown that up to 30% of patients with presumably early disease have microscopic tumor dissemination in high-risk anatomic sites such as the peritoneal fluid, the omentum, the diaphragm, and the lymph nodes. Surgery with careful examination of these sites, as was done in this case, is the mainstay of treatment for early OC (1).

Histological type and grade differentiation are indicators of prognosis in early OC. Among other indicators, DNA ploidy has proven useful. Clear-cell tumors are associated with a poorer prognosis than other histological types (2). In our series of about 400 OC patients in stage I, the 5-year survival is 60 and 88% for patients with clear-cell and non-clear-cell tumors, respectively. For clear-cell tumors in stage IA, the 5-year survival is about 80%. All of these patients received some kind of adjuvant treatment.

Adjuvant treatment with cisplatin in early OC has been shown to increase the progression-free but not the overall survival. Carboplatin has been found to be as efficacious as cisplatin in terms of overall survival when used as single drug in advanced OC, but it is less nephrotoxic, neurotoxic, ototoxic and emetogenic. Therefore, carboplatin is widely used in the adjuvant setting. In advanced OC, combination chemotherapy is widely used in the adjuvant setting. In advanced OC, combination chemotherapy is more effective than single-drug treatment and the combination of cisplatin and paclitaxel (Taxol) has proven most effective in terms of overall survival. Whether adjuvant treatment with this combination might increase the overall survival in early OC remains to be seen.

The patient in question belongs to a high-risk group, although her cancer was restricted to stage IA. We would give her adjuvant treatment with six courses of carboplatin because such treatment will reduce her risk of relapse and the risk of side effects that might interfere with her quality of life is small.

References

1. Colombo N, Chiari S, Maggioni A, et al. Controversial issues in the management of early epithelial ovarian cancer: Conservative surgery and role of adjuvant therapy. Gynecol Oncol 1994; 55:S47–S51.
2. Vergote IB, Kaern J, Abeler VM, et al. C.G. Analysis of prognostic factors in stage I epithelial ovarian carcinoma: Importance of degree of differentiation and DNA ploidy in predicting relapse. Am J Obstet Gynecol 1993; 169:40–52.

PHYSICIAN'S RESPONSE

MAUREEN JARRELL

Clear-cell carcinoma of the ovary is a rare epithelial malignancy, representing 3 to 6% of these tumors. It has a frequent association with endometriosis, which does not seem to be clinically significant except when it contributes to the surgical rupture of the tumor. It has so far been impossible to assign a grading system to this malignancy, unlike other epithelial tumors. Nuclear pleomorphism and mitoses per 10 high-power fields has not been shown to correlate with survival in retrospective studies.

The literature regarding survival and treatment of this tumor is confounded because of the lesion's rarity and the inability to grade the tumor histologically. Large studies are retrospective, spanning five decades, including many cases that were not thoroughly staged surgically. Decisions about therapy for any stage IA epithelial tumor rely on a precise surgical and pathological description of the tumor. This patient's tumor was found in only one ovary. Because of the assigned stage, it was removed without rupture and no external excrescences were found. The pathology review should discuss the presence or absence of vascular invasion. In some studies, tubulocystic and papillary histological patterns have been shown to be good prognostic indicators.

While advanced stages of ovarian clear-call cancer have survival rates comparable to those of other epithelial cell types, stage I disease as a whole does not compare favorably, with only a 50% survival at 5 years. A recent retrospective study suggests that all early-stage tumors be treated with adjuvant chemotherapy (1). However, this study did not attempt to substage the 37 stage I tumors presented.

Before the substage C was added to the classification of stage I ovarian cancers, publications often divided stage IA tumors into the subclassifications of i and ii. Stage IAi tumors were those that were unruptured and without external excrescences. Stage IAii designated those tumors that were ruptured or had evidence of tumor on the outside capsule. Therefore, in reviewing the literature regarding the type of case presented, similar cases may be called stage IA or stage IAi.

If the physician treating this patient can be assured of a stage IA tumor without evidence of lymphovascular space invasion, the patient requires no further treatment. Only stage IA tumors have been described as having a zero recurrence rate (2). Otherwise the patient should be treated adjuvantly with platinum-based combination chemotherapy.

References

1. Obrien MER, Schofield JB, Tan S, et al. Clear cell epithelial ovarian cancer (mesonephroid): Bad prognosis only in early stages. Gynecol Oncol 1993; 49:250–254.
2. Jenison E, Montag AG, Griffiths CT, et al. Clear Cell adenocarcinoma of the ovary: A clinical analysis and comparison with serous carcinoma. Gynecol Oncol 1989; 32:65–71.

PHYSICIAN'S RESPONSE

GILLIAN THOMAS

This 31-year-old woman has had an appropriate staging laparotomy for what would appear to be a stage IA clear-cell carcinoma of the left ovary. She had removal of the left adnexa but not the right adnexa or the uterus. Her CA-125 at presentation was within normal limits and there is no clinical evidence for overt residual disease in the peritoneal cavity postoperatively. No statement has been made as to the appearance of the right ovary and no biopsy of the ovary was performed, but I am assuming that the ovary appeared grossly normal.

The issue of further management for this patient is dependent on two things. The first is the possibility of relapse following this conservative surgery, and the second is the efficacy of any additional postoperative therapy with her disease as described. No comment has been made as to the patient's wishes for preservation of fertility (i.e., retention of the contralateral ovary and the uterus).

With respect to the first issue of risk of relapse following surgery, it would appear that the risk for relapse in a clear cell carcinoma is comparable to that of a grade 3 serous or undifferentiated cancer; as such, I would estimate the risk of relapse to be in the order of 30%. No study to date has shown definitively that any postoperative therapy improves survival in stage IA high-grade ovarian cancers. I do not infer, however, that therapy is necessarily ineffective. The lack of demonstrated efficacy may be related to the methodology of the clinical trials that have explored such therapy.

Because this patient is at significant risk for relapse, indeed the risk of relapse may be as high as that of many patients with stage II disease, I would offer post-operative treatment. Platinum-based chemotherapy, whole abdominal pelvic irradiation, and chromic phosphate (^{32}P) are all modalities used in the treatment of stage I disease. There are no data to determine which treatment to be preferred except that the morbidity of ^{32}P installation may be higher than that associated with chemotherapy or appropriate external beam pelvic and abdominal radiation therapy (1).

One of the issues in determining further therapy for this patient is whether or not the pelvic surgery should be completed with removal of the right ovary and uterus. There are data to suggest that the residual ovary may be a sanctuary site for disease, despite postoperative chemotherapy and possibly radiation. Because this is the case, I would recommend that the patient have the contralateral tube and ovary removed before postoperative adjuvant therapy was delivered.

While radiation therapy has not been proven to be of survival benefit in stage I disease, there is clear evidence (2) that it may have curative potential in an intermediate-risk group of patients including those with stage I high-grade lesions and stage II disease with minimal residuum in the pelvis. It also appears to achieve comparable survivals for patients with optimal stage III disease compared to the results achieved with chemotherapy. I would therefore offer this patient a course of abdominopelvic irradiation to deliver a tumor dose to the whole abdomen of 2250 cGy in 22 fractions followed with a boost to the pelvis to bring the pelvic dose to 45 Gy. The technique of radiation used would encompass the entire peritoneal cavity including the domes of the diaphragm and the peritoneal reflections. The kidneys would be suitably protected so that the dose of radiation received by the kidneys was within acceptable levels of tolerance. Following radiation therapy, the patient would be monitored clinically and further treatment in the form of chemotherapy recommended only if there were overt signs of disease progression. I would offer the patient hormone replacement therapy and recommend appropriate ongoing screening of the breasts.

References

1. Vergote IB, Vergote-De Vos LN, Abeler VM, et al. Randomized trial comparing cisplatin with radioactive phosphorus or whole-abdomen irradiation as adjuvant treatment of ovarian cancer. Cancer 1992; 69:741.
2. Thomas GM, Dembo AJ. Integrating radiation therapy into the management of ovarian cancer. Cancer 1993; 71:1710.

PHYSICIAN'S RESPONSE

GEORGE A. OMURA

Stage I clear-cell carcinoma is considered to pose a high risk of recurrence. The National Institutes of Health (NIH) Consensus Conference (April 1994) recommended adjuvant chemotherapy even though they acknowledged that it was of unproven value and they could not recommend a specific treatment.

The risk of failure for cases of stage I clear-cell carcinoma appears to be in the range of 30 to 57%, despite various adjuvant treatments. However, most reports do not give numbers for stage IA clear cell cases, so the observation by Vergote et al. (1) that only 1/15 of such cases in their series recurred (after adjuvant phosphorus 32 or cisplatin) is notable. Similarly, Jenison et al. (2) reported no recurrence in 7 patients with stage IA clear-cell histology. In that series there was a total of 22 stage I cases, so the most favorable group included only 32% (7/22) of the stage I cases, which, in turn, represented half of all the clear-cell cases described by Jenison et al. The postoperative management of their stage IA cases was not described. It is difficult, from the literature, to confirm or deny this favorable result; for example, in Young's paper (3), stages IA and IB were not separated in reporting that 3/9 with clear-cell elements recurred.

To return to the case in question, this patient is incompletely staged. The preferred option would be to complete the staging (to include a hysterectomy, right salpingo-oophorectomy, omentectomy, and node sampling on the right side). If stage IA status is confirmed, she should be considered for a protocol. If she declined to participate in a study, I would explain that the risk of recurrence is unclear and the benefit of cisplatin-based regimens is uncertain in this particular circumstance, but that, as noted above, current sentiment favors treatment and that, based on the experience of Vergote, cisplatin 50 mg/m^2 every 3 weeks for six courses could be considered. I would review with her the toxicity of cisplatin (neurotoxicity, nephrotoxicity, ototoxicity). Since the curative potential of this adjuvant therapy is unproven, I would try to have the patient participate in the decision.

After completing the staging, if the extent of disease is more than stage IA and she declines protocol therapy, I would recommend cisplatin plus paclitaxel for six courses, since the risk of recurrence is substantial and that combination is the best currently available.

If the patient declines complete staging, I would recommend cisplatin and paclitaxel, thinking that the disease might well be more than stage IA and should be treated rather than observed.

Suppose the patient insists that her primary concern is to have another child? Although a pregnancy would enormously complicate her follow-up, if she could get pregnant immediately and then complete the staging after delivery, that might be an acceptable compromise. A 1-year delay in definitive staging and treatment seems very undesirable, but we do not know that with certainty. Alternatively, she could be treated with cisplatin and paclitaxel first, but the effect of this combination on fertility is unclear.

References

1. Vergote IB, Kaern J, Abeler VM, et al. Analysis of prognostic factors in stage I epithelial ovarian carcinoma: Importance of degree of differentiation and deoxyribonucleic acid ploidy in predicting relapse. Am J Obstet Gynecol 1993; 169:40–52.
2. Jenison EL, Montag AG, Griffiths CT, et al. Clear cell adenocarcinoma of the ovary: A clinical analysis and comparison with serous carcinoma. Gynecol Oncol 1989; 32:65–71.
3. Young RC, Walton LA, Ellenberg SS, et al: Adjuvant therapy in stage I and stage II epithelial ovarian cancer: Results of two prospective randomized trials. N Engl J Med 1990; 322:1021–1027.

PHYSICIAN'S RESPONSE

ROBERT C. WALLACH

A 31-year-old woman para I with a 2-year-old child had left lower quadrant pain which led to physical examination and ultrasound revealing a 7-cm left adnexal mass, which proved to be a clear-cell carcinoma of the ovary. Appropriate sampling at the time of surgery revealed no sign of disease outside the ovary, although no specific description of the contralateral ovary is available.

Several important issues must be addressed in the management of this patient. Assuming that the retained ovary is free of disease, there are multiple choices to be made. Should the retained ovary be removed as possibly posing increased risk of a second malignancy and as the possible occult site of current malignancy? Should systemic chemotherapy, external radiation therapy, or intraperitoneal radioisotope therapy be used, regardless of the condition or surgery of the now retained ovary? In making a decision concerning management, it is most important that the patient be fully conversant with the issues at hand, as I do not believe an absolute answer is available. Since conservative management without adjuvant treatment has occasionally been advocated for a well-staged, well-differentiated epithelial carcinoma stage IA, this might be one possibility; but with a clear-cell histological type, I am reluctant to see the patient left without further treatment. I do not think there is sufficient experience with "conservative" management with this histological type, which may actually represent a more aggressive variety of endometrioid ovarian carcinoma. Without evidence of residual disease, I would also recommend against external radiation by whatever technique (moving strip, whole abdomen, etc.), as, without a specific target in such a young woman, the long-term effects of radiation therapy would be unacceptable. Again, without evidence of residual disease, I would be personally reluctant to see intraperitoneal isotopic phosphorus 32 used, although this is a reasonable consideration and might be offered at some centers. I do, however, believe that more treatment is indicated because of the possibility of occult disease despite the complete staging procedure, and I would recommend systemic chemotherapy with a combination of drugs including cisplatin, or carboplatin, and either an alkylating agent or paclitaxel (Taxol). Most of the toxicity for these drug combinations is short-term and should be tolerated easily by this young woman. With comparable response rates of platinum compounds combined with either paclitaxel or an alkylating agent, it is difficult to choose which combination to use. The potential long-term carcinogenic effect of an alkylating agent must be balanced against the relatively short total experience with paclitaxel. Also, the potential effect on ova from the platinum agents or paclitaxel is difficult to predict.

If the patient were not desirous of another pregnancy, I would recommend removal of the remaining ovary, systemic chemotherapy with carboplatin and paclitaxel, and hormone replacement therapy. If the patient wished to retain childbearing function with the unknown effects of chemotherapeutic agents on germ cells, I would recommend carboplatin and cytoxan with close surveillance (as in all situations).

The discussion of conservative management for early carcinoma of the ovary has become more complex over the past 25 years because of the availability of more active agents, but with full disclosure of the risks and hazards and unknowns to this patient, I believe an appropriate decision can be made.

Reference

1.   Munnell EW. Is conservative therapy ever justified in stage I cancer of the ovary? Am J Obstet Gynecol 1969; 103:641–653.

30

Ovarian Cancer, Epithelial (Early Disease, Unstaged)

CASE

A 44-year-old woman, gravida III, para III, had experienced some vaginal spotting and was found, by her local gynecologist, to have a pelvic mass on pelvic ultrasound. Her CA-125 was 42. The patient was taken to the operating room and a total abdominal hysterectomy/bilateral salpingo-oophorectomy (TAH/BSO) through a Pfannenstiel incision was performed with a finding of a 6 cm left pelvic mass. Postoperatively, the patient did well; 1 week after the surgery, the pathology returned as a grade 3 papillary serous carcinoma. The surgeon felt that everything seemed to be quite clear and the mass was not adherent. The surgeon said that he was not surprised by the final diagnosis since the mass, as seen grossly, did worry him. Postoperatively, an abdominal pelvic CT scan was totally normal. A chest x-ray also proved to be normal. The patient's hemoglobin was 13.5. Her electrolytes, liver function tests, and renal function tests were all normal.

PHYSICIANS' RESPONSE

N. NIKRUI
R. SAINZ DE LA CUESTA

Ovarian cancer spreads primarily via peritoneal surface extension or through the lymphatic system. Some 60 to 70% of epithelial ovarian cancers are detected in advanced stages and only 30 to 40% in stages I or II.

Patients with early-stage epithelial ovarian carcinoma tend to have a much better prognosis than those with more advanced disease. Therefore it is very important to stage the patient adequately initially. Young et al. (1) found that 28% of patients who initially were thought to have stage I and 43% of the patients with stage II disease were upstaged following restaging laparotomy. It is therefore important to surgically evaluate the entire peritoneal cavity in addition to pelvic and periaortic nodes in treating a potential epithelial ovarian malignancy. In this case, the upper abdomen was not properly evaluated and the pelvic and periaortic nodes were not sampled. It would be difficult to adequately predict the prognosis and to recommend the correct postoperative treatment to this patient. Therefore, we would recommend a restaging laparotomy/laparoscopy for this patient. Presence or absence of distant metastasis will dictate how to treat this patient. Current recommendations (2) for the treatment of high-grade stage I epithelial ovarian cancer is three to four cycles of platinum-based combination chemotherapy. For higher-stage cancers, a total of six courses is recommended. If the patient is willing to undergo a second operation, pelvic and periaortic lymph nodes should be evaluated. In addition, pelvic and abdominal cytology should be obtained, an infracolic omentectomy performed, and multiple peritoneal biopsies taken from the pelvis, gutters, and diaphragmatic surfaces. Any suspicious lesions should also be biopsied. If no disease is found during this operation, the patient should receive only three to four cycles of systemic chemotherapy. The presence of any metastatic disease would warrant the complete six cycles. If the patient decides not to undergo the second operation, the complete treatment should be given. Close follow-up of the patient with CA-125 tumor marker in addition to pelvic and abdominal examinations every 3 to 4 months for 2 years and then every 6 months for a total of 5 years should be performed. Adequate and accurate staging can help to develop a need for adjuvant chemotherapy, and it can significantly affect the patient's prognosis.

References

1. Young RC, et al. Staging laparotomy in early ovarian cancer. JAMA 1983; 250:3072–3076.
2. Piver S, et al. Five year survival for stage 1C or stage 1 grade 3 epithelial ovarian cancer treated with cisplatinum-based chemotherapy. Gynecol Oncol 1992; 46:357–360.

PHYSICIAN'S RESPONSE

HOWARD W. JONES, III

Most gynecological oncologists have recommended postoperative chemotherapy for patients with poorly differentiated stage I ovarian cancer. So, even though this patient has not been adequately staged, she would still be a candidate for platinum-based combination chemotherapy. Reexploration with definitive staging would enable you to give her a more accurate prognosis, but I do not think it would improve her chance of survival. I would recommend she be treated with carboplatin (250 mg/m^2) and paclitaxel (Taxol) (135 mg/m^2) on an outpatient basis over 3 hr every 3 weeks for six cycles.

Recently, a large cooperative study from Italy has been reported which showed no difference in median length of survival for patients with stage I and stage II epithelial ovarian adenocarcinoma of all grades, whether they were treated initially with chemotherapy or merely followed and treated with chemotherapy only if they developed recurrent cancer (1). If postoperative observation with no immediate therapy were to be considered for this patient, reexploration with definitive staging is indicated to make sure that she does not have microscopic stage III disease, undiagnosed at the time of her original surgery. Studies suggest that about 33% of such patients who are not rigorously surgically/pathologically staged will be upstaged if they are re-explored (2).

(Note: Although I believe it is inappropriate as part of the formal consultation, I would try to educate this patient's surgeon on the important effect on survival and treatment planning of careful and complete operative staging in women with early ovarian cancer and the correct interpretation of ultrasound and CA-125 in the preoperative evaluation of women with adnexal masses.)

The question of a proper incision for such patients is a difficult one. Many gynecologists would recommend a midline incision in this patient, since there might be several reasons to be suspicious that she had malignant disease. However, it might have been equally likely that she had endometriosis, causing a mass with an elevated CA-125. In the case of young patients with no ascites or any other definitive evidence of ovarian cancer, it may be reasonable to explore them through a Pfannenstiel incision, since it is possible, in many patients, to do an omentectomy and to sample the diaphragm and even take some periaortic nodes through a low transverse incision, which could be converted to a Cherney by excising the rectus muscles from their insertion on the pubic symphysis.

Another option for patients with relatively small adnexal masses would be laparoscopy. If things look benign, the adnexal mass could be removed laparoscopically. If there was concern about the possibility of malignancy, a midline incision would then be possible. When an ovarian lesion is removed, frozen-section examination is recommended in any patient where gross inspection of the ovary shows external or internal papillations, solid nodules, or adhesions. This provides an accurate diagnosis in most cases and alerts the surgeon to the necessity for adequate staging.

References

1. Sartori E, Palai N, La Face B, et al. Eur J Gynaecol Oncol 1994; 15:188–198.
2. Hoskins WJ. Surgical staging and cytoreductive surgery of epithelial ovarian cancer. Cancer 1994; 71 (4 suppl):1534–1540.

PHYSICIANS' RESPONSE

BOB TAYLOR
ROBERT PARK

This unfortunate 44-year-old patient highlights one of the most controversial management issues in gynecological oncology: the preoperative diagnosis of early-stage ovarian cancer using ultrasound and CA-125.

Although we are not privy to the details of this case regarding the ultrasound, these would be of interest, particularly if one were to consider a more appropriate incision for ovarian cancer staging and ask a pathologist to render an intraoperative frozen-section diagnosis. Nonetheless, an admittedly suspicious mass associated with an elevated albeit premenopausal CA-125 was removed through a Pfannenstiel incision. The cavalier nature of the preoperative workup and response to the intraoperative findings lead us to question that a careful inspection of all peritoneal surfaces (particularly the upper abdomen) and retroperitoneal structures (pelvic and paraaortic lymph nodes) was done, nor would it be possible to accomplish such through a Pfannenstiel incision. We are thus faced with an inadequately staged patient who will certainly require adjuvant therapy.

We would recommend reexploration of this patient for complete staging based on the published data from Young et al., who found that 16% of seemingly stage IA ovarian cancers were upstaged (1). It is unreasonable to suggest that a chest x-ray and an abdominopelvic computed tomography scan can replace surgical staging, given the possibility of subclinical and microscopic metastases. An increased likelihood of finding advanced disease is based on the tumor biology, and in this case, a poorly differentiated histological phenotype may point to an increased chance of finding metastatic spread.

Any opposition to restaging this patient would likely be predicated on the fact that she will receive adjuvant treatment regardless of restaging due to her grade 3 tumor (2). If one were to assume that the clinical findings represented a stage IA grade 3 epithelial ovarian cancer, her current treatment options would include intraperitoneal radiocolloid phosphorus or systemic cisplatin/ cytoxan or cisplatin/paclitaxel combination therapy. We would counter this position on the basis of the potential for retroperitoneal metastases and the fact that the 5-mm penetration of the beta emission of intraperitoneal radiocolloid phosphorus would not sterilize this area adequately. In the presence of retroperitoneal or upper abdominal disease, systemic cytotoxic chemotherapy would be most appropriate.

Formal reexploration and staging would provide the most accurate assessment of disease extent and thus be considered prudent and a basis for further therapy recommendations. If the surgical pathology is negative for advanced-stage disease, the patient may be counseled for either intraperitoneal radiocolloid phosphorous after an adequate peritoneal distribution study or systemic combination cytotoxic chemotherapy. The findings of advanced-stage disease would certainly result in a recommendation for systemic cisplatin/paclitaxel combination therapy.

References

1. Young RC, Decker DG, Wharton JT, et al. Staging laparotomy in early ovarian cancer. JAMA 1983; 250:3072.
2. Young RC, Walton LA, Ellenberg SS, et al. Adjuvant therapy in stage I and stage II epithelial ovarian cancer: Results of two prospective randomized trials. N Engl J Med 1990; 322:1021.

31

Progressive Cervical Cancer in a Patient Who Wants "Everything Done"

CASE

A 27-year-old woman with 2 young children and a 1-year history of cervical cancer is discovered on CT scan to have progressive disease following definitive radiation therapy. Following your examination and review of the radiographic findings, the tumor appears to remain localized to the pelvis, but you conclude it is very unlikely the patient will benefit from surgery and the performance of an exenteration. However, the patient and her family tell you that they want you to proceed with the operation and want you to be "extremely aggressive," even if there is only 1 chance in 100 that she can be "cured" with the procedure.

PHYSICIANS' RESPONSE

M.S. PIVER
J. GOLDBERG

Although cervical cancer remains the leading cause of death from cancer in women around the world, the widespread use of cervical cytology has made it an uncommon malignancy in the United States and other industrialized nations. Patients with favorable lesions confined to the cervix can expect a cure rate of 90% or better, and even patients with stage III disease have a reasonable chance for cure, especially when the paraaortic lymph nodes are shown to be histologically negative by pretherapy surgical staging. However, patients who recur following definitive therapy have a poor prognosis. Systemic disease may re-

234

spond to chemotherapy but is not curable. If the recurrence is confined to the pelvis following radical hysterectomy, radiation therapy may effect a cure. However, for patients whose disease recurs in the pelvis following radiation therapy, pelvic exenteration is the only option for curative therapy.

An important criterion for selecting candidates for this procedure is patient willingness. The advent of procedures that preserve as much body image as possible—such as vaginal reconstruction, continent urinary diversion, and rectal reanastomosis—have made the procedure more acceptable. Nonetheless, the patient must be able to tolerate a major change in body image as well as demonstrate the willingness and ability to perform self-catheterization or care for ostomy appliances. Although age and medical problems are no longer considered absolute contraindications to this procedure, younger, more motivated patients seem to fare better. In the past, operative mortality has been reported around 10%, and major morbidity can occur in 40% or more of patients. The patient must be willing to accept these risks and, most especially, to cope with the complications that may follow the procedure.

If the patient consents to proceed, a thorough evaluation must be done to exclude extrapelvic metastases or tumor extending to the pelvic side wall. In addition to a thorough physical examination, computed tomography (CT) scans of the chest, abdomen, and pelvis should be performed. If the serum creatinine is elevated, ureteral obstruction from tumor must be ruled out. The presence of unilateral leg edema or sciatic pain is generally indicative of disease fixed to the pelvic side wall and hence unresectable. The addition of a magnetic resonance imaging (MRI) scan to the patient's evaluation may be helpful, since MRI has been shown to be more sensitive than CT or physical examination in delineating the extent of tumor involvement, especially in evaluating tumor fixed to the pelvic side wall. Magnetic resonance imaging also has the ability to differentiate between radiation changes and tumor. The sensitivity of MRI for parametrial extension has been reported to be better than 90%, and sensitivity for lymph node metastases is approximately 85%. However, specificity is not quite as high, and a positive MRI in the absence of other confirmatory tests should probably not preclude attempted exenteration.

Despite sophisticated modern imaging and biopsy techniques, exploratory laparotomy is often the required final determinant of a patient's eligibility for exenteration. At the time of surgery, the abdomen and pelvis are inspected for evidence of metastatic tumor that would prevent complete resection of the patient's disease. The paravesical and pararectal spaces are defined, and the cardinal ligaments (web) are examined for evidence of parametrial extension with fixation by tumor to the pelvic side wall—usually a contraindication to proceed. However, radiation fibrosis fixed to the pelvic side wall cannot always be distinguished from tumor fixation just by examining the web. In such circumstances, intraoperative biopsies may be obtained with a Tru-Cut needle. If the central recurrence cannot be resected with clear negative margins, then the procedure most often should be abandoned. However, if the procedure is completed and frozen-section evaluation of the specimen demonstrates histological evidence of tumor on the side wall margin, intraoperative radiation to the side wall may still result in an excellent long-term outcome.

Several factors have been shown to predict cure from an exenterative procedure. Masses that recur soon (< 6 months) after definitive radiation therapy, that are larger than 3 cm, or that impinge on the pelvic side wall are associated with a lower salvage rate. Metastatic disease in the lymph nodes carries a worse prognosis, and some authorities feel that nodal disease, like pelvic side-wall involvement, is a contraindication to proceeding with an exenterative procedure. However, 5-year survival rates as high as 26% have been reported in patients with metastatic pelvic nodal disease, so clearly some patients may do quite well.

As long as the patient appears to have disease confined to the pelvis that is not fixed to the pelvic side wall, she should be considered a candidate for exenteration. If the absence of extrapelvic metastasis is confirmed at laparotomy, then en bloc resection of the uterus with adjacent parametrium, fallopian tubes and ovaries, vagina, bladder, and rectosigmoid colon would be performed with dissection carried down to the level of the levator plate. The anal sphincter and urogenital diaphragm could be preserved. Because of the patient's age, vaginal reconstructive surgery and possibly rectal reanastomosis should be performed if feasible. If the terminal ileum does not demonstrate severe radiation changes, a continent urinary pouch utilizing the ileocecal valve may be constructed. The potential morbidity of the procedure and the chances for salvage need to be carefully discussed with this patient. However, given her age and family situation, she should be offered the only possible chance for cure by pelvic exenteration.

References

1. Rutledge FN, McGuffee VB. Pelvic exenteration: Prognostic significance of regional lymph node metastases. Gynecol Oncol 1987; 26:374–380.
2. Shingleton HM, Seng-Jaw S, Gelder MS, et al. Clinical and histopathologic factors predicting recurrence and survival after pelvic exenteration for cancer of the cervix. Obstet Gynecol 1989; 73:1027–1034.
3. Hicks ML, Piver MS, Mas E, et al. Intraoperative orthovoltage radiation therapy in the treatment of recurrent gynecologic malignancies. Am J Clin Oncol 1993; 16:497–500.

PHYSICIAN'S RESPONSE

H.G. BALL

This young patient has recurrence or progression of cervical cancer within one year of completion of radiation therapy. Progression is diagnosed on CT scan, but there is no indication as to the site of the progression. On the basis of the CT scan and examination of the patient, you conclude that the patient probably will not benefit from salvage surgery.

The initial procedure in this patient should be biopsy or fine needle aspiration of vaginal or cervical lesions to confirm the clinical impression of recurrent disease. Testing for human immunodeficiency virus (HIV) before considering this patient for aggressive therapy may be indicated. With disease confined to the central pelvis and no histologically confirmed disease on the pelvic side wall or beyond the pelvis, this patient is a candidate for pelvic exenteration. Computed tomography of the pelvis, abdomen, and lungs should be performed, looking for evidence of metastatic disease to the lungs, liver, and retroperitoneum. Ureteral obstruction of recent onset is a relative contraindication to exenteration, since this is usually due to cancer extension to the side wall rather than to radiation-induced fibrosis.

The only therapy accepted as curative for recurrent cancer of the cervix following radiation therapy is pelvic exenteration. Since we lack conclusive evidence of advanced disease, I would explore this patient even if pelvic examination suggests pelvic side-wall extension. It is frequently difficult to distinguish radiation fibrosis from tumor extension in this group of patients. At the time of exploratory surgery, biopsies of any suspicious pelvic or periaortic nodes as well as any peritoneal lesions suggestive of metastatic disease should be performed. Patients who have metastatic disease to the peritoneum, periaortic nodes, or other intraabdominal sites are not candidates for exenteration due to their poor survival following surgery. Patients who have received prior pelvic radiation therapy and have metastases to pelvic nodes at the time of exenteration have an estimated median survival less than 2 years.

If the site of disease progression is on the pelvic side wall, I would agree that this patient is not a candidate for pelvic exenteration. Disease on the pelvic side wall but confined to the pelvis may be amenable to radical resection, pelvic reconstruction, and placement of interstitial radiation therapy. Although limited information is available on long-term follow-up in patients treated with this approach, I would consider this option for very select patients with localized recurrent cancer of the cervix who are not otherwise candidates for a pelvic exenteration.

Although no information is available on the potential role of chemotherapy as an adjunct to pelvic exenteration, an interesting corollary is its use in the treatment of squamous cell cancer of the cervix as an adjunct to radical hysterectomy. In patients with bulky central disease who otherwise have no evidence of disease spread beyond the pelvis, the use of a limited number of courses of cisplatin (e.g., three) might be considered before surgical exploration. This would have the potential advantage of reducing the size of the central cancer, thereby decreasing the difficulty of obtaining adequate surgical margins and of destroying micrometastatic disease.

The patient's wish for "extremely aggressive" therapy deserves a comment. Although we should attempt to salvage this patient, it is not desirable to have a physically and emotionally crippled terminally ill patient. Radical procedures using surgery, radiation therapy, or chemotherapy should be used only when there is a reasonable expectation that our patients' lives will be prolonged for a time that will be meaningful to them and their families.

References

Höckel M, Knapstein PG. The combined operative and radiotherapeutic treatment (CORT) of recurrent tumors infiltrating the pelvic wall: First experience with 18 patients. Gynecol Oncol 1992; 46:20–28.

Miller B, Morris M. Rutledge F, et al. Aborted exenterative procedures in recurrent cervical cancer. Gynecol Oncol 1993; 50:94–99.

PHYSICIAN'S RESPONSE

MANUEL A. PENALVER

This patient, a 27-year-old woman who 1 year ago had a diagnosis of cervical cancer which was treated by radiation therapy, now has been noted to have recurrent disease which, by physical examination and radiological tests, does not appear to make the patient a suitable candidate for exenteration surgery.

To make a good decision on whether to attempt a pelvic exenteration for recurrent disease one should use data obtained from the history, physical examination, and radiological tests. The history should focus on the patient's emotional stability and well-being to be able to withstand an exenteration procedure and its long recuperation. A patient with psychiatric illness may be considered to be a poor candidate for this type of surgery. In this particular patient, from the history given, it appears that both the patient and the family are highly motivated and would be able to cope with the emotional stress brought about by this kind of operation. A thorough psychological evaluation of this patient should be undertaken before the operation is considered. Other important data would include a history of recent weight loss, which is suggestive of distant disease. Weight loss unaccompanied by metastatic disease is not considered a contraindication; however, these patients should receive nutritional consultation. A thorough history of medical illnesses such as hypertension, diabetes, and pulmonary disease should be sought. Only if these conditions severely decrease patient's ability to survive the exenteration procedure should the patient not be considered a candidate for the operation.

On physical examination, one should look for signs suggestive of unresectable disease. Unilateral leg edema and/or sciatic pain usually indicate pelvic side-wall disease, and resection of these patients yields few 5-year survivors.

Radiological tests that should be ordered include a chest x-ray, abdominal pelvic CT scan, and a barium enema. A chest x-ray is helpful in establishing pulmonary metastasis and in the preoperative diagnosis of pulmonary disease. In the abdominal/pelvic CT scan one is looking for any evidence of extrapelvic disease that would contraindicate exenteration. From the CT scan, one also obtains information on the urinary tract. The status of the urinary tract can be used as a predictor of resectability. Some 60% of patients with unilateral obstruction and 90% of those with bilateral obstruction are unresectable. Obstructive uropathy is a relative contraindication to exenterative surgery. The usual cause of obstructive uropathy is radiation therapy following recurrent cancer. Studies of the colon are performed to establish the presence of coexisting disease, benign or malignant.

In this particular patient, even though the patient seems unlikely to be resectable, further studies should be done before the operation is denied her. A fine needle aspiration or a CT-directed percutaneous needle aspiration of the side-wall should be done. Sometimes what appears to be unresectable disease because of extension to the pelvic side wall turns out to be radiation fibrosis. Only if there is unequivocal evidence by either fine needle aspiration or percutaneous biopsy should the patient not be given the opportunity to be explored for possible exenteration. If the results of these tests are unequivocal, the patient should still be explored for possible exenteration, since this is her last chance of cure.

If the exploratory laparotomy is done and the operation is carried out, the newer modalities that can improve the patient's quality of life should be made available to her. Some of these techniques include a low colorectal anastomosis with a temporary colostomy to avoid a permanent colostomy and continent urinary diversion, which avoids the need for an external urinary stoma. Again, the patient's psychological condition and ability to withstand the operation with its long recuperating period and the motivation needed to handle a continent urinary stoma are conditions that must be met before the patient is offered these modalities.

PHYSICIANS' RESPONSE

BABAK EDRAKI
PETER E. SCHWARTZ

Cervical cancer is the seventh most frequent malignancy in women in the United States. Despite a progressive decline in the incidence and mortality of cervical carcinoma, which is attributable to Pap smear screening, advanced cases are still encountered at a concerning frequency. In the United States, early stage cervical carcinoma (IA-1 to IIA) is treated preferentially by surgery. This preserves vaginal function and circumvents the complications associated with radiation. More advanced cases are treated primarily with radiation therapy.

Given that this patient's primary therapy was radiation, we can only assume that she presented at an advanced stage. Recurrence correlates well with patient's stage at presentation. Although the CT scan on this patient is suggestive of a recurrence, the diagnosis needs to be based on pathological evaluation of tissue. This can be achieved through a CT-guided biopsy. Assuming that the biopsy confirms the recurrence of the patient's carcinoma, a systematic method of evaluation needs to be employed in order to determine the best management approach. The CT scan of the abdomen and pelvis, as well as a chest x-ray, should be carefully reviewed for evidence of lymph node involvement, pelvic side-wall invasion, as well as distant metastases, all of which would be absolute contraindications to curative pelvic exenteration. An exenteration is considered only if the disease is central in location and there is no evidence of lymph node or distant metastases; the pelvic side walls should be free. The patient should have a good performance status and no sacral pain.

If this patient is not deemed an appropriate candidate based on the presence of pelvic lymph node metastases or extension to the side walls, then a newly described curative procedure can be attempted. This procedure, called the combined operative radiotherapeutic treatment (CORT) (1), was developed in Mainz, Germany, and consists of five parts: an exploratory laparotomy for detection of distant metastases; maximum tumor debulking at the side wall, including resection of pelvic musculature and bones, along with exenteration of all infiltrated central pelvic organs; placement of guiding tubes into residual tumor or the tumor bed at the pelvic wall; pelvic wall plasty with muscle flaps and omentum; and surgical reconstruction of bowel, bladder, and vulvovaginal areas. It is believed that the omentum and muscle flap plasty of the pelvic side wall lead to neoangiogenesis, increasing the radiotolerance, which, in turn, allows further brachytherapy through the guiding tubes. Sixty-one percent of patients treated in such a manner were found to be without evidence of disease with a median follow-up of 15 months. This is, however, a very complicated procedure with significant associated morbidity. In the United States, this procedure is still deemed experimental and has not achieved popularity.

Some authors do advocate palliative exenteration. In Stanhope and Symmonds's experience with 59 such patients (2), the survival rates were noted to be 47% at 2 years and 17% at 5 years. Other nonsurgical approaches should also be considered. The patient's records should be carefully scrutinized for assessment of candidacy for additional radiation therapy. Interstitial needle implants may provide a better tumor dose distribution and can be combined with pelvic lid construction to minimize the morbidity from the radiation. Chemotherapy is yet another modality that may be utilized in a palliative setting. Chambers et al., (3) have reported on the efficacy of the platinum, bleomycin, methotrexate, and 5-fluorouracil protocol and have noted a 30% response rate in recurrent disease. Eighty-six percent of those who responded achieved a complete response. The median duration of response was 10.5 months and an accrued survival advantage was noted in the responders with a median of 28 months versus the nonresponders with a median of 10 months.

Our approach to this particular patient would be to extensively and rationally counsel her and her family in regard to her prognosis and the above-described possibilities, after which a plan of management based on clinical appropriateness may be formulated, taking into account the patient's wishes.

References

1. Hockel M, Knapstein PG. The combined operative and radiotherapeutic treatment (CORT) of recurrent tumors infiltrating the pelvic wall: First experience with 18 patients. Gynecol Oncol 1992; 46:20–28.
2. Chambers SK, Lamb L, Kohom EI, et al. Chemotherapy of recurrent/advanced cervical cancer: Results of the Yale University PMB-PFU protocol. Gynecol Oncol 1994; 53:161–169.
3. Stanhope CR, Symmonds RE. Palliative exenteration: What, when, and why? Am J Obstet Gynecol 1985; 152:12–16.

PHYSICIAN'S RESPONSE

FRANK MAJOR

The likelihood of obtaining a cure in this particular patient is colored by the short duration from time of original diagnosis to time of recurrence. However, at this point, we have only a high index of suspicion for recurrence of malignancy. The diagnosis must be confirmed histologically, and either a transvaginal needle biopsy may be performed or a dilation and curettage (D&C) with generous endocervical biopsy may yield results. If neither of these are feasible, I would strongly consider a CT-guided fine needle aspiration to confirm the diagnosis of recurrent disease. Once that diagnosis has been confirmed, extensive evaluation needs to be carried out to rule out any other evidence of metastatic disease within the lung. A bone scan would also be appropriate, although I would anticipate a very low yield in an asymptomatic patient. Supraclavicular biopsy may be considered, but I feel the overall yield in patients with no evidence of pulmonary disease and with no palpable adenopathy is low. Evaluation of the bladder by cystoscopy, and of the colon by colonoscopy, should also be performed to determine if there is any evidence of involvement of these organs with recurrent disease. With all of these studies showing no evidence of distant metastasis, I would then proceed to discuss with the patient the operative possibilities. The patient would understand that frozen sections of pelvic and paraaortic lymph nodes would be obtained, and should there be any evidence of nodal disease outside of the pelvis, certainly chemotherapy would be a viable option. Discussion of treatment with chemotherapy in lieu of surgery would center on the fact that we have responses for varying periods of time with chemotherapy, but we can report no cures with chemotherapy in cancer of the cervix. The patient and her family, with this understanding may choose to go with the surgical approach, and we would also mention the possibility of intraoperative radiation, which could be carried out should the surgical procedure appear to not be curative at the time of exploration. I would emphasize that we would only perform the extensive resection of pelvic organs if there were no evidence of disease beyond the margins of such resection. The use of intraoperative radiation therapy could be accomplished after selective debulking of recurrent cervical cancer and might well be directed against pelvic side-wall disease. This would be carried out in one of two modalities, either with the use of an intraoperative cone to direct a bolus of electron beam therapy to a specific area 7 cm or less in diameter during the open operation, or with polyethylene tubes that could be implanted in the bed of tumor which has been debulked on the pelvic side wall or the presacral area. Later the patient could be subjected to radiation therapy through these tubes via the high-dose-rate brachytherapy machine. The patient and family would be told that such treatment has no track record in producing a cure but has produced palliation and, coupled with subsequent chemotherapy, might provide an option for possible cure, although there are no proven data to substantiate this at present.

In summary, we would accede to the patient's desire to purse every opportunity for cure by agreeing to an exploratory procedure, with the understanding that exenteration would be carried out only in the face of frozen-section evidence of clear margins and negative lymph nodes.

References

1. Delgado G, Goldson AL, Ashayeri E, et al. Intraoperative radiation in the treatment of advanced clinical cancer. Obstet Gynecol 1984; 63:246–257.
2. Brady L, Rotman M, Calvo F. New advances in radiation oncology for gynecologic cancer. Cancer 1992; 71:1652–1654.

32

Abnormal Radiolabeled Antibody Scan in an Ovarian Cancer Patient

CASE

A 67-year-old woman is found to have stage IIIC ovarian cancer. Following laparotomy and optimal tumor debulking, she is treated with six courses of cisplatin and paclitaxel (Taxol). The CA-125, which had been 386 prior to the initiation of chemotherapy, returns into the normal range.

Six months following the completion of therapy, the patient remains asymptomatic but a repeat CA-125 increases to 97 (108 on repeat testing). Pelvic examination and repeat computed tomography (CT) are unremarkable. A radiolabeled antibody scan is performed and demonstrates uptake only in the left pelvic region.

PHYSICIAN'S RESPONSE

WILLIAM McGUIRE

This patient obviously has recurrent ovarian carcinoma 6 months after the completion of chemotherapy, based on the rising CA-125 and possibly based upon the radiolabeled antibody scan. While there remains significant controversy over the value of secondary cytoreductive surgery, there is probably adequate basis to explore this patient. This is predicated on the fact that at least one test, the Oncoscint scan, suggests disease in the left pelvis. If this is the only site of disease and it can be completely resected, most surgeons feel that these patients have a better outcome than those who are simply treated with some form of systemic therapy. It must be pointed out, however, that there are no randomized data to verify this. This belief is based on retrospective analysis of secondary cytoreductive procedures.

At exploration, it may be that the Oncoscint scan is a false positive and no macroscopic disease is discovered. At this point, multiple biopsies should be taken to look for intraperitoneal microscopic disease, and any enlarged retroperitoneal lymph nodes should be sampled. If histopathology shows persistent or recurrent microscopic disease in the peritoneal cavity and absence of disease on the basis of retroperitoneal node sampling, then consideration should be given to intraperitoneal therapy with cisplatin. A recent trial of intraperitoneal cisplatin as part of primary therapy in low-volume disease demonstrated a survival advantage over the use of the same compound intravenously. Although there are no similar randomized data in the salvage setting, there are significant phase II data suggesting that approximately 30% of patients with microscopic disease can be rendered disease-free at the time of the third laparotomy after the application of intraperitoneal therapy. Median survival in these responders is in excess of 3 years. This does not, of course, equate with cure, since it may take many months for such small-volume disease to grow to a point that it becomes clinically evident.

Should no disease be found at the time of reexploration, I would withhold chemotherapy. This is also controversial, and there seems to be greater reliance today on small changes in CA-125 as reflective of either response or progression of the tumor. There are, however, reports of discordance between tumor volume and CA-125 values, and guiding treatment solely by CA-125 analysis is not medically justified based on existing data.

Thus, in summary, I would explore this patient and resect disease only if all disease can be resected. For unresectable disease or nodal disease, the patient could be retreated with paclitaxel (Taxol) as a single agent or carboplatin as a single agent, since she has had more than 6 treatment-free months. There are few data to justify the use of combination therapy in the salvage setting, however. If the patient has microscopic disease only, consideration should be given to intraperitoneal therapy with cisplatin. If no disease is found, then a watch-and-wait approach seems appropriate.

PHYSICIAN'S RESPONSE

MICHAEL GOLDBERG

I am assuming that this patient has a stage IIIC *epithelial* ovarian carcinoma. She has been optimally debulked, had six courses of paclitaxel/platinum, and at the completion of chemotherapy had a normal CA-125, down from a preoperative value of 386. The CA-125, now 6 months later, has risen to over 100, but the patient persists in having negative pelvic exams and CT scans, although a radiolabeled antibody scan shows uptake in the left pelvic region. In such a situation we must assume that this patient has recurrent ovarian carcinoma. In a patient whose CA-125 is significantly elevated prior to initial surgical debulking and then falls to normal with chemotherapy, the demonstration of a reelevation of the CA-125 which is persistent and progressive must be assumed to be due to recurrent disease unless some other specific cause can be found. It would be of interest in this case to know how quickly the CA-125 normalized, since values that approach zero within 2 months of the initiation of treatment are usually followed by long periods of disease quiescence, as opposed to those patients in whom the CA-125 falls gradually into the upper limits of normal, where rapid recurrence of disease frequently follows the termination of active chemotherapy.

The two questions here relate to how long one wishes to observe an "asymptomatic" patient with rising CA-125s before reinitiating therapy and whether or not there is a role for secondary surgery and debulking of disease. One must naturally ask what type of operative candidate this patient at age 67 is, since the morbidity of such surgery can be quite significant. Second, one needs to know the topographical nature of the tumor at first operation, since small nodules on the diaphragm or extensive miliary disease in the abdomen and pelvis, if present at initial surgery, would almost certainly once again not be removable. If positive paraaortic nodes were present at the initial surgery, the disease, by virtue of its retroperitoneal spread, would probably contraindicate a second surgical adventure. We would also like to know if disease was present in significant bulk in the left lower quadrant and whether that represented the major focus of residual tumor at the termination of the original surgery. Perhaps the major question in this case is whether, philosophically, reoperation in patients with persistent/recurrent disease and attempts at secondary debulking plays any role in the management of epithelial ovarian carcinoma. In the present case, we are really not talking about a "second-look" operation, which is designed to determine if, after a course of chemotherapy in a patient assumed to be clinically free of disease (pelvic exams, CA-125, CT scan), the patient is biologically/histologically disease-free. The major purpose of that operation is to determine the advisability of terminating chemotherapy. In the present situation we have a patient with a presumption of disease, and surgery would be entertained only toward the option of achieving optimal secondary debulking. Unfortunately, at this point it is not possible to conclusively demonstrate that secondary cytoreduction in a patient with recurrent ovarian carcinoma alters the quality of life or influences long-term survival. Several excellent reviews are available in this regard and are referenced here. In the absence of a CT scan demonstrating disease, it is almost certain that none of the tumor nodules are more than 2 cm in maximum diameter. If we can agree on anything relative to secondary cytoreduction, it is that only an operation which renders the patient macroscopically free of disease can influence long-term survival. Because of gray areas, however, it is important for the patient to play a role in making the final decision in this type of case. In this patient, if the only major disease left at the termination of the first operation was in the left lower quadrant, if the diaphragm was essentially free of disease, the retroperitoneal nodes negative, and the patient was a good operative candidate, I would agree to surgery in an attempt to rid her of possible recurrence in that area—providing and only providing that she wanted to take an aggressive approach toward the malignancy, understood our inability to guarantee the effectiveness of secondary cytoreduction, and understood the risks of that operation. I have had this discussion with many patients and it is among the most difficult in the practice of gynecological oncology. Unless the circumstances were specifically as indicated above, it is difficult to believe that surgery would be of value. I would then repeat the CA-125 in 3 weeks, and if the expected rise occurred, would reinstitute chemotherapy, recognizing that we were now in a salvage mode. My choice of drugs would probably call for reinstitution of the same medications to which the patient had shown sensitivity. If she did not respond rapidly, I would drop the platinum combination and utilize alternatives such as ifosfamide, doxorubicin (Adriamycin), and hexamethylmelamine. A final option in this patient would be to observe her without therapy in the event that the CA-125 was rising but rising at a very slow rate. I think this is an acceptable alternative as long as the patient is informed that you do, in fact, believe the rise represents disease, but it can be continued only until the levels start jumping to where they are practically doubling every 4 to 6 weeks.

References

Potter ME. Secondary cytoreduction in ovarian cancer: Pro or Con? Gynecol Oncol 1993;
    51:131–135.
Markman M. Follow-up of the asymptomatic patient with ovarian cancer. Gynecol Oncol
    1994; 55:S134–S137.

PHYSICIAN'S RESPONSE

TATE THIGPEN

Several considerations form the basis for a proper management approach to this case. First, for a full discussion of management options, it must be assumed that the patient has no major health problems that might interfere with certain treatment alternatives. For example, renal and hepatic function should be normal. The patient should not have major cardiac problems and should not suffer from other life-threatening illnesses. She should preferably not be a diabetic and not be nutritionally depleted. Second, the patient is 67 years old. Because ovarian carcinoma appears to be a more biologically aggressive disease in older patients, any recurrence should prompt immediate and early intervention. Third, the patient was clearly a clinical complete responder to initial cisplatin/paclitaxel therapy based on lack of evidence of clinical disease at the conclusion of chemotherapy and the return of a significantly elevated CA-125 of 386 to a normal range (presumably less than 35). Fourth, the patient experienced a clinical disease-free interval of 6 months before developing evidence suggestive of recurrence. Although the evidence is entirely that of an elevated marker (CA-125 of 97), repeat testing confirms the elevation (108) and is associated with one area of abnormality on an antibody scan of the abdomen. Such an elevation of the CA-125 is virtually certain to reflect recurrence of disease.

This patient should undergo an exploratory laparotomy to look for evidence of recurrence of ovarian carcinoma. In the absence of gross disease, the surgeon should be prepared to conduct a thorough search of the entire abdominal cavity and to perform multiple biopsies of apparently uninvolved peritoneum. If gross disease is present, the surgeon should assess the possibility of complete resection of all gross disease and, if all gross disease can be resected, carry out the resection. The weight of evidence suggests that the patients who benefit from such secondary surgical cytoreduction are those who responded to initial chemotherapy (as did this patient) and who can be secondarily cytoreduced to a state of no gross residual.

Alternatives to immediate reexploration would be continued observation with repeat CA-125 and CT scanning of the abdomen and pelvis within 3 to 6 months; initiation of salvage chemotherapy on the basis of the elevated CA-125 alone without reexploration; or laparoscopy to document recurrence, followed by salvage chemotherapy. The problem with continued observation with repeat CA-125 and CT scanning is the relatively short treatment-free interval (6 months) and the age of the patient, both of which suggest that the recurrence, if present, is likely to be biologically aggressive. Even a 3- to 6-month delay could result in a deterioration of the patient's performance and nutritional status and a decreased likelihood of response to salvage therapy. The negative to initiation of salvage chemotherapy without further documentation include the possibility that the patient has not recurred (admittedly an unlikely possibility) and the loss of any opportunity to carry out secondary surgical cytoreduction. The downside to laparoscopy includes the inability to assess carefully the entire peritoneal surface should gross disease not be present and the loss of any opportunity to carry out secondary surgical cytoreduction. Although the reexploration does result in some additional risk, the potential benefits outweigh the risks and support this approach in preference to the alternatives, especially in light of the negatives cited above for the alternatives.

If recurrent disease is documented at the exploratory laparotomy, the patient should be treated with paclitaxel 135 mg/m^2 over a 24 hr followed by cisplatin 75 mg/m^2. The bases for this recommendation are the demonstrated superiority of this combination over other nonpaclitaxel regimens in previously untreated patients, the apparent initial response to chemotherapy, and the 6-month disease-free interval. The first factor, the choice of regimen, is based on a randomized phase III trial of the Gynecologic Oncology Group showing a more than 50% improvement in survival with paclitaxel/cisplatin as compared to cyclophospha- mide/cisplatin in previously untreated large-volume disease (median survival 38 months versus 24 months), thus establishing this regimen as the standard of care for advanced ovarian carcinoma. The latter two factors suggest that the disease process is still clinically sensitive to the original chemotherapy. In such a "sensitive" patient population, response rates as high as 60% have been reported in the salvage setting. The recommendation assumes that the patient experi- enced no prohibitive toxicity with the initial chemotherapy and that there is no residual nephrotoxicity or neurotoxicity that would preclude the use of one or both drugs.

Potential alternatives to paclitaxel/cisplatin include paclitaxel infusion dura- tions; paclitaxel/carboplatin; intraperitoneal therapy; high-dose chemotherapy with autologous bone marrow support or peripheral blood progenitor cells; or the use of other systemic agents such as tamoxifen, ifosfamide, or hexamethyl- melamine. With regard to the first of these, alternative paclitaxel infusion durations, both shorter (1- or 3-hr) and longer (96-hr) durations have been sug- gested. The mechanism of action for paclitaxel involves bundling of tubulin and focuses on cells in late G_2 or early M phase of the cell cycle. In theory, the drug should be more active if given as a prolonged infusion. Evidence to date shows minor differences between the 3- and 24-hr infusions in the salvage setting, but response rates as high as 28% have been reported with a 96-hr infusion in patients who have failed shorter infusion. The preference for a 24-hr infusion in this patient is based on the fact that this is the only infusion length tested to date in a major randomized trial in previously untreated patients. Although this patient has had prior exposure to paclitaxel, this prior exposure resulted in a response with a significant treatment-free interval before relapse. Until shorter or longer infusions have been tested in patients such as this in randomized trials, the infusion length should conform to results from randomized trials in front-line therapy.

With regard to the substitution of carboplatin for cisplatin in the combina- tion, randomized trials looking at nonpaclitaxel carboplatin-based combinations compared to the same regimen based on cisplatin suggest that the two drugs are therapeutic equivalents. The lack of a randomized trial of carboplatin com- bined with paclitaxel and the known success of the combination of paclitaxel and cisplatin makes the cisplatin-based combination preferable until more data are available.

As to the option of intraperitoneal therapy, both cisplatin and paclitaxel can be given intraperitoneally. A randomized trial of intravenous cyclophospha- mide/cisplatin versus intravenous cyclophosphamide plus intraperitoneal cisplatin in patients with small-volume residual stage III disease shows a survival advantage for the intraperitoneal regimen (median survival 49 months versus 41 months favoring the intraperitoneal regimen). The marked improvement in survival in large-volume disease noted with the addition of paclitaxel to front-line therapy plus the lack of data on the use of intraperitoneal paclitaxel in combination with intraperitoneal cisplatin make the preferable choice in this case the intravenous combination.

With regard to the high-dose chemotherapy option, the value of such an approach has never been tested in a randomized trial. Data available from randomized trials show no advantage to a doubling of the dose intensity. The two best drugs in ovarian carcinoma, cisplatin and paclitaxel, are not ideal candidates for further dose escalation. Additionally, high-dose chemotherapy with marrow support is associated with a small but significant mortality as well as significant morbidity. Until randomized trials show the merit of such an approach, its use should be reserved for clinical trials.

With regard to the option of alternative chemotherapy, such approaches are far less effective than repeat paclitaxel/cisplatin in the patient with disease that has responded to initial therapy and remained in remission for a period of 6 or more months. Available agents that induce responses produce response rates of 15 to 20% in resistant patients and 20 to 30% in patients with sensitive disease. By far the better approach in this patient would thus appear to be the use of repeat paclitaxel/cisplatin if in fact recurrent disease is documented.

References

1. Alberts D, Liu P, Hannigan E, et al. Phase III study of intraperitoneal cisplatin/intravenous cyclophosphamide vs intravenous cisplatin/intravenous cyclophosphamide in patients with optimal disease stage 4 III ovarian cancer: A SWOG-GOG-ECOG intergroup study. Proc ASCO 1995; 14:273.
2. Hoskins W, Bundy B, Thigpen T, et al. The influence of cytoreductive surgery on recurrence-free interval and survival in small volume stage III epithelial ovarian cancer: A Gynecologic Oncology Group study. Gynecol Oncol 1992; 47:159–166.
3. McGuire WP, Hoskins W, Brady M, et al. Taxol and cisplatin improves outcome in advanced ovarian cancer as compared to cytoxan and cisplatin. Proc ASCO 1995; 14:275.
4. McGuire WP, Rowinsky E. Old drugs revisited, new drugs, and experimental approaches in ovarian cancer therapy. Semin Oncol 1991; 18:255–269.
5. Ozols R, Young R. Chemotherapy of ovarian cancer. Semin Oncol 1991; 18:222–232.
6. Thigpen T. High-dose chemotherapy with autologous bone marrow support in ovarian carcinoma: The bottom line, more or less. Gynecol Oncol 1995; 57:275–277.
7. Thigpen T, Vance R, Puneky L, Khansur T. Chemotherapy in advanced ovarian carcinoma: Current standard of care based on randomized trials. Gynecol Oncol 1994; 55:S97–S107.

PHYSICIANS' RESPONSE

THOMAS V. SEDLACEK
MAX A. CLARK

The patient is 67 years old and is now 6 months post–initial chemotherapy; she has an elevated CA-125 and an abnormal immunoscintigraphic scan in the left pelvic region.

The immediate question is whether the patient has recurrent ovarian carcinoma. The CA-125 had been elevated prior to chemotherapy and had returned to normal with treatment. After a 6 month interval, it has again become elevated. Rubin et al. have shown that in cases such as this a secondarily rising CA-125 almost always indicates persistent disease. Other investigators have observed a 93% sensitivity with recurrent disease. The CA-125 may be elevated more than 1 year prior to the detection of clinical disease.

However, the CA-125 can be elevated in a number of other malignant conditions, such as colon cancer, breast cancer, pancreatic cancers, lung cancers, and cancers of the uterus and tube. The CA-125 may be elevated in benign conditions such as pelvic inflammatory disease, endometriosis, and inflammatory conditions of the bowel. The patient should have a colon evaluation, especially with a positive radionuclide scan in the left pelvis.

Next, the patient should undergo a reassessment laparotomy. During this restaging it can be ascertained histologically if the patient does indeed have a recurrence. Some authors rely on laboratory data and would omit a celiotomy, moving directly to treatment. However, this approach does not allow for secondary tumor debulking. While the benefits of secondary cytoreductive surgery have not been clearly established, approximately 10 to 30% of patients can be successfully cytoreduced. Leusley et al. have shown that there seems to be little survival advantage for patients who have been secondarily cytoreduced to microscopic disease when compared to patients cytoreduced to macroscopic disease. However studies by Hoskins have revealed a 5-year survival rate of greater than 50% when disease is reduced to microscopic levels. The use of whole abdominal radiation has been shown to be effective, especially with small-volume disease, which this patient seems to exhibit. Dembo has reported long-term survivors using whole abdominal radiation doses of 2000 to 3000 cGy in patients with microscopic disease.

Another advantage of laparotomy is the ability to use intraoperative radiation for any localized disease. If the tumor cannot be treated intraoperatively, then any localized disease can be marked for later postoperative radiation boosts to the area. After the patient has recovered postoperatively, our recommendation would be to start treatment with whole abdominal radiation with a boost to any localized areas. This is usually well tolerated, but up to 14% of patients will have posttreatment bowel obstruction requiring resection.

Second-line chemotherapy has produced few long-term survivors. However, ovarian cancer patients who have a disease-free interval of 6 months or longer after initial treatment with a cisplatin-based regimen will respond approximately 30% of the time to retreatment with cisplatin or carboplatin. If peripheral neuropathy was noted with the initial cisplatin treatment, the carboplatin should be considered. If severe hematological toxicities were noted with the initial cisplatin treatment, the carboplatin should probably be avoided and retreatment with cisplatin considered.

Ifosfamide has shown an overall 20% response rate when used as salvage chemotherapy in ovarian cancer patients. Other agents such as VP-16, 5-fluorouracil, mitomycin-C, and vinblastine have all shown low response rates when used as salvage chemotherapy. When salvage chemotherapy regimens have been combined, they have been found to be more toxic and no real survival advantage has been noted.

Newer therapies may offer some hope to patients with recurrent disease. High-dose chemotherapy with autologous bone marrow transplantation (ABMT) has been shown to achieve complete remission in over 40% of patients with persistent disease at second-look laparotomy. This treatment, while terribly expensive, may offer salvage and long-term survival to some patients. A cheaper and equally effective approach utilizes high-dose chemotherapy and autologous stem-cell transfusion.

Recommendations:

1. Exploratory laparotomy with cytoreduction if possible
2. Intraoperative radiation therapy if appropriate
3. Intraoperative marking of any localized areas of tumor for postoperative radiation boost
4. Postoperative whole abdominal radiation therapy
5. Consideration of postradiation high-dose chemotherapy with autologous stem-cell transfusion

References

Berek JS, et al. Survival of patients following secondary cytoreductive surgery in ovarian cancer: Obstet Gynecol 1983; 61:189.

Dembo AJ. Abdominopelvic radiotherapy in ovarian cancer: 10 year experience. Cancer 1985; 55:2285.

PHYSICIAN'S RESPONSE

R. GERALD PRETORIUS

There is little controversy over the initial treatment of this 67-year-old woman with stage IIIC epithelial (I assume) ovarian cancer who had an elevated CA-125 prior to therapy. Current standard treatment includes tumor debulking followed by cisplatin or carboplatin and paclitaxel. If, at the conclusion of six courses of chemotherapy, the CA-125 had normalized and the patient was clinically without evidence of disease, I would follow her.

(The case presentation does not state whether the patient underwent second-look surgery. I have not found that the literature supports the notion that second-look surgery influences survival in women with epithelial ovarian cancer.)

If, 6 months later, the patient's CA-125 increased to 97 (108 on repeat) and her examination and CT scan were unremarkable, I would presume that she had persistent ovarian cancer and would treat her with megestrol acetate (Megace) 40 mg qid. I would not perform the radiolabeled antibody scan because it would not provide me with any additional information. Knowing the location of the recurrence would not change the subsequent treatment. When and if the patient progressed on megestrol, I would encourage her to enter a hospice program. If she desired further therapy, I would suggest that she enter one of the Gynecologic Oncology Group (GOG) phase I trials (e.g., protocol 124 with high-dose carboplatin and ifosfamide/mesna with bone marrow rescue).

Second-line therapy in women with advanced epithelial ovarian cancer who have early failure following platinum-based chemotherapy is not particularly effective. Second-line therapy with intraperitoneal chemotherapy, intravenous chemotherapy, hormonal manipulation, whole abdominal radiation, reoperation with the intent of secondary debulking, or high-dose chemotherapy with bone marrow rescue all appear equally ineffective. It appears that the second-line therapy more often simply selects the population with less aggressive cancers rather than significantly affecting survival.

Megestrol would be my choice of therapy because a small portion of patients will respond to it as second-line therapy and it is the least toxic of these treatments. If the recurrence had appeared later (for example, 3 years following chemotherapy) and seemed to be resectable, I would perform laparotomy with an attempt at removing the tumor. I would probably follow this surgery with retreatment with platinum-based combination chemotherapy.

Reference

Giesler HE. Megestrol acetate for the palliation of advanced ovarian carcinoma. Obstet Gynecol 1983; 61:95.

PHYSICIANS' RESPONSE

JOHN T. COMERCI
CAROLYN D. RUNOWICZ

This patient's rise in CA-125 suggests that she has recurrent or persistent small-volume disease. The positive predictive value of a rising CA-125 following first-line chemotherapy approaches 100% for patients with ovarian cancer. It is not surprising that the pelvic examination and computed tomography (CT) scan are reported as negative, as epithelial ovarian carcinoma frequently recurs or persists as diffuse implants (< 1 cm) over the peritoneal surfaces. The sensitivity of CT for disease detection is directly proportional to lesion size. A negative CT scan does not exclude microscopic disease or macroscopic tumor (< 1 cm). Radioimmunoscintigraphy may be more sensitive than CT in detecting occult recurrent disease. A laparoscopy or an exploratory laparotomy to confirm persistent disease is unnecessary in view of the abnormal radioimmunoscintigraphy and elevated tumor marker. The question then becomes: What type of salvage therapy should be offered to the patient with small-volume recurrent/persistent disease following treatment with first-line paclitaxel and cisplatin?

The balance of evidence suggests that treatment results with radiation therapy, either external or intraperitoneal chromic phosphate (^{32}P) are disappointing. This is probably due to cross-resistance between platinum-based chemotherapy and irradiation as well as an accelerated proliferation of resistant clonogenic tumor cells following cytoreductive chemotherapy. Furthermore, most studies of abdominopelvic radiotherapy following chemotherapy have reported significant complication rates.

Patients who progress during platinum-based treatment, those with stable disease, and those who relapse within 6 months are considered to have platinum-refractory disease. Patients who respond and have a progression-free interval of greater than 6 months off treatment are defined as platinum-sensitive. Response rates of less than 10% are observed for patients with a treatment-free interval of less than 6 months. The observed response rate rises as the treatment-free interval lengthens, with rates as high as 90% for patients with an interval greater than 21 months.

The fact that this patient has evidence of recurrence within 6 months following platinum-based induction chemotherapy indicates that she most likely has platinum-refractory disease. Unfortunately, this patient's disease may also have developed resistance to paclitaxel. With respect to retreatment with paclitaxel, there are no data using standard paclitaxel doses and schedules for patients with ovarian cancer. At present, we do not know if the antitumor effect of paclitaxel may be improved with longer infusion times. In patients with breast cancer resistant to anthracyclines, a 50% response rate has been reported using a 96-hr paclitaxel infusion. A 33% response rate has been demonstrated with 96-hr paclitaxel infusion in breast cancer patients who had progressive disease on a 3-hr paclitaxel infusion schedule. Longer infusion schedules are being studied in patients with ovarian cancer.

Currently available chemotherapies in this setting (ifosfamide, etoposide, hexamethylmelamine) have response rates of approximately 15 to 20%. In view of these poor response rates, this patient would be enrolled in a phase II study evaluating topotecan at our institution. Phase I studies have shown activity in platinum-resistant patients with ovarian cancer. Topotecan, CPT-11, and 9-amino-camptothecin are topoisomerase I inhibitors.

Other drugs being evaluated in phase I/II settings include gemcitabine, pyra-zoloacridine, treosulfan, and new platinum analogs. Therapies focusing on novel molecular targets, such as antiangiogenesis agents, antimetastatic agents, and signal transduction inhibitors are in phase I testing.

Patients with recurrent disease should be enrolled in clinical trials so that new drugs can be identified in ovarian cancer.

33

Recurrent Ovarian Cancer 4 Years After Initial Diagnosis

CASE

A 64-year-old completely asymptomatic woman with a history of ovarian cancer is referred to you for a second opinion concerning management of recurrent disease. She was diagnosed as having stage IIIB ovarian cancer 4 years ago, having achieved a clinically defined complete response following treatment with 6 monthly courses of cisplatin and cyclophosphamide. On a routine follow-up visit, a 3- by 4-cm movable, nontender, pelvic mass is noted. This was not appreciated on an examination performed 6 months earlier. CA-125, which had been normal since after the third course of chemotherapy, has risen to 49. A computed tomography (CT) scan of the abdomen and pelvis confirms the presence of the pelvic mass, a small amount of ascites, and a suspicious 1- by 1-cm defect in the right lobe of the liver but is otherwise unremarkable. No prior CT is available for comparison.

PHYSICIANS' RESPONSE

THOMAS J. RUTHERFORD
JOSEPH T. CHAMBERS

The crux of the problem in deciding upon an approach to this patient is whether or not the lesion in the liver represents metastatic ovarian carcinoma. A biopsy of this is best performed under ultrasound or CT direction.

Although not firmly established, there is evidence that secondary tumor debulking for recurrent epithelial ovarian cancer confers a survival advantage provided that the patient has a good performance status, the recurrence is isolated and mobile, and the disease-free interval exceeds 1 year. In one study, following initial aggressive cytoreductive surgery and platinum-based chemotherapy, 100 patients with recurrent or progressive epithelial ovarian cancer underwent a secondary cytoreduction. Sixty-one patients were left with residual disease less than 2 cm in diameter. The median survival was 27.1 months in the optimally debulked group versus 9.0 months for others ($p = 0.0001$). Other factors found significant for improved survival included age (< 55 years), interval from initial diagnosis (more than 12 months), residual disease at initial staging surgery (less than 2 cm), and a complete clinical response to a form of platinum-based front-line chemotherapy.

Presumably this patient has an excellent performance status and is a good surgical candidate. Although nothing is known about her initial surgery, we assume on the basis of her initial response, that she was optimally debulked. The pelvic mass is mobile and she has had a prolonged disease-free interval. If the biopsy of the liver lesion was negative for carcinoma, then surgical exploration should be considered for secondary debulking, to be followed by additional systemic therapy.

Many patients with recurrent disease demonstrate isolated lesions on imaging studies but upon laparotomy have diffuse intraabdominal disease. If the surgeon is skilled, a laparoscopic approach might be attempted. If there is diffuse nondebulkable disease, the surgical approach should be aborted and the patient offered alterative therapy. If the liver biopsy was positive for carcinoma, the concern is that optimal debulking could not be achieved in this patient. An aggressive surgical approach would be a liver resection if all other disease could be resected. However, if surgery is performed and the liver lesion is the only remaining disease, an experimental approach might be cryosurgery, although its efficacy has not been established.

If the patient refuses surgical exploration but desires further therapy or additional therapy is indicated, then chemotherapy is an option. This patient's tumor should be platinum-sensitive and could be retreated on a platinum-based regimen anticipating up to a 59% response rate, since the disease-free interval has been longer than 2 years. In a Gynecologic Oncology Group (GOG) trial, patients treated with paclitaxel (Taxol) as a salvage regimen had a 30% overall response rate; more importantly, in patients who were platinum-sensitive, the overall response rate was 50%. In this patient, we would recommend a combination of platinum and paclitaxel.

On the other hand, if the liver biopsy was positive for metastatic disease, there is an argument for not offering any therapy until the patient becomes symptomatic. Since she has a good quality of life, surgical intervention or chemotherapy could have detrimental effect on her quality of life with no realistic chance for cure. When she becomes symptomatic, one could institute palliative therapy.

References

Markman M, Rothman R, Hakes T, et al. Second-line platinum therapy in patients with ovarian cancer previously treated with cisplatin. J Clin Oncol 1991; 9:389–393.

Segna RA, Dottino PR, Mandeli JP, et al. Secondary cytoreduction for ovarian cancer following cisplatin therapy. J Clin Oncol 1993; 11:434–439.

PHYSICIAN'S RESPONSE

R.F. OZOLS

The treatment of recurrent ovarian carcinoma is dependent upon several factors. Among the most important are the nature of the initial response to chemotherapy and the duration of the disease-free interval. In this particular case, the patient had an excellent response to initial chemotherapy and rapidly achieved a clinical complete remission with normalization of her CA-125 after three cycles of chemotherapy. She did not undergo second-look laparotomy and remained disease-free for 4 years, at which time there was physical and radiological evidence of a recurrence. In addition, the CA-125 has risen to 49. The first step would be to obtain tissue confirmation of recurrent ovarian cancer. CT-directed biopsy is a safe, reliable way to obtain adequate tissue to compare with the original histology. Late recurrences from ovarian cancer unfortunately are not uncommon; however, it is possible that this represents metastatic disease from another primary. Mammography and breast palpation are indicated in this patient to rule out breast cancer, which has an increased risk in patients with ovarian cancer.

In all probability the histological diagnosis will confirm that this is recurrent ovarian cancer. With such a long disease-free interval and an excellent response to cisplatin, the patient has a very high probability of having a secondary response of cisplatin or carboplatin. Prior to the availability of paclitaxel, the treatment of choice would have been with carboplatin, because of its more favorable toxicity profile. The addition of cyclophosphamide to carboplatin to treat patients with a long disease-free intervals has not been shown to be beneficial. However, some investigators may feel that this represents a second primary peritoneal tumor; consequently combination chemotherapy with carboplatin and cyclophosphamide, theoretically, at least, would be superior to the treatment with single-agent carboplatin.

However, the advent of paclitaxel has changed the landscape, and this drug certainly should be included in the salvage therapy of this patient. Unanswered questions in this clinical situation include: What is the optimum dose and schedule of paclitaxel to be used, and should paclitaxel be combined with a platinum compound? On the basis of the European-Canadian trial that examined two different doses and schedules of paclitaxel in recurrent ovarian cancer, a 175 mg/m^2 3-hr infusion has been accepted by many clinicians to be the standard dose and schedule of paclitaxel for recurrent ovarian cancer. Other investigators have recommended 250 mg/m^2, which usually requires granulocyte colony-stimulating factor (G-CSF), on the basis of nonrandomized studies showing a higher response rate (48%) in previously treated patients compared to results reported with lower doses of paclitaxel. The GOG is performing a prospective randomized trial of different doses of paclitaxel to help resolve this issue. Furthermore, in this situation, with such a long disease-free interval, one could make the argument that the patient be treated as a chemotherapy-naive patient and that therefore paclitaxel should be combined with a platinum compound, thereby taking advantage of any potential synergy between these agents. If combination chemotherapy is to be used, the physician has a choice of paclitaxel plus carboplatin or paclitaxel plus cisplatin. An acceptable dose and schedule of carboplatin plus paclitaxel would be carboplatin dosed to an area under the curve (AUC) of 7.5 and paclitaxel at a dose of 175 mg/m^2 over 3 hr. This may be the preferred alternative to cisplatin plus paclitaxel in this patient, due to the possibly increased risk of neurotoxicity from cisplatin (due to her previous exposure to six cycles of cisplatin, which could have sensitized her to neurotoxicity from more cisplatin).

I would not recommend surgical debulking prior to chemotherapy, even though the patient has what is most likely a "debulkable" mass in the pelvis. Secondary debulking has been recommended by some in patients who have had a long disease-free interval. If secondary cytoreduction has an impact upon survival, it is only in the group of patients who can be maximally cytoreduced, so that they are left with microscopic disease. This particular patient has liver metastases and consequently, while the pelvic mass can be surgically removed, she is very unlikely to be left with only microscopic disease. If she was symptomatic and had a pending bowel obstruction, the argument for surgery would be strengthened. This not being the case, I would institute chemotherapy once a needle biopsy confirmed recurrent ovarian cancer.

The probability of a clinical complete remission with paclitaxel and carboplatin is high; unfortunately, however, the patient is likely to suffer a subsequent relapse. The second disease-free interval is likely to be shorter than the first.

At the subsequent relapse I would reinstitute paclitaxel, but this time as a single agent. If she were to achieve another response with such a second-line salvage approach, a platinum compound would still be available for a third recurrence. Ovarian cancer can have a long course, and in this patient it may be better to think of it as a chronic illness. Consequently the judicious use of chemotherapy, and surgery to deal with specific problems such as a bowel obstruction, and even radiation to palliate symptoms when chemotherapy is no longer effective, can provide this patient reasonable quality of life during this protracted illness.

Of course, other available chemotherapeutic regimens such as ifosfamide, hexamethylmelamine, oral etoposide, and tamoxifen can also provide some benefit when patients become platinum-refractory. However, toxicity considerations become exceedingly important with some of these agents in the terminal stages of this disease.

References

Eisenhauser EA, ten Bokkel Huinink WW, Swenerton KD, et al. European-Canadian randomized trial of paclitaxel in relapsed ovarian cancer: High-dose versus low-dose and longer versus short infusion. J Clin Oncol 1994; 12:2654–2666.

Gore ME, Fryatt I, Wiltshaw E, Dawson T. Treatment of relapsed carcinoma of the ovary with cisplatin or carboplatin following initial treatment with these compounds. Gynecol Oncol 1990; 36:207–211.

Markman M, Rothman R, Hakes T, et al. Second-line platinum therapy in patients with ovarian cancer previously treated with cisplatin. J Clin Oncol 1991; 9:389–393.

Ozols RF. Carboplatin and paclitaxel (Taxol®) for the treatment of advanced ovarian cancer. Int J Gynecol Cancer 1994; 4 (suppl 1):13–17.

PHYSICIANS' RESPONSE

JOHN CARLSON
CHARLES DUNTON

Managing recurrent ovarian cancer is challenging and requires a rational balance between our desire to help and a realization that, in almost all cases, intervention is only palliative. However, appropriate intervention can prolong survival, and we believe this is a classic case for aggressive management of recurrent disease.

The favorable aspects of this case are as follows:

1. The relatively young age of this patient
2. Her long disease-free interval
3. Her excellent clinical response to prior treatment, evidenced by a 4-year disease-free survival
4. The probably isolated recurrence described as a 3- by 4-cm cm pelvic mass

Our initial plan would be to evaluate the patient for surgery, anticipating optimal cytoreduction and then reinstituting chemotherapy. Based on the literature, evidence of successful retreatment with platinum-based drugs in this setting and the addition of paclitaxel to our chemotherapy regimen, we would anticipate a postoperative chemotherapy regimen of paclitaxel/platinum. However, we might obtain a tumor sample at surgery for chemosensitivity assay in case the patient failed to respond to these agents.

Obviously, our initial assumption that our patient now has recurrent and isolated disease must be further investigated. For example, is the 3- by 4-cm pelvic mass truly a pelvic recurrence or a second primary of the large bowel? We would recommend a barium enema study to evaluate this. While a colonoscopy would also answer the question, a barium enema will inform us about the extent of the serosal involvement and provide us with information about the need to perform a colon resection at the time of surgery.

Assuming that the barium enema revealed only serosal involvement of the rectosigmoid, the liver lesion should be evaluated. Since the lesion is "suspicious" by CT and unlikely to be a cyst or hemangioma, a needle aspiration is appropriate. If there is a confirmed liver metastasis, we would further assess the liver with an enhanced magnetic resonance imaging. If the hepatic lesion is unifocal, we would consider resecting the liver metastasis with the pelvic tumor resection unless other significant disease were identified at surgery that was not anticipated on the basis of preoperative imaging.

PHYSICIAN'S RESPONSE

WILLIAM HOSKINS

In this patient with a prior history of advanced epithelial ovarian cancer who has an elevated CA-125 and a pelvic mass, the most likely diagnosis is recurrent ovarian cancer. An apparent pelvic mass of only 4 cm or an elevation of CA-125 of only 49 might be inconclusive and require further observation, but the combination of findings is highly suspicious and requires tissue confirmation without further delay. Factors that point to the possibility of successful therapy of this patient include a long treatment-free interval and no prior paclitaxel therapy. Because of this likelihood of successful retreatment, prompt intervention is warranted.

Tissue diagnosis could be obtained by needle biopsy of the pelvic mass or by exploratory laparotomy. In this patient, I would favor exploratory laparotomy for secondary cytoreduction prior to institution of chemotherapy. The chances of success for secondary cytoreduction are influenced by a variety of factors, but two of the most important are the treatment-free interval and the histological grade. It would be important to review the original histology to determine the cell type and grade of the tumor. Some would argue that laparoscopy might be indicated to determine extent of disease prior to full surgical exploration.

While I would not recommend tissue diagnosis of the pelvic mass by needle aspiration and avoidance of surgical exploration, I do think the liver lesion should be evaluated, and this may require needle biopsy. The first step would be a liver ultrasound to rule out a liver cyst. If the lesion is not a simple cyst, a tagged red blood cell scan can rule out a hemangioma. If the lesion is neither a simple cyst nor a hemangioma, needle biopsy is indicated. The presence of a tissue diagnosis of a 1-cm metastasis to the liver does not contraindicate surgical exploration to remove the pelvic disease but might prepare one for the possible need to resect the lesion if this can be done without a major liver resection. Since there is obvious disease other than in the liver, a major liver resection would not be indicated. Patients with extensive liver metastases should go directly to chemotherapy based on the results of the needle biopsy alone.

The long treatment-free interval in this patient makes it quite likely that she will respond to a platinum compound with a degree of success similar to that of her initial therapy. Since she has not received prior paclitaxel therapy, I would recommend chemotherapy with a combination of paclitaxel and either cisplatin or carboplatin. Some might recommend therapy with a platinum drug with or without cyclophosphamide, saving paclitaxel for the possibility of platinum failure, but I would recommend using the best therapy available initially. There is little doubt that optimum therapy would be a combination of paclitaxel and a platinum drug.

Intraperitoneal therapy is another option for this patient, provided that the liver does not contain metastases and one can surgically resect all disease to less than 1 cm. One could consider intraperitoneal cisplatin alone or a combination of intraperitoneal cisplatin and intravenous paclitaxel. While paclitaxel has been evaluated in phase I trials by the intraperitoneal route, there are no reported phase II data at this time. There are in vitro data indicating that cisplatin and paclitaxel cannot be mixed in an intraperitoneal solution without inactivation of the cisplatin.

In summary, this is a patient with a probable recurrence of ovarian cancer 4 years following successful initial therapy. She should be treated aggressively with surgical cytoreduction and combination chemotherapy with paclitaxel and a platinum compound. Secondary therapy will be most effective in a patient with minimal disease and, if the disease can be completely resected, one could consider the possibility of intraperitoneal therapy provided that the workup rules out liver metastases.

References

Alberts DS, Liu PY, Hannigan EV, et al. Phase III of intraperitoneal cisplatin, intravenous cyclophosphamide vs intravenous cisplatin and cyclophosphamide in patients with optimal disease stage III ovarian cancer: A SWOG-GOG-ECOG intergroup study (abstr). Proc ASCO 1995; 14:273.

Markman M, Rothman R, Hakes T, et al. Second-line platinum therapy in patients with ovarian cancer previously treated with cisplatin. J Clin Oncol 1991; 9:389–393.

McGuire WP, Hoskins WJ, Brady MF, et al. Taxol and cisplatin improves outcome in advanced ovarian cancer as compared to cytoxan and cisplatin (abstr). Proc ASCO 1995; 14:275.

Thigpen JT, Blessing JA, Ball H, et al. Phase II trial of paclitaxel in patients with progressive ovarian carcinoma after platinum-based chemotherapy: A Gynecologic Oncology Group study. J Clin Oncol 1994; 12:1748–1753.

Vaccarello L, Rubin SC, Vlamis V, et al. Cytoreductive surgery in ovarian carcinoma patients with a documented previously complete surgical response. Gynecol Oncol 1995; 57:61–65.

PHYSICIANS' RESPONSE

MAURICE J. WEBB
HARRY J. LONG
JOHN H. EDMONSON

This 64-year-old woman with late relapsing ovarian carcinoma needs further therapy for what appears to be late pelvic (and possibly hepatic) recurrence of her cancer. The treatment ordinarily would be planned following surgical reassessment of her status with the potential of secondary total gross excision of all residual disease. The long free interval preceding this relapse suggests that she probably could again respond favorably to a platinum based regimen (1).

Assuming that the patient's medical status permitted abdominal surgery, the patient might be rendered free of all macroscopically visible ovarian cancer, including excision of even the hepatic nodule, prior to secondary aggressive cytotoxic drug treatment with a combination of paclitaxel and cisplatin (2) (or carboplatin) for at least 6 months. This patient has an excellent opportunity for another clinically complete tumor regression, which could lead to a third-look surgery if a reasonable consolidation therapy can be identified for use at that time.

References

1. Christina MC, Trimble EL. Salvage chemotherapy for epithelial ovarian carcinoma. Gynecol Oncol 1994; 55:S143–S150.
2. McGuire WP, Hoskins WJ, Brady MF, et al. A phase III trial comparing cisplatin/cytoxan and cisplatin/Taxol in advanced ovarian cancer (abstr). Proc ASCO 1993; 12:255.

34

Stage IIC Ovarian Cancer Which Is Completely Resected

CASE

A 56-year-old woman notes the gradual onset of abdominal bloating. On physical examination she is found to have a moderate amount of ascites and a left-sided ovarian mass. Computed tomography confirms the presence of ascites and the ovarian mass. Preoperative CA-125 is 61.

At surgery the patient is found to have a left-sided ovarian cancer and two pelvic implants. There is no gross disease in the upper abdomen and all macroscopic cancer is resected.

Pathology reveals moderately well differentiated papillary serous adenocarcinoma of the left ovary. The pelvic implants contain cancer and the washings are positive for cancer cells. The omentum reveals no cancer and all nodes are negative for the presence of malignancy.

PHYSICIAN'S RESPONSE

DAVID GERSHENSON

This patient appears to have stage IIC, grade 2 carcinoma of the ovary with no gross residual disease. In general, her prognosis is relatively favorable based on the fact that the tumor did not extend to the upper abdomen or retroperitoneum and no bulky residual tumor is present. Stage II accounts for only about 15% of all epithelial ovarian cancers. Of patients referred to a tertiary center after primary surgery and a stage designation of II, approximately one-third will be upstaged at the time of reexploration.

Options that should be considered for this patient include single-agent chemotherapy, intraperitoneal chromic phosphate, radiotherapy, intraperitoneal chemotherapy, and systemic combination chemotherapy. In my opinion, stage II invasive epithelial ovarian cancer should be treated the same as stage IIIA and IIIB tumors. As stated by some of the senior members of our discipline, "There is no lid on the pelvis." In other words, although a locoregional approach may seem attractive for this patient, it places too much confidence in surgical staging. Although radiotherapy—either delivered using a pelvic field or an abdominal-pelvic field—is an attractive option, there are no prospective randomized trials comparing radiotherapy with contemporary combination chemotherapy. Lacking such information, I would definitely select combination chemotherapy for this patient. I would not choose intraperitoneal chromic phosphate because I believe that its role is extremely limited or nonexistent and its potential for gastrointestinal toxicity is unacceptable. I would also not select intraperitoneal chemotherapy for this patient, since there are no convincing data that it is superior to systemic chemotherapy and its cost and potential for complications are greater.

I would select the combination of cisplatin and paclitaxel for this patient. By doing so, I am clearly extrapolating from the results of GOG study #111, which showed a progression-free survival and overall survival advantage for the paclitaxel/cisplatin regimen over the cyclophosphamide/cisplatin regimen in patients with suboptimal stage III and IV epithelial ovarian cancer. In addition, we currently do not know the optimal dose and schedule for the use of paclitaxel. Until such information is available from randomized trials, I would start with a dose of 175 mg/m^2 and deliver the paclitaxel over a period of 24 hr. Standard therapy would include six cycles of chemotherapy, during which I would monitor the patient using physical examination and serum CA-125 determinations (although serum CA-125 does not appear to be a very good marker for this patient). After completion of chemotherapy, I would reassess the patient with a CT scan of the abdomen and pelvis. If the serum CA-125 and CT are negative, I would observe the patient without recommending second-look surgery. Five-year survival rates for patients with stage II epithelial ovarian cancer range from 50 to 80% in more recent reports.

Reference

McGuire WP, Hoskins WJ, Brady MF, et al. A Phase III trial comparing cisplatin/cytoxan (PC) and cisplatin/taxol (PT) in advanced ovarian cancer (AOC). Proc ASCO 1993; 12:255.

PHYSICIANS' RESPONSE

MICHAEL FRIEDLANDER
NEVILLE F. HACKER

This 56-year-old woman has a moderately differentiated stage IIC ovarian cancer and all macroscopic disease has been resected. The aim of treatment in stage II ovarian cancer is cure and the available data suggest 5-year survival rates that range from 50 to 80% depending on the series.

The optimum approach to treatment is still debated, but we would recommend six cycles of chemotherapy with cisplatin ($75mg/m^2$) and cyclophosphamide ($750mg/m^2$) at 3-week intervals commencing on about the 10th postoperative day. Carboplatin has less toxicity, particularly with respect to emesis, neurotoxicity, and nephrotoxicity, and has been demonstrated to have equivalent efficacy to cisplatin in randomized trials of patients with *advanced* ovarian cancer. We personally favor cisplatin over carboplatin when treating patients with curative intent, as in the case of this patient, and there are limited data supporting this approach. In most patients toxicity associated with cisplatin is manageable, particularly when using 5HT3 antagonists and dexamethasone as antiemetics. However, if the patient develops evidence for neurotoxicity or grade 4 nausea and vomiting, we would substitute carboplatin (AUC5) for cisplatin. The role of paclitaxel (Taxol) in combination with cisplatin as first-line treatment in patients with early ovarian cancer is unknown, and we await results of randomized trials before using paclitaxel combinations in this setting.

Although the patient's preoperative CA-125 level will almost certainly fall to normal following surgical resection of all visible tumor, we would recommend that she have a CA-125 level prior to each cycle of treatment in order to detect the unlikely event of tumor progression while on treatment. At the completion of chemotherapy, we would not routinely recommend a second-look laparotomy, as the likelihood of this being positive would be very low in an asymptomatic patient with no macroscopic disease following initial surgery. In addition, the effect on survival is questionable.

Stage II tumors are relatively uncommon and account for only about 3% of ovarian cancers. In view of their rarity, they have usually been grouped with stage I tumors with adverse prognostic features or included with stage III tumors that have been completely resected in various randomized trials that have addressed treatment issues.

The GOG (protocol 7602) study of melphalan versus intraperitoneal phosphorus 32 (^{32}P) included 141 patients with both stage II ovarian cancer as well as stage I with adverse prognostic features and the survival in both arms was approximately 80% (1). In a more recent study from Norway, 347 patients with stages 1 (adverse features), II, and III (no macroscopic residuum) were randomized to ^{32}P or cisplatin. The 5-year survival was similar in both arms and approximated 80%. The 5-year survival in 48 patients with stage II tumors in this study was 55% in the ^{32}P arm compared to 68% in the cisplatin group ($p = .015$) (2).

Although most people are advocating platinum-based chemotherapy, radiotherapy is also a treatment option (3). There are data from Toronto demonstrating that whole abdominal radiotherapy is associated with 5-year survival in stage II ovarian cancer ranging from 50 to 90%, depending on grade and volume of residuum. These data are superior to most other radiotherapy series but there is still some debate regarding the efficacy of whole abdominal radiotherapy as compared to chemotherapy. The toxicity of whole abdominal radiotherapy has been significant in a number of studies, although this has not been the case in the Toronto series. While we have opted for chemotherapy, it should be said that whole abdominal radiotherapy may also be an option, particularly for patients treated in those centers with significant experience using this modality in ovarian cancer.

References

1. Young RC, Walton LA, Ellemberg SA, et al. Adjuvant therapy in stage I and II epithelial ovarian cancer. Results of two prospective randomized trials N Engl J Med 1990; 332:1021–1027.
2. Vergote IB, De Vos LN, Abeler VM, et al. Randomized trial comparing Cisplatin with radioactive phosphorus or whole abdominal irradiation as adjuvant treatment of ovarian cancer. Cancer 1992; 69:741–749.
3. Thomas GM. Radiotherapy in early ovarian cancer. Gynecol Oncol 1994; 55:573–579.

PHYSICIAN'S RESPONSE

GILLIAN THOMAS

This 56-year-old woman has had a laparotomy revealing a grade 1, stage II ovarian cancer. From the description at surgery, the tumor appeared to be grossly confined to the pelvis, with macroscopic disease in at least the left ovary and the presence of pelvic implants. I am assuming that bilateral salpingo-oophorectomy and hysterectomy were performed as well as resection of the two pelvic implants. There was moderate ascites at the time of the laparotomy and the washings were positive for cancer cells. At the operation, it sounds as if a partial omentectomy was performed and some nodes, presumably from the paraaortic region, were dissected. Both of these latter sites revealed no evidence of tumor. Thus, at the end of the operation, the patient had no macroscopic residual disease and no apparent evidence for macroscopic disease in the abdomen outside of the pelvis. It is highly unlikely that this operation has been curative; I would estimate that without adjuvant therapy, this patient's risk of relapse is probably in the order of 90%. Thus, I would recommend adjuvant therapy.

Many patients have been treated with whole-abdominopelvic radiation therapy for ovarian cancer and it has been determined that certain subgroups of patients, constituting about one-third of the total patient population with ovarian cancer, have experienced substantial cure rates when whole-abdominopelvic radiation therapy is used. This patient with stage II, grade 1–2 cancer with no gross residual disease falls into the category of patients that we have determined as at "intermediate" risk when treated with radiation. They have a more than 67% chance of remaining alive and disease-free 10 years after treatment with minimal late morbidity (1,2). Thus, I would recommend that this patient be offered abdominopelvic radiation therapy as the sole postoperative adjuvant therapy.

She would have a tumor dose prescribed to the whole abdomen of 2250 cGy in 22 fractions, followed by a boost to the pelvis to bring the pelvic dose to a total of 45 Gy. The technique of radiation would encompass the entire peritoneal cavity including the domes of the diaphragms and the peritoneal reflections. The kidneys would be suitably protected so that the dose of radiation received was within acceptable levels of kidney tolerance. Following radiation therapy, the patient would be monitored clinically and further treatment in the form of chemotherapy would only be recommended for overt signs of disease progression.

I would anticipate that the probability of her being able to complete the treatment course is close to 100%. I would inform the patient that the risk of her having serious bowel damage from treatment is less than 5%. While some degree of nausea, anorexia, and diarrhea occurs during the acute phase of radiation treatment, this is transient and often well controlled by appropriate medication.

References

1. Dembo AJ. Epithelial ovarian cancer: The role of radiotherapy. Int J Radiat Oncol Biol Phys 1992; 22:835–845.
2. Carey M, Dembo AJ, Fyles AW, Simm J. Testing the validity of a prognostic classification in patients with surgically optimal ovarian carcinoma: A 15-year review. Int J Gynecol Cancer 1993; 3:24–35.

PHYSICIAN'S RESPONSE

DAN SMITH

With the findings outlined in the case, further therapy will be required for this patient. Historically, a patient with stage IIC disease should have an expected 5-year survival of around 45%. This patient presents with an additionally favorable factor, complete resection of macroscopic disease. Therefore her survival may exceed the traditional expectation somewhat. The choice of further therapy may also be a determinant in her survival.

Standard treatment for a patient with stage IIC disease has not been clearly defined. Options for treatment range from whole-abdomen radiation to chemotherapy or combinations of the two modalities. Despite relative successes in limited trials, the role of whole-abdomen radiation with or without intraperitoneal radionuclide would not be my first choice for this patient. Difficulties in shielding and adequacy of treatment fields compound the concerns of complications that can be avoided by using other modalities.

A standard of care for the treatment of patients with advanced ovarian cancers is multiagent chemotherapy using a platinum-based compound as one component. Cyclophosphamide and paraplatin is the most common choice. An alternate regimen would be one using the agent paclitaxel in conjunction with cisplatin/carboplatin. At this writing, studies are under way to test the hypothesis that this second regimen is more effective than the first. There also exist study protocols for patients with stage IIC disease. An intergroup study involving the Gynecologic Oncology Group (GOG) and the Southwest Oncology Group (SWOG) randomizes patients to therapy with intraperitoneal phosphorus 32 (^{32}P) or cyclophosphamide/cisplatin. The purpose of the study is to compare progression-free and overall survival.

Considering available regimens, I would recommend the use of cyclophosphamide and paraplatin for this patient. The usual course of treatment would be six cycles. During the therapy, the patient would be monitored for toxic effects and evidence of progressive disease. Barring any evidence of progression, a complete evaluation—including physical /pelvic exam, blood testing (including CA-125), and CT/MRI examinations of the abdomen and pelvis—would be performed at the end of chemotherapy.

If the patient had no clinical evidence of disease, she would be a candidate for either careful observation or a protocol of clinical investigation, which may or may not include further surgery and/or chemotherapy. Should the post-treatment evaluation reveal evidence of disease, further diagnostic and therapeutic procedures would be indicated.

Before beginning therapy, baseline assessments of the patient should be made. These data include body surface area, performance status, and renal function. When the patient has reasonably recovered from the surgery (1 to 3 weeks postoperatively), selected chemotherapy can begin.

Reference

Williams CJ. Systematic overview of randomized trials in advanced ovarian carcinoma: Results and implications for future trials. Proc Int Gynecol Cancer Soc 1991; 3:49.

PHYSICIAN'S RESPONSE

HUGH BARBER

The clinical picture is typical for a common epithelial ovarian carcinoma. The gastrointestinal unrest is often present for several months before the diagnosis of ovarian cancer is made. Unfortunately, the common epithelial ovarian cancer is usually found in stages III and IV in 70% of the patients. Tumor markers are obtained as baselines, but since they are neither specific nor sensitive, their greatest value is in monitoring treatment.

The patient should have a preoperative evaluation, including an intravenous pyelogram, barium enema, and CT scan of the pelvis and abdomen. After a bowel preparation, the patient should have an examination under anesthesia, a curettage, and an exploratory laparotomy. The ascitic fluid should be sent for cytology and cytology must be obtained from the upper abdomen and the pelvis. This should be carried out before exploratory examination is performed. The left-sided mass should not be palpated until the infundibulopelvic ligament on that side has been ligated. The reason for this is that the tumor is often very vascular and hemorrhage may result. Having secured the infundibulopelvic ligament, the mass is excised and sent for frozen section. While waiting for the report of the frozen section, the uterus, tubes, and ovaries should be removed and biopsies of any nodules identified. If the frozen section is positive for cancer, the omentum and appendix should be excised and paraaortic node sampling done to help in staging the disease. The findings as listed place the carcinoma in stage IIC. Overall, stage II common epithelial ovarian cancers are associated with an elevated level of CA-125 in 90% of the patients.

It is assumed that all gross disease has been removed. Since the patient is staged as IIC and ascites is present, chemotherapy is indicated. Patinol and cyclophosphamide are recommended for the first line of chemotherapy. Paclitaxel is an excellent second-line drug.

In monitoring patients after initial therapy, it has been reported that levels over 100 µg/mL of CA-125 are associated with a median survival of 7 months; if the level is 10 µg/mL or less, there is a 5-year survival of 50%. Intermediate levels are associated with median survival of 22 months. Progressively higher levels after remission indicate recurrence, and this occurs at least 3 months before other noninvasive methods detect it.

After six chemotherapy treatments at 1-month intervals, the patient should be carefully evaluated with tumor markers, CT scan, and careful pelvic examination. If all this proves to be negative, the patient should be counseled and given the option of a second-look operation. It is estimated that up to 50% may have some evidence of persistent disease; in those where all biopsies and washings are negative at second-look operation, it is anticipated that 33% will recur within 5 years. Second-look operations had little to offer until paclitaxel proved to be a very potent second-line drug.

It is important to explain to the patient at the beginning of therapy that, following six courses of chemotherapy, she will have a careful workup and, assuming that everything is negative, the role of second-look will be presented and explained. This is important, because the discussion with the patient after six treatments may give the patient the impression that nothing is working and she is doomed. Paclitaxel is an excellent second-line drug and produces remissions in 30 to 40% of those found to have disease at second-look operation.

The second-look operation must be done as carefully as the initial operation, with washings for cytology from the upper abdomen and the pelvis; if no gross disease is identified, biopsies should be taken from the peritoneum on the back of the bladder, from the cul-de-sac, the omental site along the transverse colon, and the pelvic side walls as well as biopsies or scraping of the diaphragm and sampling of periortic and pelvic lymph nodes. If no disease is found, the biopsies are negative, and cytology is negative, it is recommended that the patient have one more treatment with cyclophosphamide and platinol, best given about 5 days after surgery. OncoScint CR/OV is a diagnostic tool effective in determining both the location and extent of recurrent ovarian adenocarcinoma and may eventually replace second-look surgery. The follow-up regimen should be the same as that outlined after the initial surgery.

References

McGuire WP. Primary therapy of epithelial ovarian malignancies. Cancer 1993; 71:1541.
Qazi F, McGuire WP. The treatment of epithelial ovarian cancer. 1995; 45(2):88.

35

Recurrent Ovarian Carcinoma: Bowel Obstruction

CASE

A 59-year-old woman was diagnosed $3^1/_2$ years ago with a stage IIIC papillary serous carcinoma of the ovary. It was a high-grade tumor that responded initially to platinum cytoxan chemotherapy. She underwent a second-look procedure, which was positive, and was then treated with paclitaxel (Taxol). After more than a year of being disease-free, she recurred, with a palpable mass at the apex of the vagina. She then received some pelvic radiotherapy. The 4-cm mass seemed to resolve clinically and her CA-125—which prior to radiation therapy was 350—fell to 44. Approximately 6 months later, however, the CA-125 began to rise and the patient was placed on single-agent carboplatin. During the interval after her first course of chemotherapy, she began experiencing some episodes of gas pain and started to lose weight. She felt that the weight loss was primarily due to her inability to eat. Her stools were not pencil-thin, but she felt they were slightly thinner than normal. A short time after being counseled concerning her diet, she began vomiting and developed some abdominal distention. An acute abdominal series showed one dilated loop of bowel in the upper abdomen but not many air-fluid levels. There is no evidence of stool to suggest an impacted colon on the x-ray.

PHYSICIANS' RESPONSE

LARRY J. COPELAND
JAMES L. NICKLIN

This patient is presenting with gastrointestinal symptoms probably secondary to her neoplastic process. However, the possibility of an irradiation injury to the bowel or an independent gastrointestinal (GI) problem should not be overlooked. Retrospectively, one should question whether the most recent rise in CA-125 could not be related to the current GI problem, and it would be important to better document tumor status with a CT or OncoScint scan. However, more urgent is the need to evaluate and manage the GI problem. Acute management steps would include nasogastric decompression and intravenous support. The initial GI evaluation should include upper and lower GI endoscopy. Should the lower GI endoscopy be unsatisfactory, a barium enema is also indicated and, depending on the results of these preliminary tests, an upper GI series with follow-through may yield useful information with regard to the possibility of an irradiation injury to the bowel. If there is no imaging evidence of tumor and there is imaging or endoscopic evidence of a GI obstruction, it would be appropriate to proceed with surgical intervention directed at the GI problem. Given the patient's history, it is very probable that persistent tumor will be encountered, and appropriate aggressiveness toward the concept of tumor debulking will require tempered clinical judgment. Indeed, given her history, we would predict that a comprehensive evaluation would reveal evidence of persistent tumor and an associated GI obstruction. This would require surgical intervention, and the procedure could vary from a simple diverting colostomy to an attempt to debulk tumor and resolve the obstruction with or without an ostomy.

Beyond the acute management of the GI problem, the clinical essence of this clinical problem is the issue of secondary tumor debulking. The role of secondary tumor debulking attracts considerable controversy. If universally applied to all patients with ovarian cancer, one could not support secondary debulking as a reasonable therapeutic approach. However, there are select situations where aggressive secondary debulking does have the potential for extended progression-free survival. In our clinical experience, features that encourage intervention include: (a) extended duration of disease (this patient is about 42 months from her diagnosis, and this is relatively favorable); (b) previously demonstrated excellent response to chemotherapy, with extended intervals off treatment (this patient has demonstrated a reasonable previous response to her chemotherapy and she was off treatment for one year; both of these features are relatively favorable and suggest she may derive some continued benefit from additional chemotherapy); (c) limited but symptomatic disease (the last imaging information provided was a description of a 4-cm mass in the pelvis, which resolved with pelvic irradiation; the disease characteristics at the primary and second-look surgery would also shed light on what one would most likely find at repeat laparotomy); (d) low-grade, clinically indolent tumor (unfortunately this patient is characterized as having a high-grade tumor despite surviving now for about 3.5 years); (e) absence of stage IV disease characteristics (no parenchymal metastasis, no pleural effusion, and no extraabdominal disease); and (f) initial surgical endeavor limited due to surgeon's capabilities rather than disease process (unevaluable in the current case).

Overall, given the current clinical setting and assuming that a comprehensive GI evaluation confirmed my clinical suspicion, we would consider an exploratory laparotomy to address the probable obstruction. The extent of the secondary tumor debulking effort would be influenced by the nature of the intraabdominal tumor and by the patient's desire for such an aggressive surgical attempt. In the face of very extensive metastatic disease, a diverting or bypass procedure to relieve the obstruction would be appropriate. On rare occasions no bypass or diversion is feasible and a gastrostomy may be one's only therapeutic contribution. However, if this patient's disease appeared to be limited and potentially resectable, we would consider the potential benefits of surgical debulking. Extended survival will be dependent on identifying an active chemotherapy program, and consideration should be given to submitting tumor from this surgery for chemosensitivity/resistance testing and hormone receptor testing. Since two forms of genetic therapy based on the presence of either the her/2neu or p53 gene are on the brink of translational application, it would not be inappropriate to also include testing for their presence. It is interesting that the case presented is almost identical to that of a patient managed by one of us a number of years ago, actually a niece of a gynecological oncologist. Following aggressive surgical debulking and additional chemotherapy, the patient was clinically disease-free 8 years later. We mention this not to justify a routine attitude of surgical aggression but only to point out that sometimes, given the right circumstances and a little luck, outcomes can be surprising.

PHYSICIAN'S RESPONSE

GREG SUTTON

First, it is very likely that this woman has recurrent ovarian cancer and that she is in the final months or perhaps weeks of her illness. The most important aspect of care is to meet with her and her family to discuss the implications of her recent symptoms if this has not been done already. We know that women who develop small bowel obstruction *after* aggressive treatment for ovarian cancer have a poor prognosis, regardless of therapy. Decisions at this point must be rational ones and should take into consideration the end-of-life wishes of both the patient and her family. It is important to discourage heroics and to take measures that will place the patient in a home or hospice environment if at all possible. "No code" or "do not resuscitate" orders should be written for both inpatient and outpatient settings; this is simplified if discussions about a living will have been held with the patient and her family following the initial diagnosis of recurrent ovarian cancer.

On a more practical note, few people in this situation refuse volume resuscitation and gastrointestinal decompression. Although it is unlikely that the above symptoms are related to a postsurgical obstruction or radiation enteritis, it is still possible that they will resolve with simple measures. If the patient and her family understand that short-term intervention may be effective and are willing to try, nasogastic decompression and intravenous fluids for 3 or 4 days may provide relief. During this time, a thorough abdominal, nodal, and pelvic examination should be done and CA-125 level drawn. A transferrin level and total lymphocyte count are probably sufficient to evaluate nutritional status. If a recurrence is not identified clinically, computed tomography may be indicated; if there is no evidence of disease on tomography, exploratory surgery could be considered. My guess is that some evidence of disease will be identified, however, and that surgery would be of little benefit.

A scoring system such as that of Krebs and Goplerud (1) or Clarke-Pearson (2) may be employed to assess surgical risk. In that of the first authors, a risk score of 2 is assigned for age > 65 years, severe nutritional depletion, tumor in distant sites or liver, severe ascites, unsuccessful combination chemotherapy, or previous whole abdominal radiotherapy. A score of 1 is assigned to age between 45 and 65, moderate nutritional depletion, palpable intraabdominal masses, moderate ascites, resistance to single-agent chemotherapy, or previous pelvic radiotherapy. A cumulative score of 7 or greater was associated with an 8-week survival projection of only 20% in the experience of these authors.

If there is evidence of persistent ovarian cancer and the small bowel obstruction does not respond to nasogastric decompression or if there is convincing evidence of a substantial recurrence (e.g., a large, palpable pelvic mass, CA-125 level in excess of 300 to 400 U/mL, or radiographic findings of a large mass in the abdomen), a percutaneous gastrostomy is in order. In our institution, gastrostomies may be placed by either the interventional radiologists or by the gastroenterologists. The former group is usually utilized, since they can complete the procedure without endoscopy.

The use of hyperalimentation in this patient poses a difficult ethical situation. The decision to employ this expensive therapy should be individualized and should be made after suitable interaction with the patient, her family, social work, nursing, and clergy.

The resumption of chemotherapy in such a situation also poses many ethical concerns, assuming that the tumor in question has become refractory to carboplatin. Although paclitaxel may be effective in 35% of patients failing first-line platinum therapy, little is known regarding the effectiveness of paclitaxel in platinum-refractory tumors previously exposed to this agent. After careful consideration of the clinical and social situation, a brief trial of paclitaxel or another drug such as ifosfamide, leuprolide acetate, or phase I or II agents, when available, may be warranted. It would certainly be difficult to advocate aggressive chemotherapy in a non-investigational situation, however.

References

1. Krebs HB, Goplerud DR. Surgical management of bowel obstruction in advanced ovarian carcinoma. Obstet Gynecol 1983; 61:327–330.
2. Clarke-Pearson DL, Rodriguez GC, Boente M. Palliative surgery for epithelial ovarian cancer. In: Ovarian Cancer. McGraw-Hill, New York: Rubin SC, Sutton GP, eds. 1993.

PHYSICIAN'S RESPONSE

J. M. CAIN

This patient has recurrence of her epithelial ovarian cancer after prior treatment with cisplatin and cytoxan and then paclitaxel chemotherapy and presents with an assumed partial small and/or large bowel obstruction or ileus. This is not an uncommon situation in the course of stage IIIC ovarian cancer.

Background information is lacking in this patient and should be sought, as treatment planning will differ depending on chemotherapy and radiation specifics. For example, if the paclitaxel received after her second-look laparotomy was two cycles we cannot assume that she has any relative resistance or sensitivity to that agent. We assume that she received a standard six-cycle course of platinum/cytoxan, but that must be documented. The assumption that she was sensitive to platinum-family chemotherapy is reasonable given the interval of disease-free survival, but this may have been attributable to paclitaxel rather than the platinum-based therapy. This assumes importance, because the potential success of further treatment possibilities must play an important role in the level of response to the present clinical situation. An extensive surgery for debulking and resolution of small or large bowel obstruction may have value if additional therapy of value exists (1). Furthermore, differentiation of the fields and types of radiation therapy may be of significant value in planning this patient's therapy, as the location and level of radiation may point the clinician toward a significantly increased risk of fistula formation (with prior bowel radiation) as well as a potential site of partial small bowel obstruction at the distal ileum secondary to pelvic radiation rather than progressive disease.

For this patient, an interval attempt to passively treat partial obstruction of the small bowel with a nasogastric, Baker, or other long suction tube is the appropriate first attempt. A significant number of patients will have resolution with this nonoperative means alone (2). Additionally, evaluation of status of disease should be initiated. First and foremost, a careful clinical examination should be done, including a pelvic examination to evaluate the status of the previously treated disease at the vaginal apex. A computed tomography may be of great value in this patient, both to elucidate the site of partial obstruction (3) but also to evaluate for disease volume and location (such as spleen or liver metastases). Based on the status of disease, the response to conservative management, and careful evaluation of prior therapy and responses, possible further treatment could include surgical debulking/relief of obstruction and further chemotherapy with single-agent carboplatin. If disease is progressing on carboplatin by evaluation operatively or nonoperatively, a first consideration would be to use both paclitaxel and a platinum-containing drug. Additionally, hexamethylmelamine may be an appropriate agent to further chemotherapy in this patient.

References

1. Janicke F, Holscher M, Kuhn W, et al. Radical surgical procedures improves survival time in patients with recurrent ovarian cancer. Cancer 1992; 70:2129–2139.
2. Butler JA, Cameron BL, Morrow M, et al. Small bowel obstruction in patients with a prior history of cancer. Am J Surg 1991; 162:624–628.
3. Frager D, Medwid SW, Baer JW, et al. CT of small-bowel obstruction: Value in establishing the diagnosis and determining the degree and cause. Am J Roentgenol 1994; 162:37–41.

PHYSICIAN'S RESPONSE

KENNETH D. WEBSTER

This case suggests the natural course of disease in ovarian carcinoma. Fortunately, with platinum-based chemotherapy and the addition of paclitaxel, many patients have very good palliation and longer clinically disease-free intervals.

The question arises as to what other sites of disease were detected at the time of pelvic radiotherapy for the vaginal apex recurrence. If no other sites were detected, I would not argue with pelvic irradiation for small-volume pelvic recurrence. If disease were detected elsewhere by CT scan, I would recommend chemotherapy by resuming paclitaxel or carboplatin/paclitaxel. If CT at that time was inconclusive, laparoscopy could have been considered to detect other disease sites. This history suggests that the cancer was sensitive to paclitaxel, but information regarding sites and amount of persistent disease at the second-look procedure is not available. Also, the number of courses of paclitaxel is unknown.

Symptoms presently suggest either a partial small bowel obstruction secondary to pelvic irradiation or multiple sites of bowel involvement with progressive carcinoma. A CT scan of the abdomen and pelvis is indicated to assess amount and location of disease. If the CT is not informative as to the degree of bowel involvement, I would do an upper GI series with small bowel follow-through.

If the site of obstruction is the distal small bowel, I think this patient deserves exploration with a a possible bypass procedure with or without resection of the involved segment. The integrity of the large bowel should also be assessed prior to surgery. If the CT study or small bowel series suggested multiple sites of intestinal involvement with metastatic ovarian carcinoma, I would not operate on this patient. I would reinstitute paclitaxel chemotherapy in an effort to further palliate the patient.

PHYSICIAN'S RESPONSE

JOHN MIKUTA

This patient presents some of the dilemmas noted in individuals with advanced, persistent, partially therapeutically responsive ovarian carcinomas. With her present status, it is advisable that she have a long intestinal tube placed to see if it can be carried down to the point of obstruction for the purpose of decompression and reduction of the edema of the bowel wall, in hopes that the obstructive area may be opened up. If radiographic improvement is noted, one may then attempt clamping the tube and trying clear liquids orally. If the symptoms recur, it may be helpful to identify the degree of blockage by the use of a radiopaque liquid material to see if it is localized to a small area or if other sites of luminal compromise may be present. It may be possible to identify serosal implants of tumor in the opacified bowel. Radiological study of the colon is also helpful in this regard.

If conservative management of this patient does not provide a resumption of bowel activity, then it may be necessary to carry out an exploration with lysis of adhesions if found. This may be all that is necessary. In the presence of extensive involvement of the bowel with tumor, particularly in multiple areas of the peritoneal cavity, efforts at relieving obstruction through adhesiolysis or bowel resection have never been demonstrated to provide satisfactory long-term results and are, at best, only palliative for a short time. It is important to observe the fact that the patient has had prior radiation therapy and that excessive handling or lysis of adhesions surrounding such an intestine may create further problems, such as enteroperitoneal fistula and peritonitis, leading to a need to reexplore the patient.

The patient is obviously not in the best nutritional state, and I would recommend an evaluation by the nutritional service with a view toward consideration of intravenous hyperalimentation until the obstruction is relieved. Continued treatment at this point must be the decision of the patient and her family.

36

Bulky Stage III Ovarian Cancer with Excellent Response to Chemotherapy

CASE

A 52-year-old woman presents with massive ascites and extensive intraabdominal tumor. Pelvic exam reveals a fixed nodular mass extending from side wall to side wall and filling the cul-de-sac. Chest x-ray reveals small bilateral pleural effusions. Computed tomography (CT) confirms the physical findings and reveals a large left ovarian mass. There is no evidence of a pancreatic or gastric mass. The CA-125 value is 9750. A laparoscopy is performed for diagnostic purposes, but it is decided the disease cannot be resected.

The patient is started on chemotherapy with carboplatin and paclitaxel (Taxol). Following two courses of treatment, her ascites has decreased dramatically and pelvic exam demonstrates significant improvement. The CA-125 has decreased to 115.

PHYSICIAN'S RESPONSE

ALEXANDER W. KENNEDY

The patient presented has been treated with neoadjuvant chemotherapy for presumed ovarian cancer determined to be unresectable at the time of laparoscopy (1). I would like to have further information regarding any cytological or histological specimens obtained from this patient at the time of surgery. I would presume, for the purposes of this consult, that pathology revealed high-grade adenocarcinoma consistent with primary epithelial ovarian carcinoma, that lapa-

278

roscopy revealed diffuse intraabdominal carcinomatosis, and that the patient's general medical status is excellent now, given her initial response to chemotherapy and her young age.

The judgment to be made at the time of this consultation is essentially whether to advise this patient to undergo laparotomy for resection of her undoubtedly persistent cancer or whether to delay surgery until additional further courses of chemotherapy have been administered.

I recommend at this time that chemotherapy be continued for an additional four cycles. During this time, I advise continued monthly clinical examination and CA-125 determinations. If at any time there is the suggestion of chemotherapy resistance and progressive disease, I would immediately intervene surgically and perform a laparotomy. If there is evidence of continuing response to chemotherapy, I would plan to perform surgery after the sixth course of chemotherapy.

Prior to surgery, I advise repeating this patient's CT scan to exclude any obvious nonresectable tumor (e.g., parenchymal liver metastases) and would perform a bowel prep preoperatively. At the time of surgery, my goals would be to perform a total abdominal hysterectomy, bilateral salpingo-oophorectomy, and infracolic omentectomy. A complete examination of the peritoneal cavity would be performed, looking for any other evidence of macroscopic persistent cancer as well as to assess the extent of peritoneal adhesions. If no macroscopic cancer is remaining at the completion of this procedure, I would advise that paraaortic lymph node biopsies be performed and then a peritoneal catheter with a subcutaneous reservoir inserted. Following recovery from surgery, I recommend proceeding with three courses of intraperitoneal cisplatin (100 mg/m^2). If macroscopic residual disease other than small miliary seeding remains at the time of the laparotomy that is judged nonresectable, the patient, unfortunately, is then in a strictly palliative situation and I would advise continuing monthly single-agent paclitaxel (175 mg/m^2) until there is clinical evidence of disease progression.

Reference

1. Schwartz PE, Chambers JT, Makuch R. Neoadjuvant chemotherapy for advanced ovarian cancer. Gynecol Oncol 1994; 53:33–37.

PHYSICIAN'S RESPONSE

WILLIAM McGUIRE

This is a patient with poor-prognosis ovarian carcinoma based on large tumor volume, large-volume ascites, and the possibility, although not verified, of stage IV disease based on bilateral pleural effusion. With the dramatic response to two cycles of chemotherapy, there is a strong temptation to simply continue this chemotherapy. This approach is incorrect, since the patient probably has significant amounts of tumor still present, with the larger masses likely containing dually drug-resistant clones. Thus, the proper approach to this patient is laparotomy and complete tumor debulking. It is important that this procedure be done after two and no more than three cycles of chemotherapy, so that there is still capability, in terms of end-organ toxicity, for three to five additional cycles of chemotherapy following surgical debulking. The significant decline in CA-125 has obvious important, positive prognostic factors for this patient, and—if the patient can be made macroscopically free of disease at the time of her surgical procedure—her chances for long-term survival are *probably* better than those of a patient who is suboptimally debulked at a primary surgical procedure. This concept of interval debulking has been put to a randomized trial, by a group of European clinical trialists, in which patients similar to this one either received six cycles of chemotherapy following minimal surgery or three cycles of the same chemotherapy followed by an interval debulking procedure and three additional cycles of chemotherapy. Statistical analyses suggested benefit for the latter procedure. This concept is currently being tested in the United States with a similar patient population and similar study design, but with the use of paclitaxel and cisplatin as the treatment regimen.

If this patient, in fact, is made NED at the time of her surgical procedure, I would strongly encourage the treating physician to make certain that the paclitaxel is given as a 24-hr infusion to be followed by cisplatin. The data showing that paclitaxel/cisplatin is significantly better in terms of all outcome parameters than the previous regimen of cytoxan/cisplatin stemmed from the use of 24-hr paclitaxel/cisplatin. Unfortunately, many physicians in this country have substituted carboplatin for cisplatin prior to any publication of this drug combination in a phase I trial and have also shortened paclitaxel infusion to 3 hr. This is potentially dangerous in terms of abrogating efficacy, since in vitro data strongly suggest that, in ovarian cancer cell lines, duration of exposure to paclitaxel is important in cell kill. Additionally, there are anecdotal reports of patients failing short paclitaxel infusions who subsequently responded to longer infusions.

Thus, in summary, this patient should have an immediate interval debulking procedure followed by three to five additional cycles of paclitaxel given as a 24-hr infusion at a dose of 135 mg/m^2 and cisplatin immediately following the taxol at a dose of 75 mg/m^2.

PHYSICIAN'S RESPONSE

WIM TEN BOKKEL HUININK

This case of an ovarian cancer patient stage IV elicits the following remarks.

The half-life of the patient's CA-125 seems to be in a steep decline. On the basis of the publication of Van der Burg et al. (1), this is related to a fair prognosis.

The referred investigators showed that a half-life of < 20 days of CA-125 in a patient treated with cisplatin-based chemotherapy suffering from ovarian cancer is far better than when a half-life of > 20 days. Therefore chemotherapy applied in this patient seems to be highly effective. It seems most likely that this is related by the combination used in this patient. Preliminary evaluation of a multicentric study performed within the Gynecologic Oncology Group (GOG) in the United States revealed that the combination of cisplatin and paclitaxel (Taxol) achieves superior response and survival figures than those achieved in patients treated with the so-called standard treatment cisplatin and cyclophosphamide. Since carboplatin has been shown to be equal to cisplatin, one may assume that treatment results with the combination of carboplatin and paclitaxel are equal to those achieved with cisplatin and paclitaxel. Dose-finding studies, currently under way or soon to be completed, seem to support this hypothesis.

However, this case history points to another important problem: should secondary cytoreductive surgery be performed in this patient? In my opinion, it should. The same author, Van der Burg showed in a recent publication (2) that debulking surgery after induction chemotherapy has a beneficial effect on the prognosis in advanced epithelial ovarian cancer. Notwithstanding the lack of confirmative studies, the improved survival in patients in whom surgery has been performed points to a role for secondary cytoreductive surgery in these patients.

I therefore would strongly advise continued treatment with the combination of carboplatin and paclitaxel after a secondary attempt to reduce the tumor mass by surgical means. By doing so, even in this patient with a stage IV ovarian cancer, a favorable treatment outcome is not unlikely.

References

1. Van der Burg MEL, Lammes FB, Van Putten WLJ, Stoter G. Ovarian cancer: The prognostic value of the serum half-life of CA-125 during induction chemotherapy. Gynecol Oncol 1988; 30:307–312.
2. Van der Burg MEL, Van Lent M, Buyse M, et al. The effect of debulking surgery after induction chemotherapy on the prognosis in advanced epithelial ovarian cancer. Engl J Med 1995; 332:629–634.

PHYSICIAN'S RESPONSE

JONATHAN BEREK

As a rule, laparoscopy should not be performed in the presence of massive ascites. Under these circumstances, the procedure is essentially useless in determining whether or not the ovarian cancer can be resected. A proper laparotomy should be the standard of care, and it should be performed prior to the initiation of chemotherapy so that a proper diagnosis can be made, and, if ovarian cancer is found, metastatic disease can be appropriately debulked. One of the principal disadvantages of starting the chemotherapy prior to surgery is that one could be treating something other than ovarian cancer and, also, one might miss the optimal opportunity for resecting any bulk disease so that the proper chemotherapy has the best chance to be effective.

There are two acceptable choices for a patient who has not been started on platinum chemotherapy—either initiate the so-called "induction" chemotherapy or perform a proper laparotomy. Because the data support that a proper cytoreductive (debulking operation) should be initially performed, this should be the standard of care for such women unless there is an appropriate reason to defer. If a patient has medical contraindications to the surgery, chemotherapy may be given; however, such contraindications tend to persist after two to three cycles of chemotherapy.

If this particular patient had been referred to me prior to her chemotherapy, I would have recommended immediate reexploration. However, in the situation in which two or three cycles of chemotherapy had already been given, I would then re-explore the patient and perform a "interval debulking." There is evidence that interval cytoreductive surgery in such patients is beneficial (1). Patients who successfully undergo such interval debulking operations have a longer disease progression–free and overall survival than those who do not. Therefore this patient should definitely be explored by someone capable of doing such operations, that is, a gynecological oncologist (2).

References

1. van der Burg MEL, van Lent M, Buyse M, et al. The effect of debulking surgery after induction chemotherapy on the prognosis in advanced epithelial ovarian cancer. N Engl J Med 1995; 332:629–634.
2. Berek JS. Interval debulking of ovarian cancer—An interim measure. N Engl J Med 1995; 332:675–677

PHYSICIAN'S RESPONSE

ERNEST W. FRANKLIN, III

Impression

Carcinoma of the ovary responsive to systemic chemotherapy.

Recommendation

Continued clinical evaluation by physical examination and CA-125 to assess further response to chemotherapy. Surgical exploration for resection should be considered when the mass becomes mobile and it is deemed probable that the surgery can reduce remaining disease to an optimal category, i.e., less than 1 cm of residual disease. Surgery will probably be necessary after three to four courses of chemotherapy. Repeat physical examination and CT scan will assist in this decision.

Discussion

The management of this patient with clinical presentation consistent with ovarian carcinoma, presumably confirmed on the laparoscopy by biopsy, does not follow the usual clinical pathways of management with laparotomy for resection of the ovarian mass, perhaps still leaving suboptimal disease. Some experience has been accumulated with primary chemotherapy treatment after biopsy only for confirmation of diagnosis. This has been used initially in elderly and more debilitated patients or those with current medical contraindications such as deep venous thrombophlebitis. Such a program of primary chemotherapy allows in essence for an in vivo evaluation of the chemosensitivity of the malignancy.

In view of the data accumulated regarding the advisability of minimizing tumor burden in determining optimum response to chemotherapy, surgical intervention to debulk disease is still appropriate. The exact timing has to be determined by the physical examination of the patient in conjunction with further CT scan or magnetic resonance imaging.

Subsequent to surgical resection, the same chemotherapy would be continued, as the malignancy appears to be quite responsive to this combination of medication. At the time of surgery, it is possible to obtain tissues for clonogenic assay to determine any second-line chemotherapy that may be necessary.

PHYSICIAN'S RESPONSE

MALCOLM G. IDELSON

After two courses of neoadjuvant cytotoxic chemotherapy, there has been clear-cut objective evidence of a fine response. I would now prepare the patient promptly for surgery, thereby not delaying for more than several days her continued postoperative chemotherapy. By doing surgery now, one would hope to maximize the opportunity to successfully and optimally cytoreduce this patient's tumor burden before persistent but resectable tumor masses lead to drug resistance.

Following an aggressive, radical, and hopefully total or maximal macroscopic tumor-debulking effort (during which tumor specimens were sent for estrogen and progesterone receptor assay as well as clonogenic assay for drug resistance), I would continue with the same chemotherapy for a total of six or seven courses (including the two neoadjuvant courses).

If the patient then was determined to be without evidence of persistent disease,

I would recommend a reassessment laparotomy with all its meticulous detail, including the excision of all intraperitoneal adhesions, redebulking if found necessary and possible, and the implantation of an intraperitoneal Portacath system.

If the second-look procedure was pathologically negative or microscopically positive, the following day, 15 mCi of radioactive chromic phosphate (^{32}P) in 2 L of lactated Ringer's would be administered into the peritoneal cavity rapidly, utilizing proper safeguards and turning-mixing procedure. Several days later as well as 4 weeks later, a second and third intraperitoneal instillation utilizing cisplatin (100 mg/m^2) and etoposide (200 mg/m^2) would be given. In addition, a fourth and fifth intraperitoneal therapy with mitoxantrone (10 mg/m^2), 2 to 3 weeks apart would complete the intraperitoneal therapy.

Moreover, with a pathologically negative second-look operation, two courses of systemic chemotherapy utilizing the same drugs (carboplatin and paclitaxel) would be given concomitant with the intraperitoneal mitoxantrone chemotherapy and perhaps a third systemic cycle of the same drugs if lymph nodes were originally positive. If the reassessment laparotomy is microscopically positive, two or three additional systemic chemotherapy cycles (using carboplatinum and cytoxan) would be given, concomitant to and after the intraperitoneal mitoxantrone, but four or five cycles if nodes are involved.

If the second-look procedure is macroscopically positive but cytoreductive efforts lead to a resection of *all* macroscopic disease, this situation would be treated exactly as a microscopically positive second-look laparotomy as outlined above.

Finally, if the original surgical event following two courses of neoadjuvant chemotherapy or the reassessment laparotomy result in a suboptimally debulked patient, I would tend to treat continuously, as long as I could, utilizing any and all active chemotherapy agents available. Doses would be therapeutic but less than aggressive, with the hope of manipulation of agents and the use of supportive measures in order to maintain stability of the disease and safety with comfort for the patient. Under these circumstances, the patient and her family would have a realistic disclosure and outlook in order to help with any and all therapeutic plans.

Reference

1. Hatch KD. Published discussion regarding neoadjuvant chemotherapy in heavy-burden stage III ovarian carcinoma. Symposium on controversies in Ovarian Cancer. Cleveland Clinic Cancer Center, July 1994.

37

Second-Look Laparotomy in an Ovarian Cancer Patient Responding to Chemotherapy

CASE

A 56-year-old female is diagnosed as having stage IIIB ovarian cancer. After initial staging and tumor debulking, she is treated with six courses of cisplatin and cyclophosphamide. Her prechemotherapy CA-125 was 162; it has now decreased into the normal range following her second course of chemotherapy.

Following the six courses of chemotherapy, the pelvic examination is normal and a CT scan of the abdomen and pelvis is unremarkable. CA-125 is 9.

PHYSICIAN'S RESPONSE

JAMES SPEYER

This patient received appropriate chemotherapy for a stage IIIB ovarian cancer. Today perhaps she would receive a paclitaxel-based regimen up front, based on the results of the randomized GOG 111 study. We are faced here with the question of the role of second-look exploratory surgery and how patients with no apparent residual disease should be followed.

The main questions are: (a) Should further laparoscopic or surgical restaging be offered to this patient? (b) Should additional chemotherapy be offered to this patient? and (c) What is the appropriate way to monitor these patients?

The first question addresses the issue of second-look surgery. Clearly surgical restaging is more accurate than even the combination of a good physical exami-

285

nation, negative CT scan, and normal CA-125. Several studies show that laparoscopic or surgical restaging with a formal exploratory laparotomy would indicate otherwise nondetectable disease in approximately 30% of patients. Many clinical trials have adopted this form of evaluation as the best way to determine treatment efficacy. For a period of time, this procedure was widely advocated. Two issues, though, are raised. First, is the outcome different for patients with negative second-look evaluations? While the information provided by a negative second-look laparotomy is reassuring, it does not necessarily guarantee a perfect outcome. Even with a negative pathological result, up to 50% of patients will eventually recur. In addition, investigators at the M.D. Anderson Hospital have presented data suggesting that the rate of intraperitoneal recurrence is similar for patients with minimal residual disease found at second-look surgery compared to those with negative second-look laparotomies. This might argue against doing second-look surgeries. It would, however, bias against the outcome in patients in whom residual disease is found, since unless one is prepared to give additional therapy to all patients beyond six cycles (hardly a standard of practice), additional and perhaps effective therapy will be delayed in the disease-positive patients until the disease progresses enough to be detectable clinically.

Second, if you find disease, does it make a difference? That is, do you have effective therapy to offer that may alter the patient's outcome? If there is residual disease, it is unlikely that more cytoxan/platinum or, for that matter, switching to cytoxan and carboplatin is likely to add much. The patient has not, however, received paclitaxel, an active agent. In addition, there are new and investigational agents that are showing considerable promise. At N.Y.U., we have had a number of responses with 21-day infusions of the topoisomerase I inhibitor topotecan. Trials with a related analog, 9-aminocamptothecin, have also begun.

Since this patient has not "seen" paclitaxel and since other second-line therapies are becoming available, I would favor a surgical restaging procedure. If disease is found, I would begin paclitaxel-based therapy.

The related question is: What do you do if the surgery demonstrates a complete pathological remission? That is, is there a role for additional chemotherapy, given that up to half of these patients will recur and must therefore have microscopic residual disease? While this is attractive conceptually, there are no published data to support additional therapy in this group of patients. We await the results of the Southwestern Oncology Group trial of intraperitoneal Fudr in patients with clinically complete responses. Outside of a study, additional therapy at this point cannot be justified, based on lack of proven efficacy and the expected additional morbidity and cost.

Finally, if the decision is made to follow the patient, what is the best way? I would follow with physical examinations every three months, CA-125 determinations, and twice-yearly CT scans for at least 3 years. The period of observation can be less frequent after that. Clearly this is a pattern of practice. The best way to follow patients is not known. Even though we believe that patients with recurrence detected earlier have a better chance of responding to therapy, this has not been definitely demonstrated. The effect on survival is even less certain.

References

Colombo N, Maggioni A, Vignali M, et al. Options for primary chemotherapy in advanced ovarian cancer: The European Perspective. Gynecol Oncol 1994; 55:S108–S113.

Creasman WT. Second-look laparotomy in ovarian cancer. Gynecol Oncol 1994; 55:S122–S127.

Gershenson DM, Copeland LJ, Wharton JT, et al. Prognosis of surgically determined complete responders in advanced ovarian cancer. Cancer 1985; 55:1129–1135.

McGuire WP, Hoskins WJ, Brady MF, et al. A Phase III Trial comparing cisplatin/cytoxan and cisplatin/Taxol in advanced ovarian cancer (abstr). Proc ASCO 1993; 12:255.

Podratz KC, Cliby WA. Second-look surgery in the management of epithelial ovarian carcinoma. Gynecol Oncol 1994; 55:S128–S133.

Thigpen T, Vance R, Puneky L, Khansur. Chemotherapy in advanced ovarian carcinoma: Current standard of care based on randomized trials. Gynecol Oncol 1994; 55:S97–S107.

Trimble EL, Arbuck SG, McGuire WP. Options for primary chemotherapy of epithelial ovarian cancer: Taxanes. Gynecol Oncol 1994; 55:S114–S121.

PHYSICIANS' RESPONSE

A. MENZIN
S. RUBIN

This patient is among the two-thirds of patients with ovarian cancer who are found to have advanced-stage disease at the time of diagnosis. She is also one of the 50 to 70% of women who achieve a complete clinical response following primary cytoreductive surgery and platinum-based chemotherapy. Before addressing the issue of the appropriate next step for this patient, several points should be made regarding additional information not included in the clinical summary.

The importance of a thorough surgical staging cannot be overstated. Though this woman must have presented with gross disease in the abdomen less than 2 cm in maximal diameter, one must consider whether or not there was an evaluation for the presence of nodal metastases. Some 60 to 70% of patients with advanced disease will have nodal disease detected if thorough sampling is performed. Furthermore, this woman's residual disease status following cytoreduction is not given. Was her stage documented by a single omental nodule that was completely resected or by carcinomatosis, leaving numerous nodules in situ? Did she have bulky, unresectable residual in the pelvis? This information would be of value in considering whether or not to recommend a reassessment exploration or second-look laparotomy (1).

Although approximately half of patients with advanced-stage ovarian cancer will be clinically free of disease after five or six treatments with platinum-based therapy, as determined by clinical examination and radiological evaluation, 50 to 60% of these women will be found to have persistent disease at the time of second-look surgery. Seventy-five percent of patients with a positive second-look will have macroscopic evidence of persistence. Tumor stage and grade, amount of residual disease following primary cytoreduction, and other factors may predict persistence. Serum CA-125 level is a good positive predictor but a poor negative predictor; more than 60% of patients with normal CA-125 values will have evidence of persistence at second-look surgery. Radiographic evaluation, whether by sonography, CT scanning, or magnetic resonance imaging, has been shown by several authors to have suboptimal accuracy and significant false-negative rates. Second-look laparotomy allows for direct determination of the response to chemotherapy, documentation of the extent and location of residual disease, and assessment of the condition of the peritoneal cavity—factors that can be important in subsequent treatment decisions. Additionally, second-look laparotomy provides an opportunity for tumor debulking if indicated.

Though no evidence exists to document an improved survival due to the second-look operation itself, several authors have reported the feasibility of secondary cytoreduction with an acceptable rate of morbidity and a mortality of well under 1%. Approximately 70% of women with positive second-look laparotomies can be debulked to microscopic disease, yet a survival advantage from secondary cytoreduction has not been consistently shown. Hoskins and colleagues from the Memorial Sloan-Kettering Cancer Center found that patients found with or cytoreduced to microscopic disease at second-look surgery had a 50 to 60% 5-year survival, as opposed to those with gross residual who have less than a 10% survival rate (2). A critical factor in predicting a benefit from secondary cytoreduction appears to be patient selection. Patients with progressive disease are least likely to experience improved survival even in the setting of a technically feasible cytoreductive procedure. However, those patients with good responses to therapy noted at second-look laparotomy or identified by a prolonged recurrence-free interval will have a substantially better chance to benefit. The advantage offered by this aggressive surgical approach will clearly be enhanced when salvage regimens used in recurrent or persistent ovarian cancer are improved.

It is noteworthy, in this era of "minimally invasive" surgery, that laparoscopic evaluation is being considered as an alternative to second-look laparotomy. This may provide, in skilled hands, a means to identify persistence and avoid the morbidity and cost of a laparotomy. However, caution should be exercised, given false-negative rates of up to 55% and the "learning curve" associated with complicated operative laparoscopy.

Our recommendation is for a reassessment laparotomy with secondary cytoreduction if a good response to chemotherapy is documented despite persistent disease.

References

1. Morgan MA, Rubin SC. Secondary cytoreduction in epithelial ovarian cancer. Crit Rev Oncol/Hematol 1995; 18:1–8.
2. Hoskins WJ, Rubin SC, Dulaney E, et al. Influence of secondary cytoreduction at the time of second-look laparotomy on the survival of patients with epithelial ovarian carcinoma. Gynecol Oncol 1989; 34:365–371.

PHYSICIANS' RESPONSE

CORNELIUS O. GRANAI
WALTER GAJEWSKI
STEPHEN FALKENBERRY

This case represents a common and perplexing problem for clinicians caring for women with epithelial ovarian cancer—what to recommend once primary treatment is completed and the patient is NED. In this case, after laparotomy with surgical cytoreduction, the patient received six cycles of cisplatin combination chemotherapy with an excellent response as judged by physical examination and CA-125 regression. Paclitaxel, which has largely replaced cytoxan as part of first-line therapy for epithelial ovarian cancer, was not available at the time and thus not employed. The question now is how to proceed. Background may be helpful.

Following optimal surgical cytoreduction, (residual tumor diameter less than 2 cm) and six to eight cycles of platinum-based chemotherapy, approximately two-thirds of patients starting with stage III disease will achieve a complete clinical response. Indeed, the physical examination, radiographic studies, and serum CA-125 will all be normal. Unfortunately, despite these negative studies, 40 to 50% will have disease identified if a second-look laparotomy is performed. Although second-look laparotomy (SLL) is able to detect persistent disease when other means cannot, studies have failed to show that SLL results in improved outcome. Presumably, failure to extend survival reflects the limited efficacy of the "second-line" chemotherapy called for after surgery. Further limiting the rationale for SLL is the fact that even among the most optimistic group, those patients with pathologically negative SLL, approximately 50% will have recurrent disease within 5 years, as will most of the others over time. Because of these considerations, today SLL is generally not recommended outside the research protocol setting. This particular case may be an exception, however, Since paclitaxel was not used as first-line therapy, it remains a therapeutic option to be employed after SLL. Whether having an active chemotherapy (paclitaxel) for second-line use justifies the morbidity of the operation in this case remains uncertain.

When recurrent disease is diagnosed after completion of platinum-based chemotherapy, the subsequent management is influenced by a number of factors such as disease-free interval, symptomatology, extent and location of recurrence, and the patient's overall clinical condition, including nutritional status. Patients with long disease-free intervals (greater than 1 to 2 years) are more likely to benefit from aggressive reintervention to include secondary cytoreductive surgery in select cases. A longer disease-free interval is also predictive of a second response to platinum-based chemotherapy. In contrast, less survival benefit is expected from second-line treatment where the disease-free interval has been short.

Another clinical dilemma is in determining the best management strategy for patients in complete clinical remission following chemotherapy. For example, how much is enough, or should additional alternative drugs be administered? Because of evolving resistance of residual tumor cells to chemotherapy, no advantage to prolonged platinum-based treatment beyond the standard six to eight cycles seems likely. Moreover, the few relevant studies find no survival advantage for continuing "maintenance" chemotherapy once standard treatment is done. Nevertheless, concepts of maintenance treatment with drugs such as hexamethymelamine are appealing and being investigated. The role of intraperitoneal chemotherapy, chromic phosphate (^{32}P) and whole abdominal radiation as consolidation treatments in this setting remains to be proven by its proponents.

As a practical matter then, for patients who have completed first-line treatment and are NED, it has been our policy to offer participation in thoughtful clinical trials to those who are eligible. Until more evidence is available, however, patients who decline or are ineligible for research protocols are counseled regarding the seemingly inevitable risk of relapse and the need for follow up. Generally, such patients not on protocols have no second-look surgery, are off chemotherapy, are followed by physical examinations and CA-125s, and encouraged to engage fully in life. During follow-up, radiographic studies add little to surveillance in otherwise asymptomatic patients.

Although ovarian cancer remains a lethal disease for most, still, as this case demonstrates, quality of life and disease-free survival is improved by modern treatment strategies, even if imperfect. Separating this patient from some others facing comparable decisions is the availability of paclitaxel to be employed upon recurrence. Whether or not its use accelerated by SLL, would benefit the patient's overall survival is unknown but seems dubious. After careful consideration, only she can choose from among the available options the strategy she feels is best.

References

NIH Consensus Conference. Ovarian cancer: Screening, treatment, and follow-up, JAMA 1995; 273:.

Roberts W, et al. Second-look laparotomy in the management of gynecologic malignancy. Gynecol Oncol 1982; 133:345.

PHYSICIAN'S RESPONSE

GEORGE A. OMURA

In a patient with stage IIIB disease following six courses of cisplatin and cyclophosphamide, further intervention is of uncertain value; the patient can be observed.

However, it is very probable that residual microscopic or macroscopic cancer is still present. If a protocol is available and the patient consents, that would be the best solution to this quandary. Such a protocol (or protocols) would likely require a second-look laparotomy, with different intervention depending on the pathological findings.

A current study of the Gynecologic Oncology Group (GOG) randomizes patients with no residual to intraperitoneal chromic phosphate (^{32}P) or observation; a Southwest Oncology Group study of intraperitoneal interferon versus observation is also being conducted. No results are available at present from these trials. Studies of systemic or intraperitoneal chemotherapy need to be done with appropriate controls. Whole abdominal irradiation would be appropriate for study as a "consolidation" therapy, again with concurrent controls in a randomized trial. Microscopic residual could be studied in the same way.

For the patient with gross residual disease, debulking could be attempted but is of unproven value. Systemic chemotherapy can be considered, but there is no agreement about the drug regimen, dose, or duration. A GOG trial of paclitaxel at two dose levels (GOG 134) recently completed accrual, but no results are available.

Second-line chemotherapy with doxorubicin, hexamethylmelamine, fluorouracil, ifosfamide, alpha interferon, or tamoxifen has not been predictably helpful. Studies of new agents are appropriate for consenting patients. Megadose chemotherapy with marrow rescue is a legitimate area of study but must be regarded as investigational.

Should this patient be treated longer with cyclophosphamide and cisplatin? Two randomized trials (1,2) failed to show a significant advantage for more than five or six courses of cisplatin-based chemotherapy. Actually, those trials did allow partial responders in the short arm to receive more therapy, confounding the study design. There was a slight (not significant) improvement in median survival for the longer planned treatment, but there was clearly more toxicity.

Although the question about longer treatment has not been completely settled, I would not give this patient more of the same chemotherapy.

Since paclitaxel has emerged as a very active drug both first- and second-line, what about skipping the second-look operation and switching this patient to paclitaxel now? That approach raises several unanswered questions. How long to treat, at what dose? Would treating at relapse produce the same long-term result?

To summarize: If the patient were ineligible for a study or did not consent, I would recommend observation at this point. If the patient found that plan unacceptable, I would consider six courses of paclitaxel (175 mg/m^2 over 3 hr every 3 weeks) while reiterating that its value as a consolidation therapy is unproven.

References

1. Bertelsen K, Jakobsen A, Stroyer I, et al. A prospective randomized comparison of 6 and 12 cycles of cyclophosphamide, Adriamycin, and cisplatin in advanced epithelial ovarian cancer: A Danish Ovarian Study Group trial (DACOVA). Gynecol Oncol 1993; 49:30–36.
2. Hakes TB, Chalas E, Hoskins WJ, et al. Randomized prospective trial of 5 versus 10 cycles of cyclophosphamide, doxorubicin and cisplatin in advanced ovarian carcinoma. Gynecol Oncol 1992; 45:284–289.

PHYSICIAN'S RESPONSE

HOWARD D. HOMESLEY

By definition, a stage IIIB patient has involvement of one or both ovaries with histologically confirmed abdominal peritoneal implants, none exceeding 2 cm in diameter, and negative lymph nodes, Thus, this is an optimal patient of unknown tumor grade who should have a median relapse-free interval of at least 18 to 24 months. The dilemma is whether any treatment at this time would alter the outcome. Long-term survival is low (15 to 20%) and improvement in therapy for advanced-disease patients is essential; thus, intervention on protocol therapy at this time is advised.

In addition to having optimal disease, this patient responded rapidly with normalization of the CA-125, which is indicative of being platinum-sensitive. The normal pelvic examination means little other than that no disease is palpable within the pelvis, while the CT scan of the abdomen may be at most 70 to 80% accurate in establishing no persistent disease.

Because of the availability of a number of protocol approaches, it may be worthwhile to consider at least operative second-look laparoscopy to discover macroscopic disease. Laparotomy would be necessary to find microscopic disease in order to establish whether the patient has persistent tumor at this particular time. The operative morbidity should be minimal for this patient.

There is no indication that continuing chemotherapy beyond six cycles is beneficial (1). Over 200 stage III and IV epithelial ovarian patients were randomized to six more courses of cyclophosphamide, doxorubicin, and cisplatin. The complete pathological response at second-look laparotomy was 23% at six cycles versus 25% for 12 cycles, when the median 3-year survival was 29% for six cycles and 35% for 12 cycles, with none of the differences statistically significant.

Yet, there is a plethora of approaches available for women in this age group who have persistent disease following first-line therapy. In the 1980s, highly active agents such as paclitaxel were not available to these patients, so it is truly unknown at this time what the benefit of early intervention with different active agents may be in patients with minimal or microscopic persistent disease after first-line therapy.

Immediately available to the patient would be intraperitoneal chemotherapy with paclitaxel, which is being assessed in an ongoing Gynecologic Oncology Group trial. This may have significant benefit to the patient with macroscopic (< 5 mm) or microscopic persistent disease. Systemic paclitaxel therapy could be offered to this patient as well.

Another agent possibly soon to be available to the patient would be topotecan which is undergoing phase II testing and may be of benefit. Camptothecins belong to a group of anticancer agents with the unique mechanism of action of poisoning eukaryotic DNA topoisomerase 1. Topotecan is one of the two camptothecin derivatives—topotecan and CPT-11—that are promising chemotherapeutic agents and may have value in second-line therapy.

Although this patient was platinum-sensitive with evidence of rapid response to first-line therapy, there appears to be minimal activity for intensification by using intraperitoneal carboplatin, as in a recent series the overall response was 12% (2). After second-look laparotomy with discovery of persistent disease 2 cm or less in diameter, there seems to be no advantage to consolidation therapy with whole abdominal radiation therapy.

Even in platinum-resistant epithelial ovarian cancer, there is some indication that oral etoposide will have a moderate response rate of about 25%. Hexamethylmelamine chemotherapy has demonstrated an objective response of at least 20% only in platinum-sensitive patients.

Unfortunately, if the second-look laparotomy is negative and the patients are consolidated with intraperitoneal chemotherapy with either cisplatin or mitoxantrone, there is a recurrence rate of about 25% as early as 24 months later. A randomized GOG study in second-look–negative patients will clarify the role of chromic phosphate (^{32}P) in this setting.

There are many potentially beneficial treatment alternatives available to the patient with a "clinical complete response." A second-look procedure definitely establishes the disease status. Protocol approaches hopefully will offer leads to improved outcome.

References

1. Bertelsen K, Jakobsen A, Stroyer J, et al. A prospective randomized comparison of 6 and 12 cycles of cyclophosphamide, Adriamycin, and cisplatin in advanced epithelial ovarian cancer: A Danish Ovarian Study Group trial. Gynecol Oncol 1993: 49:30–36.
2. Guaslla J, Lhomme C, Kerbrat P, et al. Phase II trial of intraperitoneal carboplatin in ovarian carcinoma patients with macroscopic residual disease at second-look laparotomy: A multicentre study of the French Federation Nationale des Centres de Lutte Contre le Cancer. Ann Oncol 1994; 5:127–132.

PHYSICIAN'S RESPONSE

JAMES NELSON

This 56-year-old woman with stage IIIB ovarian carcinoma, after initial surgical staging/debulking and six courses of platinum-based chemotherapy, is clinically free of disease based on physical exam, CT scan, and serum CA-125. What is the next step in managing this patient?

Radiological assessment is used both preoperatively to aid in staging and postoperatively to screen for gross recurrence. Ascites, most large omental masses, retroperitoneal adenopathy, and hepatic lesions are seen easily on CT scans, but this imaging technique has limited value in detecting subclinical disease. The false-negative rate of CT scans in picking up persistent or recurrent ovarian cancer is 45%.

This patient's serum CA-125 level is decreased from the preoperative level and is now in the normal range. When used to follow ovarian cancer patients after surgery and during and after chemotherapy, serum CA-125 has a positive predictive value for recurrence of almost 100% but a negative predictive value of only 56%. This assay is not sensitive enough to exclude subclinical disease. Although still under study, cancer-associated serum antigen (CASA) is a tumor marker shown to be sensitive to ovarian cancer (1). When used in conjunction with CA-125, the negative predictive value of tumor marker studies improved markedly, and the CASA assay detected 50% of positive second-look laparotomies.

Zorlu et al. (2), in April 1994, found that one-third of 46 patients with epithelial ovarian cancer who were clinically free of disease after initial surgical debulking and six courses of CAP chemotherapy had positive second-look laparotomies; they concluded that a routine second-look is still important in the management of advanced-stage disease.

Second-look laparotomy is necessary to determine response to therapy. Through a low midline vertical incision, one accomplishes thorough inspection, washings for cytology, resection of macroscopic disease, multiple biopsies of all peritoneal surfaces, and lymphadenectomy if not previously done. Although second-look laparotomy (SLL) has not been shown to influence patient survival, it does provide important prognostic information. The findings on SLL correlate with prognosis based on initial tumor stage and grade, on type of chemotherapy used, and on the degree of surgical effort on initial laparotomy.

Laparoscopy is a less invasive mode to evaluate the abdominal cavity. The open technique is recommended for use in the patients at risk for intraperitoneal adhesions, i.e., previous laparotomy and presence of cancer. Through the laparoscope, good visualization of peritoneal surfaces can be accomplished, cytological and histological specimens are easily obtained, and resectability of any recurrence can be evaluated. Laparoscopic lymphadenectomies are now performed regularly in most large centers. However, a recent study showed 35% false-negative laparoscopies when immediate laparotomy was done. The role of laparoscopy in second-look evaluation of ovarian cancer still needs to be defined.

We recommend SLL in this patient. It will provide prognostic information and indicate the possible need for intraperitoneal chemotherapy. The only reason not to proceed with second-look surgery is the failure of studies to show a benefit. The reason we recommend this approach is that all of the large studies have lumped all epithelial ovarian carcinomas together and refer to them as a single entity. Whether this is valid or not we do not know. In this case we do not know the histological type of this cancer. Certainly we do not know with any certainty whether SLL is a good procedure or not. We do know that platinum-based regimens are followed by the highest rate of recurrence after a complete clinical response.

References

1. Ward BG, McGuckin MA, Ramm LE, et al. The management of ovarian carcinoma is improved by the use of cancer-associated serum antigen and CA 125 assays. Cancer 1993; 71:430.
2. Zorlu CG, Cobanoglu O, Caglar T, et al. How does negative clinical evaluation of ovarian carcinoma after full course of chemotherapy correlate with second-look laparotomy findings? J Surg Oncol 1994; 55:255.

38

Secondary Surgical Cytoreduction in a Patient Responding to Chemotherapy

CASE

A 42-year-old woman is found to have bulky stage III ovarian cancer at an exploratory laparotomy. Minimal tumor debulking is achieved. The postlaparotomy CA-125 is 4350.

The patient is treated with six courses of cisplatin and paclitaxel (Taxol) with a decline of the CA-125 into the normal range following the fifth course of chemotherapy. Pelvic examination following the completion of chemotherapy reveals a 2- by 2-cm movable left-sided pelvic mass. The remainder of the physical examination is unremarkable. An abdominal and pelvic CT scan confirms the physical findings but demonstrates no other disease.

PHYSICIANS' RESPONSE

POLLY VAUGHAN
WELDON E. CHAFE

This 42-year-old woman with an ovarian cancer presents a difficult management dilemma. We are charged with the goal of providing her with the longest disease-free survival possible coupled with the optimal quality of life possible during any treatment recommended. A thorough attempt needs to be made to obtain her operative note and pathology report from her previous surgery. What was it that made her essentially inoperable at her first laparotomy? The extent of

296

residual disease left after that laparotomy and the cell type and grade of her tumor all impact upon her survival and any recommendation for future management. It is presumed that this information may not be available.

Because of the suboptimal debulking at her initial surgery and the fact that she has had an excellent response to induction chemotherapy with paclitaxel and cisplatin, she is a good candidate for a repeat laparotomy. Guidelines for choosing a patient for this procedure vary, but generally her younger age, normal CA-125, and essentially the clinical absence of disease by examination and radiographic studies. No prospective randomized trials have been done to demonstrate an increase in survival for those undergoing secondary cytoreduction with subsequent chemotherapy versus continued chemotherapy alone. Hoskins et al. (1) have reported increased disease-free survival and survival times within the subgroup undergoing secondary cytoreduction. That is, those with only microscopic residual disease had significantly increased survival times compared with those with macroscopic disease.

In this patient a repeat surgical procedure would determine the nature of this 2- by 2-cm movable left-sided pelvic mass. The surgery also offers the advantages of assessing directly the response to induction chemotherapy. A complete restaging procedure could be done, including total abdominal hysterectomy, bilateral salpingo-oophorectomy, omentectomy, appendectomy, nodal sampling, and so on. If the mass felt represents persistent disease, tissue samples can be obtained for in vitro studies to determine sensitivities to chemotherapeutic agents. This may allow the selection of agents with a greater probability of disease response.

If the second-look procedure is negative (no evidence of disease), several management options are available. Relapse is expected to occur in 50% of women with ovarian cancer having a negative second-look surgery. Therefore, adjunctive treatment is recommended in an attempt to improve survival. Five-year survivals with intraperitoneal chromic phosphate (^{32}P) after a negative second-look laparotomy have been reported as high as 85 to 90%.

If the laparotomy is positive for disease, all possible attempts at cytoreductive surgery should be made. Continued intravenous chemotherapy with the patient's previous regimen of platinum and paclitaxel or with other agents are both reasonable choices in this patient, given her good initial response. Drug resistance assay studies would be helpful in drug selection. The number of courses of additional chemotherapy would be dependent in part on the agents used and their side effects. For continued platinum-based regimens, an additional six to eight courses may be acceptable (toxicity limited) with intermittent CA-125, physical examination, and radiographic studies used to follow response and/or evidence of recurrence.

Another option to consider is whole abdominal radiation after minimal volume disease has been obtained at her second laparotomy. There are no reports available comparing whole abdominal radiation versus chemotherapy in patients who have undergone secondary cytoreductive surgical procedures following induction chemotherapy. Some investigators have reported good results in small series of patients treated with whole abdominal radiation. Morgan et al. (2) have reported on the utilization of hyperfractionation of dosing for whole abdominal radiation, pointing out that it is associated with significant, long disease-free intervals and minimal short- and long-term toxicities in selected patients.

Intraperitoneal chemotherapy provides another option for management after both negative and positive laparotomies. The results seem to be institution- and investigator-dependent.

In summary, although this patient had large-volume residual disease following initial surgery, her young age and rapid response to induction chemotherapy are good prognostic factors. We would recommend a reassessment laparotomy at this time with subsequent therapy based on surgical findings and pathological assessment.

References

1. Hoskins WJ, Rubin SC, et al. Influence of secondary cytoreduction at the time of second-look laparotomy on the survival of patients with epithelial ovarian carcinoma. Gynecol Oncol 1989; 34:365.
2. Morgan L, Chafe WE, et al: Hyperfractionation of whole abdomen radiation therapy: Salvage treatment of persistent ovarian carcinoma following chemotherapy. Gynecol Oncol 1988; 31:122–134.

PHYSICIAN'S RESPONSE

HANS KREBS

The patient presented in this case has an advanced, biologically aggressive ovarian carcinoma and faces a very poor prognosis. This assumption is based on the following observations:

1. Only minimal tumor debulking was carried out at the time of the primary exploratory laparotomy. Assuming that a competent surgeon was present at the operation, inadequate cytoreductive surgery is often related to unfavorable growth characteristics of the ovarian carcinoma.

2. The CA-125 level fell into the normal range only after the fifth course of chemotherapy. This reflects a relatively slow regression of the tumor in response to the chemotherapy. Long-term remissions are uncommon unless the CA-125 level decreases to normal after the *second* course of chemotherapy.

3. Following completion of chemotherapy with six courses of cisplatin and paclitaxel, the patient is found to have a 2- by 2-cm mass. If cancerous, the mass signals chemotherapy failure. The fact, however, that the CA-125 was quite high (4350 µg/mL) following the primary laparotomy strongly suggests that the

CA-125 is a very sensitive tumor marker in this case. Hence, a CA-125 value in the normal range may indicate that the palpated mass is not malignant. The patient being only 42 years old and having a single mass without any evidence of tumor elsewhere appears to be an excellent candidate for secondary cytoreductive surgery.

Unfortunately, there is currently no clear evidence to suggest that secondary debulking offers any substantial survival advantage to patients with partial responses to chemotherapy. This is because of lack of effective salvage therapy after firstline chemotherapy failure (1). Nonetheless, secondary cytoreduction may well render this patient free of all visible tumor and thus improve her chances of responding favorably to second-line chemotherapy, intraperitoneal chemotherapy, intraperitoneal chromic phosphate (^{32}P), or whole abdominal radiation therapy. As the tumor is mobile, a primary laparoscopic approach for evaluation and possible resection of the mass may be preferable to laparotomy in this particular situation.

Theoretically, removal of poorly perfused, devascularized, and necrotic bulky tumor will increase the fraction of actively dividing cells and make them more susceptible to cytotoxic agents. This is a major argument why the patient may have fared better altogether had a secondary debulking procedure been carried out earlier, i.e., after the second or third course of chemotherapy, when persistence of the CA-125 above normal projected suboptimal response to chemotherapy and ultimate treatment failure. This approach, often referred to as "interval debulking" after induction chemotherapy, has recently been shown to significantly lengthen progression-free and overall survival in patients who had mostly bulky, unresectable tumor at initial surgery (2).

References

1. Williams L. Secondary cytoreduction of ovarian malignancies. In: Markman M, Hoskins WJ, eds. Cancer of the Ovary. New York: Raven Press, 1993:187–203.
2. Van der Burg MEL, van Lent M. Buyse M, et al. The effect of debulking surgery after induction chemotherapy on the prognosis in advanced epithelial ovarian cancer. N Engl J Med 1995; 332:629–634.

PHYSICIAN'S RESPONSE

ED PARTRIDGE

This patient presents an interesting dilemma in which there are a number of potential options, none of which has a well-established survival advantage over any other. This patient has a number of poor prognostic factors influencing ultimate survival; stage III suboptimally resected disease at initial surgery, failure of the CA-125 to return to normal after the first two to three courses of chemotherapy, and lack of complete response to paclitaxel/cisplatin combination therapy, thereby limiting effective second-line chemotherapy interventions. Current options for this patient include:

Continue paclitaxel/cisplatin. She has had an obvious response to this combination, although apparently not complete. An argument could be made for continuing for several more cycles, although there is little likelihood that this would eventually result in a complete pathological response.

Change to another chemotherapy regimen. The response to currently available standard second line agents in paclitaxel/cisplatin failures is not well documented, since this is a relatively new combination. The response rate would be expected to be quite low and ultimate cure unlikely. Options would include hexamethymelamine, ifosfamide, or cyclophosphamide. Since these standard second-line therapies would be expected to have only a modest response rate, a more attractive option, if a change in therapy is to be made, would be to offer investigational second-line therapy to this patient with measurable disease.

Secondary debulking surgery. A reexploration with intent to secondarily debulk this presumed isolated area of persistent disease is also a consideration in this patient. The impact of secondary debulking upon ultimate survival is very controversial. (1,2) An OncoScint scan to evaluate the extent of persistent disease may be very appropriate in this situation. If multiple areas of uptake are found, there would be very doubtful benefit from surgery, as complete elimination of residual disease would be unlikely. A secondary laparotomy would, however, be more attractive if the patient were willing to undergo investigational therapy, particularly intraperitoneal investigational protocols.

Discontinuation of therapy. The last option would be discontinuation of therapy with follow-up only. Since there is unconvincing evidence that any second-line therapy will ultimately result in total eradication of the cancer, a perfectly reasonable option is to follow the patient and consider second-line therapy (conventional or investigational) only when there is progression of disease and/or the patient is symptomatic.

If the patient is ineligible or unwilling to participate in an investigational therapy, this latter option is perhaps the most attractive. The patient would be spared the burden of therapy until there is a clear benefit, such as relief of symptoms.

References

1. Redman CW, Blackledge G, Lawton FG, et al. Early second surgery in ovarian cancer–Improving the potential for cure or another unnecessary operation? Eur J Surg Oncol 1990; 16:426–429.

2. Carson LF, Rubin SC. Secondary cytoreduction—Thoughts on the "pro" side. Gynecol Oncol 1993; 51:127–130.

PHYSICIANS' RESPONSE

EDWARD PODCZASKI
RODRIGUE MORTEL

Management of advanced ovarian epithelial carcinomas has emphasized optimal cytoreductive surgery (debulking) followed by cytotoxic chemotherapy employing a platinum-based regimen with paclitaxel (Taxol). Clinical studies have demonstrated that response rates and survival rates are significantly improved in those patients who complete initial surgery with small tumor burdens. Since a substantial number of patients complete initial surgery with bulky residual disease, neoadjuvant or "cytoreductive" chemotherapy has been used, followed by interval debulking surgery. In this approach two or three cycles of intensive cytotoxic chemotherapy are administered, followed by repeat debulking surgery. The European Organization for Research on Treatment of Cancer prospectively evaluated such an approach in 299 patients completing primary surgery with tumor implants greater than 1 cm in diameter. After three cycles of cisplatin/cyclophosphamide chemotherapy, patients without progression were randomized between interval debulking or no further surgery, followed by at least three cycles of chemotherapy. Interval debulking surgery resulted in a significant improvement in both progression-free and overall survival.

In the present situation, the patient underwent minimal debulking surgery followed by six cycles of chemotherapy. Despite initially bulky disease, the patient was left with only a small, mobile 2-cm mass. The CA-125 had normalized and there was no evidence of other disease by radiological studies. Despite advances in imaging and tumor markers, these diagnostic methods leave limitations in demonstrating residual disease.

Under the circumstances presented, we would recommend a reassessment laparotomy in order to document disease status with hysterectomy, bilateral salpingo-oophorectomy, and tumor debulking in the presence of residual disease. The findings noted after completion of chemotherapy may represent benign pathology. The patient obviously experienced an excellent response to initial chemotherapy. If residual disease were found, we would perform a secondary cytoreductive procedure. The subject of secondary debulking remains controversial; however, second-look data have shown that patients completing surgery with minimal disease have had extended survival with further chemotherapy. Furthermore, such observations are supported by calculations of tumor volumes and doubling times. If one or more spherical tumor implants measuring 2.5 cm in diameter are aggressively reduced to diameters of 5 mm, the residual tumor would require six doublings to achieve its original size. Assuming a doubling time of 50 to 90 days for ovarian carcinoma, the prolongation of life would be estimated to be 6 to 18 months, even without the benefit of further chemotherapy. If residual disease were documented, we would continue with a platinum-based paclitaxel regimen, as toxicity permits. In light of some deterioration of kidney function, we would switch to carboplatin or high-dose paclitaxel chemotherapy. Although the slow fall in CA-125 beyond the third cycle of chemotherapy is concerning, this patient is young and no doubt wants an aggressive therapeutic approach.

References

Podratz KC, Cliby WA. Second-look surgery in the management of epithelial ovarian carcinoma. Gynecol Oncol 1994; 55:S128–S133.

van der Burg MEL, van Lent M, Kobierska A, et al. Intervention debulking surgery (IDS) does improve survival in advanced epithelial ovarian cancer (EOC); An EORTC Gynecological Cancer Cooperative Group (GCCG) Study. Proc ASCO 1993; 12:258.

PHYSICIAN'S RESPONSE

JOHN WEED

The patient has achieved an excellent response to combination chemotherapy with cisplatin and paclitaxel. Notwithstanding the high probability of encountering residual carcinoma, one should recommend cytoreductive surgery. The advantages of this approach are definition and documentation of disease, cytoreduction, tumor cell harvest for chemosensitivity testing, and the opportunity for bone marrow harvest.

Since we assume the patient has persistent disease and needs further cytotoxic therapy, we can take advantage of this situation by performing a bone marrow aspiration to look for malignant seeding, which may be present in 1.9% of ovarian cancer patients. A negative marrow aspirate would allow us to consider a high-dose marrow replacement protocol.

A second advantage of cytoreductive surgery would be tumor harvest for chemosensitivity assay. This patient has received the two most active available agents for the treatment of advanced ovarian malignancy. Any help received from the assay to guide our choices and to possibly reduce toxicity would be very helpful.

We recommend reexploration for cytoreduction following bone marrow aspirate and mechanical bowel preparation under the cover of prophylactic antibiotics. We favor this approach over a laparoscopic evaluation for the ability to optimally cytoreduce and because of the options for marrow harvest and/or the implantation of a peritoneal access device for intraperitoneal therapy.

PHYSICIAN'S RESPONSE

EDDIE REED

Although this is a very controversial area, this consultant strongly supports secondary cytoreduction surgery in a patient who fits the following criteria: (a) a presentation of bulky disease that has responded well to initial chemotherapy; (b) reasonable evidence that tumor debulking can now be done safely; (c) good patient performance status; (d) reasonable evidence that the tumor may still retain chemosensitivity; (e) patient acceptance that postoperative chemotherapy (either intraperitoneal or intravenous) will be implemented after surgery.

If cytoreduction is to be performed, it might be approached by initial laparoscopic evaluation. If laparoscopy shows disease that is probably amenable to debulking, then general anesthesia with full laparotomy can be implemented at the same sitting. If laparoscopy shows disease that is probably not amenable to debulking, the risk of general anesthesia has been avoided, along with avoidance of delay of the next cycle of chemotherapy.

The goal of cytoreduction is to eliminate all visible disease. Under this circumstance, it is clear that the patient should benefit from such surgery. Surgery should be followed by intraperitoneal chemotherapy (preferably cisplatin-based), or possibly by intravenous chemotherapy. The most experience is with intraperitoneal chemotherapy, although several research centers (including the National Cancer Institute) are investigating the role of intravenous consolidation with paclitaxel-based chemotherapy. One advantage of paclitaxel-based therapy (paclitaxel alone or given with cyclophosphamide), is the ability of such therapy to induce continued tumor regression after six, or eight, or ten cycles of treatment.

This patient has shown dramatic reduction of the CA-125 level (from 4350 to normal), suggesting a dramatic reduction in tumor bulk. This occurred over five cycles of chemotherapy, and the patient received a sixth cycle. The current comparatively low volume of disease suggests that it is certainly possible that debulking could now be done and that chemosensitivity might still be present. However, it has been reported that induction of DNA repair gene expression occurs in ovarian tumor tissues with time while patients are receiving platinum-based chemotherapy. If a secondary cytoreduction is to be performed, it should be done by an experienced gynecological or surgical oncologist. Although this may seem obvious, it is a point that should be stressed.

Some physicians believe that youth (this patient is 42 years old) is an important factor in the decision-making process. I personally agree with that philosophy. I believe that the decision should be made based on patient performance status and the presence or absence of comorbid disease. At this institution, we have had good anecdotal success, using this approach, with several patients above the age 65.

References

Bicher A, Kohn E, Sarosy G, et al. The absence of cumulative bone marrow toxicity in patients with recurrent adenocarcinoma of the ovary receiving dose intense Taxol and G-CSF. Anti-Cancer Drugs 1993; 4:141–148.

Chambers SK, Chambers JT, Kohorn EI, et al. Evaluation of the role of second-look surgery in ovarian cancer. Obstet Gynecol 1988; 72:404–408.

Dabholkar M, Bostick-Bruton F, Weber C, et al. ERCC1 and ERCC2 expression in malignant tissues from ovarian cancer patients. J Natl Cancer Inst 1992; 84:1512–1517.

Hoskins WJ, Rubin SC, Dulaney E, et al. Influence of secondary cytoreduction at the time of second-look laparotomy on the survival of patients with epithelial ovarian carcinoma. Gynecol Oncol 1989; 34:365–371.

Markman M, Howell SB, et al. Intraperitoneal chemotherapy with high dose cisplatin and cytarabine for refractory ovarian carcinoma and other malignancies principally involving the peritoneal cavity. J Clin Oncol 1985; 3:925–.

Podratz KC, Schray MF, Wiegand HS, et al. Evaluation of treatment and survival after positive second-look laparatomy. Gynecol Oncol 1988; 31:9–24.

Reed E, John ED, Sarosy G, et al. Paclitaxel, cisplatin, and cyclophosphamide in human ovarian cancer: Molecular rationale and early clinical results. Semin Oncol 1995; 22:90–96.

39

Advanced Borderline Tumor of the Ovary

CASE

A 36-year-old woman is found to have a left-sided ovarian mass on an infertility evaluation. Computed tomography (CT) confirms the presence of the mass. The CA-125 is 12.

At laparotomy, performed by a gynecologist assisted by a general surgeon, the patient is found to have a borderline tumor of the left ovary. The patient undergoes a left salpingo-oophorectomy, omentectomy, and complete debulking of multiple pelvic implants.

PHYSICIAN'S RESPONSE

TATE THIGPEN

Borderline tumors of the ovary (or tumors of low malignant potential) constitute a small percentage of patients with coelomic epithelial carcinoma of the ovary. These lesions are distinguished pathologically by a lack of invasion. They are distinguished clinically by an indolent course with little tendency to behave aggressively. These facts determine the appropriate management for this patient. Before a final course of action is set, several questions should be answered.

First, is the lesion truly a borderline tumor of the ovary? The pathological specimens should be reexamined by an experienced gynecological pathologist for any evidence of invasion. Should such evidence be found, the patient will require chemotherapy in the form of paclitaxel plus cisplatin. In the absence of evidence of invasion, the diagnosis of a tumor of low malignant potential can be confirmed and further management decision made.

Second, what is the extent of disease? The data provided suggest that this patient has at least a stage II tumor. In the absence of a careful exploration of the abdominal cavity, which is not mentioned in the case description, there is a significant likelihood that at least microscopic evidence of disease outside the pelvis is present and that the patient has stage III disease. The case description suggests that all gross disease in the pelvis was resected at the initial surgery; but, in the absence of an adequate staging laparotomy, residual gross disease may well be present outside the pelvis. Does this in fact matter to management decisions? In the case of invasive carcinoma, a reexploration should be carried out. For borderline lesions, however, no further surgery is indicated at this point because of the indolent nature of the disease. Even in the presence of gross residual disease, the patient may experience years of progression-free survival.

Third, based on the answers to the first two questions, what further therapy is indicated at the present time? Assuming that a borderline lesion has been confirmed, this patient requires observation only regardless of the stage of disease. The fact that the initial CA-125 was normal means that this marker will probably be of little value in monitoring for recurrence and progression of disease. A baseline postoperative CT scan of the abdomen and pelvis should be done. The patient should thereafter be followed at 3-month intervals for any evidence of disease recurrence or progression by clinical examination. There is no need to repeat the CT scan unless the patient develops symptoms suggestive of recurrence.

Fourth, if recurrence or progression should occur at a later time, what therapy would be indicated? There is little scientific evidence on which to base such a decision. There are anecdotal reports of responses to both alkylating agents and the platinum compounds. Some have advocated the use of a single alkylating agent upon progression, in the belief that such an approach produces low risk and a reasonable chance for disease remission. If, on the other hand, the disease is clearly progressing, the use of the best chemotherapy regimen to offer the patient an optimal chance for disease response would seem to be the preferred course of action. The patient should, in fact, be treated with paclitaxel plus cisplatin at the time of progression but not before. The disease should clearly be behaving in a more aggressive manner.

In summary, the diagnosis of a borderline tumor should first be confirmed by an experienced gynecological pathologist. If confirmed, observation is all that is required until the disease process behaves in a clearly more aggressive manner, as manifested by disease progression. At that time, chemotherapy in the form of paclitaxel plus cisplatin should be used.

Reference

Trimble C, Trimble E: Management of epithelial ovarian tumors of low malignant potential. Gynecol Oncol 1994; 55:S52–S61.

PHYSICIANS' RESPONSE

MICHAEL RODRIGUEZ
BERND-UWE SEVIN

The patient presents with a stage II epithelial ovarian neoplasm of low malignant potential (LMP). All gross residual tumor was removed at the time of initial surgery. Fortunately, ovarian tumors of low malignant potential generally have an excellent prognosis and tend to follow an indolent disease course. For all stages, overall 5-, 10-, and 20-year survivals are 97, 95, and 89%, respectively.

Pathological criteria needed for the diagnosis include epithelial budding, multilayering of epithelium, mitotic activity, and nuclear atypia in the absence of stromal invasion, which is critical in distinguishing this entity from an invasive carcinoma of the ovary. Serous and mucinous are the two most common histological types, with serous types having a higher prevalence of bilateral ovarian and extraovarian involvement.

Interestingly, this patient has a history of infertility and possibly has used ovulation-inducing agents, which have been shown to be a risk factor for LMP ovarian neoplasms. Conversely, pregnancy, breast-feeding and the use of oral contraceptives all have been found to have protective effects against the development of LMP ovarian neoplasms.

Stage is the only prognostic factor that has definitely been correlated with survival. For stages I and II, long-term survival rates range between 94 and 100% whether adjuvant chemo/radiation therapy is included or not. For stage III patients, long-term survival rates reported range between 50 and 70%. Residual disease and conservative fertility-preserving surgery have been correlated with higher rates of recurrence and may impact on survival in more advanced-stage lesions. Mixed results have been obtained using DNA ploidy as an indicator for prognosis and invasiveness. We recommend that DNA flow cytometry should be obtained on ovarian neoplasms of LMP to identify patients with aneuploid (potentially more aggressive) tumors.

The presence of peritoneal implants in this patient is an important and interesting finding. Three types of peritoneal implants have been described in the literature: benign, noninvasive, and invasive. Benign implants have histological features of endosalpingosis. Noninvasive implants are glandular proliferations whose histological features are similar to those of borderline ovarian tumors. Invasive implants have similar histologic features with the presence of infiltration of the desmoplastic stroma and irregular borders at the margins of the implants.

The significance of the different types of implants is unclear. It is agreed that benign implants should be considered as such; however, the impact on survival and recurrence of noninvasive and especially invasive implants is controversial, with mixed reports in the literature.

The surgical management of this patient may have been optimized slightly by the addition of an ipsilateral pelvic and paraaortic lymph node sampling. If positive, this would upstage this patient from a stage II to stage IIIC. Though of academic interest, we would not recommend a repeat surgical procedure to restage this patient because the minimal information it would render would not change our clinical management. The preservation of the reproductive organs was appropriate, with removal of all gross tumor in patients desiring fertility. Most of these patients will be long-term survivors and many will go on to become pregnant. Thus, in patients desiring fertility, we recommend peritoneal washings for cytology, unilateral salpingo-oophorectomy, omentectomy, and peritoneal and diaphragmatic biopsies with ipsilateral pelvic and paraaortic lymph node sampling. To ensure adequate evaluation of the upper abdomen, we recommend the use of a midline vertical incision versus a low transverse incision for the staging procedure.

The question of adjuvant chemotherapy in patients with ovarian neoplasms of LMP has been an elusive one to answer. Clearly patients with stage I disease do not benefit from adjuvant therapy. In addition, most oncologists would agree that patients with stage II disease do not need further treatment. However, because of the mixed data suggesting poorer long-term survival in patients with invasive implants, if the peritoneal implants in this patient were invasive, we would recommend three to six courses of standard chemotherapy using the combination of a platinum-containing compound and paclitaxel or cyclophosphamide. In patients with stage III disease with no residual tumor after primary surgery or without invasive implants, adjuvant therapy has not been shown to affect long-term survival, and we would not recommend adjuvant chemotherapy in such patients.

References

Gershenson DM, Silva EG. Serous ovarian tumors of low malignant potential with peritoneal implants. Cancer 1990; 65:578–585.

Trimble CL, Trimble EL. Management of epithelial ovarian tumors of low malignant potential. Gynecol Oncol 1994; 55:S52–S61.

PHYSICIAN'S RESPONSE

FRANCO MUGGIA

This patient has had an adequate cancer operation and has also undergone apparently definitive treatment in view of the pathological findings. Chemotherapy or radiotherapy is not warranted in patients with resectable borderline (low-malignant-potential) tumors even with apparent pelvic spread of carcinoma that has been resected. Studies by the Gynecologic Oncology Group support less than 5% recurrence rates in resectable borderline tumors.

Current efforts utilizing molecular biology and DNA-ploidy analysis by flow cytometry are attempting to identify those patients with borderline tumors at high risk of recurrence and tumor progression at resection. Some indication that tumors with aneuploidy (1), her2/neu overexpression (2), and p53 and K-*ras* mutations (3,4) are associated with a higher incidence of recurrences has been obtained. Additional studies utilizing the patient material from the Gynecologic Oncology Group Protocol #72 with 456 entries are ongoing.

Two additional aspects in management should be discussed in the context of this patient: (a) use of additional tests or monitoring methods and (b) the pros and cons of administering chemotherapy—often advised by overly zealous oncologists abetted by overanxious patients. Experimental monitoring techniques might include positron emission tomography. A laparoscopy 6 months after the initial surgery could be considered appropriate. This might be preceded by one repeat CA-125 and a CT scan at that time. Subsequent assessments could be confined to physical (pelvic) exams semiannually. Chemotherapy is not indicated. Alkylating agents may not be effective against borderline cancers, and inadequate information exists for platinum compounds. In any event, treatment may promote a false sense of security as well as expose the patient to unnecessary toxicity and theoretically promote resistance.

References

1. Friedlander ML, Russell P, Taylor IW, et al. Flow cytometric analysis of cellular DNA content as an adjuvant to the diagnosis of ovarian tumors of borderline malignancy. Pathology 1984; 16:301–306.
2. Seidman J, Frisman DM, Norris HJ. Expression of the HER-2/neu protooncogene in serous ovarian neoplasms. Cancer 1992; 70: 2857–2860.
3. Mok SC, Bell DA, Knapp RC, et al. Mutations of K-ras protooncogene in human ovarian epithelial tumors of borderline malignancy. Cancer Res 1993; 53:1489–1492.
4. Kohler MF, Kerns BJ, Humphrey PA, et al. Mutation and overexpression of p53 in early-stage epithelial ovarian cancer. Obstet Gynecol 1993; 81:643–650.

PHYSICIANS' RESPONSE

HOLLY H. GALLION
EDWARD L. TRIMBLE

This infertility patient with an advanced borderline tumor of the ovary presents a challenging clinical dilemma. Although most borderline ovarian tumors occur in women of reproductive age, the majority are confined to the ovary at the time of diagnosis. In women who desire to retain their childbearing function, stage I borderline ovarian tumors can be safely managed with cystectomy or oophorectomy and surgical staging. In contrast, total abdominal hysterectomy and bilateral salpingo-oophorectomy is the recommended treatment for more advanced-stage disease. The value of adjuvant chemotherapy or radiotherapy in patients with advanced disease remains unproved. Overall, the prognosis for patients with serous and mucinous borderline ovarian tumors is excellent, with 20-year survival rates ranging from 90% with stage I disease to 70% for more advanced-stage disease.

Prior to any clinical decision making in this case, a careful pathological review of the primary ovarian tumor is needed to rule out the presence of frankly invasive disease. In addition, histological assessment of the peritoneal implants should be performed, and these implants should be classified as either benign, noninvasive, or invasive. Patients with benign peritoneal implants that contain areas of epithelium resembling the fallopian tube (endosalpingiosis) should be considered to have stage I disease and treated accordingly (1). However, patients with invasive peritoneal implants have a higher risk of recurrence and should be treated accordingly (2,3). It is possible that invasive implants may actually reflect the presence of primary peritoneal carcinoma rather than a borderline ovarian tumor. Although there are little data in the literature regarding the optimum treatment of borderline ovarian tumors with invasive implants, the general consensus is that these patients should be treated with adjuvant platinum and paclitaxel chemotherapy.

In the present case, if the diagnosis of borderline ovarian tumor is confirmed and the patient's implants are found to be benign, the patient should be reassured that her prognosis following conservative therapy is excellent. On the other hand, if the implants are not benign, the decision making is more difficult. The patient must be thoroughly educated regarding the clinical behavior of advanced-stage borderline ovarian tumors. She should be advised that the recurrence or progression rate for stage II and III borderline tumors is approximately 30% but that many patients with recurrent tumors are clinically well. It should also be emphasized that surgery is the mainstay of therapy and that although most investigators recommend adjuvant chemotherapy in the face of invasive peritoneal implants, the value of such therapy has not been demonstrated.

If, after careful consideration of these issues, the patient elects to give up her fertility, removal of the contralateral ovary, uterus, appendix, and complete staging should be performed. Alternatively, if she desires to continue her attempts at pregnancy, close monitoring of the residual ovary with transvaginal sonography and serum CA-125 determinations should be performed and definitive surgery delayed until the completion of childbearing.

References

1. Gershenson DM, Silva EG. Serous ovarian tumors of low malignant potential with peritoneal implants. Cancer 1990; 65:578–585.
2. Bell DA, Weinstock M, Scully RE. Peritoneal implants of ovarian serous borderline tumors: Histologic features and prognosis. Cancer 1988; 62:2212–2222.

PHYSICIAN'S RESPONSE

JONATHAN M. NILOFF

This case presents several problems. I will assume, based on the history, that this patient has a stage II borderline ovarian tumor and that all gross disease was resected. Issues that must be addressed include (a) the need for further surgery, (b) the need for adjuvant chemotherapy, and (c) appropriate follow-up.

a. The classic management for patients with stage II or greater border-line epithelial tumors of the ovary would include total abdominal hysterectomy and bilateral salpingo-oophorectomy with a complete cytoreductive procedure. If this patient is not interested in further fertility, then I would recommend proceeding with such surgery. If the patient strongly desires further fertility (which I assume she does based on her description as an infertility patient) and her fertility evaluation suggests that there is a realistic possibility that she might become pregnant, one might consider a more conservative management. However, the patient would have to understand that this would represent a departure from standard therapy and be willing to assume the unquantifiable potential risk of such an approach (informed consent). Borderline tumors, even when advanced in stage, are associated with very favorable prognoses, typically exceeding 80% at 5 years. Therefore, in the interest of fertility, one could consider no further surgery and follow the patient very carefully. However, borderline tumors are commonly estrogen-receptor-positive (1), and this patient likely has persistent microscopic disease. The magnitude of the potential increased risk for recurrence from the use of pharmacological agents to induce ovulation or the hormonal milieu of pregnancy is unknown.

b. Borderline epithelial tumors of the ovary are typically not responsive to cytotoxic chemotherapy. There is no evidence in the literature to suggest that survival is improved with such therapy. Therefore, given the favorable prognosis associated with this tumor and its lack of chemosensitivity, I would not recommend adjuvant chemotherapy regardless of the surgical approach selected.

c. This patient will require careful follow-up. Recurrences with border-line tumors often occur several years after their initial presentation. Follow-up modalities should include pelvic examination and infrequent radiologic imaging. CA-125 levels should also be obtained. However, borderline tumors typically do not manifest CA-125 elevations of the same magnitude observed among patients with invasive epithelial tumors. This patient's normal preoperative CA-125 level is consistent with this. Therefore, CA-125 in this patient may prove to be an insensitive marker for the early detection of recurrence, inasmuch as a large tumor burden may be required before the serum CA-125 level becomes elevated.

Reference

1. Jacobs TW, Cannistra S, Niloff J, Abu-Jawdeh GM. Immunohistochemical expression of estrogen receptors in ovarian serous and mucinous borderline tumors. Mod Pathol 1995; 8:91A.

PHYSICIAN'S RESPONSE

PEYTON T. TAYLOR

The "borderline" ovarian tumors were once viewed with circumspection and suspicion in the community of surgeons, especially among general surgeons. They are now internationally recognized as distinct histological types that are morphologically and biologically intermediate between obviously benign and obviously malignant ovarian neoplasms (1). Before making a prognostic statement and providing therapeutic advice, *all* of the histological material in this case will need to be reviewed by a pathologist interested and skilled in ovarian pathology. The distinction between a tumor of low malignant potential and a well-differentiated carcinoma is not easy, especially on frozen-section evaluation, and requires detailed study of multiple permanent sections.

Essentially all borderline ovarian tumors are either serous or mucinous in type and occur with roughly equal frequency. Serous tumors of low malignant potential (LMP) are bilateral in about 15% of patients, prompting careful inspection and, usually, wedge biopsy of a retained normal-appearing contralateral ovary. Mucinous LMP tumors are more commonly confined to the ovary. The presence of any appendiceal abnormality and a mucinous ovarian tumor (especially if there are visible extraovarian foci) requires appendectomy. The appendix is suspected to be the origin of most intraperitoneal low grade mucinous tumors involving the ovary, appendix, and distant intraperitoneal sites (2). Although LMP endometrioid and clear-cell tumor types exist, precise criteria for their diagnosis have not been generally established.

The multiple pelvic "implants" described do not necessarily imply malignant clinical behavior, a poor outcome, or the need for subsequent chemotherapy. In one large series, extraovarian disease was present at presentation in almost 20% of patients. In spite of this, nearly 90% of all patients with LMP (all histological types) were alive after 10 years, including those with extraovarian foci (3). Many of these patients received some type of postoperative treatment but often only localized pelvic radiation.

There are three patterns of extraovarian foci, and distinction between the types may have important prognostic and therapeutic implications. This point is also disputed. The types are (a) benign (endosalpingiosis), (b) LMP (borderline), and (c) invasive, well-differentiated carcinoma. Some consider the implants to represent metastases; others consider them to represent synchronous extraovarian proliferations arising from surface coelomic epithelium (mesothelium). Spontaneous "regression" of benign and borderline extraovarian foci has been reported following resection of the ovarian "primary." From cumulative reports, I am unclear as to whether subsequent radiation therapy or chemotherapy significantly alters the natural history of the disease.

In the absence of invasive foci, I believe the decision not to remove the uterus and apparently normal contralateral ovary, especially based on the frozen-section report, is entirely appropriate; the patient does not immediately need further surgery or chemotherapy and can pursue attempts for pregnancy. Because some patients do die with progressive/recurrent disease, many authors have advised hysterectomy and removal of the remaining ovary after completion of childbearing, hopefully to prevent subsequent relapse. There are few data to support or refute the concept or an advantage of "completion hysterectomy/ovariectomy"; it remains a highly individual decision.

References

1. Hart WR. Ovarian epithelial tumors of borderline malignancy (carcinomas of low malignant potential). Hum Pathol 1977; 8:541–549.
2. Young RH, Gilks CB, Scully RE. Mucinous tumors of the appendix associated with mucinous tumors of the ovary and pseudomyxoma peritonei. Am J Surg Pathol 1991; 15:415–429.
3. Aure JC, Høeg K, Kolstad P. Clinical and histological studies of ovarian carcinoma: Long-term follow-up of 990 cases. Obstet Gynecol 1971; 37:1–9.

40

Microscopic Residual Ovarian Cancer at Second-Look Laparotomy

CASE

A 47-year-old woman presents to her internist with increasing abdominal girth of 1 month's duration. Physical examination reveals massive ascites and a large pelvic mass.

The patient subsequently undergoes an exploratory laparotomy, which reveals stage IIIC papillary serous ovarian cancer. The patient is left with suboptimal residual disease following surgery. The postoperative CA-125 is 976.

The patient is treated with eight courses of carboplatin and paclitaxel (Taxol) with complete disappearance of ascites and other physical findings of disease. The CA-125 is < 7. The CT scan is unremarkable.

At second-look laparotomy, no gross disease is discovered but several biopsies reveal papillary serous cancer.

PHYSICIAN'S RESPONSE

ROBERT A. BURGER

The prognosis for patients with stage IIIC epithelial ovarian cancer depends on several variables, including age and performance status at diagnosis, tumor grade, extent of residual disease following initial debulking surgery, and completeness of response to platinum-containing chemotherapy found at reassessment surgery. The reported 5-year survival rate for patients whose greatest residual tumor diameter after primary surgery exceeds 1 cm (suboptimal disease) is only 10 to

20%. As these unfavorable survival statistics suggest, most patients with suboptimal disease following initial surgery will have gross residual disease found at surgical reassessment. On the other hand, women with microscopic disease following chemotherapy, as in the case presentation, will have an expected 5-year survival of 35%, while those with a negative second-look operation will have a 5-year survival of 60 to 70%. Thus, even a negative second-assessment operation does not assure a favorable outcome. The unfavorable prognosis for women who present with stage IIIC disease has been attributed primarily to chemotherapeutic drug resistance. Clinical trials directed at overcoming drug resistance are under way in a number of institutional and cooperative group protocols.

While six cycles of cisplatin and paclitaxel have been adopted by the Gynecologic Oncology Group as the standard regimen for suboptimally resected stage III or IV epithelial ovarian cancer, the results of several recent prospective randomized studies suggest that carboplatin and cisplatin have equivalent efficacy in this disease. Thus the choice of chemotherapy agents in this case should be viewed as the "gold standard."

With many cytotoxic agents, including the platinum compounds, demonstrating steep dose-response curves both in vitro and in preclinical testing, several dose-intensification approaches have been investigated in patients with platinum-refractory ovarian cancer in an effort to overcome drug resistance. Extensive experience has been gained from phase II trials of intraperitoneal cytotoxic agents, biological response modifiers or radioisotopes, and of dose-intensive systemic chemotherapy with autologous hematopoietic support. With these modalities, complete pathological responses have been observed principally in patients with microscopic or minimal macroscopic disease after achieving objective responses to initial platinum-based therapy (1,2).

Whole abdominal radiotherapy in the management of minimal residual disease has also been attempted as salvage treatment. Limited phase II data suggest that this modality is associated with few long-term survivors and an unacceptably high morbidity rate. Finally, new systemic agents with either novel mechanisms of action or the ability to reverse chemotherapeutic drug resistance are currently under phase I and II investigation.

Given the youth of the patient and her excellent response to first-line chemotherapy, we believe that continued aggressive chemotherapy is warranted. Nevertheless, the choice of salvage therapy is not clear-cut because (a) the theoretical pharmacokinetic advantage of intraperitoneal over systemic administration has not been confirmed by randomized trials, and (b) while a number of phase II studies of high-dose systemic therapy for patients with residual disease at second look have demonstrated pathological response rates of 70 to 80% (2), such responses have been short-lived and associated with substantial toxicity and cost. Accordingly, we believe that the preferred choice of treatment in this setting is a peer-reviewed, randomized trial that employs either intraperitoneal cytotoxic therapy and/or established cytotoxic agents of proven efficacy in the treatment of epithelial ovarian cancers. We believe that high-dose chemotherapy with autologous bone marrow support should be considered only in the investigational setting in view of the associated morbidity and cost. Such a phase II trial, currently under way by the Southwest Oncology Group (SWOG 9106), employs one of two high-dose chemotherapy regimens, each with autologous bone marrow support for all enrollees. In the absence of an available protocol, we currently prefer a regimen of weekly intraperitoneal paclitaxel at a dose of 60 mg/m^2 for a total of 12 weeks. We do not advocate a third-look procedure following this or any other salvage regimen except for patients on investigational protocols.

References

1. Markman M. Salvage therapy in ovarian cancer: Is there a role for intraperitoneal drug delivery? Gynecol Oncol 1993; 51:86–89.
2. Shpall EJ, Jones RB, Bearman SI, Purdy MP. Future strategies for the treatment of advanced epithelial ovarian cancer using high-dose chemotherapy and autologous bone marrow support. Gynecol Oncol 1994; 54:357–361.

PHYSICIAN'S RESPONSE

H.G. BALL

This patient with advanced suboptimally cytoreduced serous carcinoma of the ovary has had an excellent response to chemotherapy with carboplatin and paclitaxel. This is manifested by a fall in the CA-125, negative physical examination and CT scan, and a second-look laparotomy with microscopic residual disease. The decision we must now make is between expectant observation with no treatment or continued treatment.

Patients with microscopic residual disease at second-look have a better prognosis than those with gross residual disease, and their progression-free interval approaches that of patients with negative second-look operations. There has been no randomized study comparing no further treatment until disease progression with continued chemotherapy in this group of patients. Therefore, we cannot tell this patient which is the best course of action.

If therapy is continued, several options can be considered for this patient, including additional carboplatin and paclitaxel, intraperitoneal chromic phosphate (^{32}P), whole abdominal radiation therapy, intraperitoneal chemotherapy, intraperitoneal alpha-interferon, and high-dose chemotherapy with stem-cell rescue. Unfortunately, limited information is available on the efficacy of these options.

This patient has had an excellent response to primary therapy and continued chemotherapy with three to six courses of carboplatin and paclitaxel could be considered. This should be viewed as palliative, since patients with any amount of residual disease at second look are rarely cured with further treatment.

Intraperitoneal ^{32}P and whole abdominal radiation therapy have not been shown to prolong survival in this group of patients. If an ongoing Gynecologic Oncology Group protocol randomizing patients who have negative second-look operations to no further therapy versus intraperitoneal ^{32}P shows a survival advantage for patients receiving ^{32}P, then future studies should evaluate ^{32}P in patients with microscopic residual at second-look operations. Whole abdominal radiation therapy may be associated with troublesome bowel complications, particularly in patients who have had multiple previous surgeries.

Although high-dose chemotherapy with stem-cell rescue is appealing on theoretical grounds, there is no evidence to suggest that this approach is superior to conventional therapy. For this patient, I would favor intraperitoneal chemotherapy using either single-agent platinum, platinum-based combination therapy, or alpha-interferon. This is a young patient who has had an excellent response to primary treatment and might respond to additional intensive therapy. Ideally, I would prefer to treat this patient on an investigational protocol, since our knowledge of optimal therapy in this circumstance is meager.

References

Braly PS, Berek JS, Blessing JA, et al. Intraperitoneal administration of cisplatin and 5-fluorouracil in residual ovarian cancer: A phase II Gynecologic Oncology Group trial. Gynecol Oncol 1995; 56:164–168.
Copeland LJ, Gershenson DM, Wharton JT, et al. Microscopic disease at second-look laparotomy in advanced ovarian cancer. Cancer 1985; 55:472–478.

PHYSICIANS' RESPONSE

PABLO J. CAGNONI
ELIZABETH J. SHPALL

This 47-year-old woman's clinical course is quite representative of the results achieved today with conventional-dose therapy for stage II epithelial ovarian cancer. After optimal debulking surgery and state-of-the-art chemotherapy, 50% of the patients will have residual disease at the time of second-look laparotomy. There is currently no treatment option with certain possibility of cure in these patients.

We will comment upon three treatment options available for patients like yours who have residual disease documented at second-look laparotomy; they include standard, intraperitoneal, or hematopoietic stem-cell supported high-dose chemotherapy.

1. Standard chemotherapy. This patient received eight cycles of a platin

analog in combination with paclitaxel (Taxol). If the doses of carboplatin administered were appropriate, the chances for further standard chemotherapy to produce a sustained remission in this patient are very small.

2. Intraperitoneal chemotherapy. The role of intraperitoneal chemotherapy is still unclear, but it may be useful for patients like this, who initially respond to platin-containing chemotherapy and have small-volume residual disease. The reported response rates using intraperitoneal cisplatin and etoposide are as high as 50%, with up to 12 months of disease-free interval. Randomized trials have not been performed to confirm this data.

3. High-dose chemotherapy with autologous hematopoietic progenitor cell support (AHPCS). There are strong preclinical and clinical data to support the rationale for dose intensity in the treatment of ovarian cancer. Two prospective randomized trials testing dose intensity in advanced cancer patients demonstrated a significant survival advantage for those patients who received the higher-dose regimen.

The vast majority of studies using high-dose chemotherapy with AHPCS were made up of patients with bulky and/or refractory disease at the time of transplant. Table 1 describes results from a world survey of high-dose chemotherapy regimens employing AHPCS for ovarian cancer patients (1).

This report, published in 1993, included 277 transplants for ovarian cancer from five countries. The vast majority of patients had refractory bulk disease at the time of transplant. The patients from France and Japan, who had the least prior therapy and extent of disease when treated with high-dose therapy, had the longest median follow-up (> 40 months) and the best survival rates, while the remaining studies included patients followed for 2 years or less.

As of January 6, 1995, 249 transplants for ovarian cancer have been reported to the Autologous Blood and Marrow Transplant Registry from 51 U.S. centers

Table 1 High-Dose Chemotherapy with AHPCS for Poor-Prognosis Ovarian Cancer: World Survey

	N	Response Rate %	Median Duration (mo)	Median Survival (mo)
United States	146	71	6	12
Netherlands	21	60	10	NR
Italy	13	82	NR	NR
France	55	NE	NE	40
Japan	42	NE	NE	48
Total	277			

Key: AHPCS: high-dose chemotherapy with autologous hematopoietic progenitor cell support; NE: not evaluable; NR: not reported; mo: months.

(Table 2) (2). Of these patients 83% had measurable disease and 17% were in clinical complete remission at the time of transplant.

The 100-day mortality for this group of patients treated with a variety of regimens was 6 to 9%. The 2-year probability of survival was 33% for patients transplanted with measurable disease and 68% for those patients who were transplanted in complete remission.

These studies in refractory ovarian cancer patients demonstrate a higher response rate with stem-cell-supported high-dose therapy than any reported response rates for standard-dose therapy in a similar population. However, as we have learned by treating high-risk breast cancer patients, the maximal benefit of this therapy will be demonstrated in patients who have a poor prognosis with standard therapy but have minimal disease and minimal prior therapy at the time of transplant. The Southwestern Oncology Group has designed and initiated such a trial (SWOG 9106, Figure 1).

In this randomized phase II study patients with residual disease < 1.0 cm after cisplatin/carboplatin-based induction chemotherapy will receive either thiotepa/cyclophosphamide/cisplatin (Duke/University of Colorado regimen) or mitoxantrone/cyclophosphamide/carboplatin (Loyola regimen). Considering the poor re-

Table 2 High-Dose Chemotherapy with AHPCS in Ovarian Cancer: American Blood and Marrow Transplant Registry[a]

Patients	249
Centers	51
Disease status at time of transplant	
No disease evident	17%
Disease evident	83%
Source of AHCS	
Bone Marrow	48%
PBPC	25%
BP + PBPC	27%
100-day mortality	9%
Probability of survival at 2 years	
No disease evident	68%
Disease evident	33%

[a]These data have not yet been approved by the Advisory Committee of the ABMTR.
Key: AHPCS: high-dose chemotherapy with autologous hematopoietic progenitor cell support; PBPC: peripheral blood progenitor cell; BM: bone marrow.

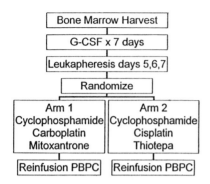

Figure 1 SWOG 9106: High-dose therapy with AHPCS for advanced ovarian cancer. (*Key*: SWOG = Southwestern Oncology Group; AHPCS = autologous hematopoietic progenitor cell support; G-CSF = granulocyte colony-stimulating factor; PBPC = peripheral blood progenitor cell.)

sults with the current standard treatment in patients with a positive second-look laparotomy, we recommend that this patient be enrolled on SWOG 9106.

References

1. Shpall EJ, Stemmer SM, Bearman SI, et al. High-dose chemotherapy with autologous bone marrow support for the treatment of epithelial ovarian cancer. In: Markman M, Hoskins WJ, eds. Cancer of the Ovary. New York: Raven Press, 1993; 327–339.
2. Horowitz MM. Personal communication. These data have not yet been approved by the Advisory Committee of the ABMTR.

PHYSICIAN'S RESPONSE

DAVID ALBERTS

Numerous therapeutic options are available to this patient, who has several disease features that convey a guarded prognosis. Specifically, the diagnosis of stage IIIC suboptimally debulked disease, treated first-line with paclitaxel/carboplatin, suggests a median survival of approximately 3 years (1). Although the serum CA-125 concentration is extremely low (i.e., < 7 U/mL), the presence of microscopic disease at second-look surgery is associated with progressive disease in virtually all patients within a 12- to 36-month period, depending on the aggressiveness of the cancer (e.g., tumor grade, which would invariably be moderately to poorly differentiated in this patient, who had suboptimal disease following initial exploratory laparotomy). In discussions with this patient concerning therapeutic options, I would subdivide potential treatments into standard, FDA-approved drugs for salvage treatment of ovarian cancer; standard, FDA-approved drugs for other indications; and experimental therapies as follows:

1. Standard, FDA-approved drugs for salvage therapy of ovarian cancer.
   a. Carboplatin. Since the patient has already received eight courses of carboplatin (dose not given but assumed to be between 500 and 600 mg/m^2 or, using the Calvert equation (1), AUCs of 5 to 7.5 mg/mL min), continued carboplatin therapy would eventually be limited by cumulative bone marrow damage and resulting grade 4 neutropenia and thrombocytopenia. Pretreatment with amifostine could reduce these toxicities.
   b. Paclitaxel. Since the patient had an outstanding response to carboplatin/paclitaxel and carboplatin would not be a good treatment choice because of its high potential of cumulative bone marrow damage, paclitaxel treatment would be a high priority, administered as a salvage agent at a dose of 175 mg/m^2 over 3 hr in the outpatient department every 3 weeks. Recent evidence suggests that standard doses of paclitaxel are associated with little or no cumulative toxicities and thus can be administered for as long as 2 years. In this patient's case, I would recommend six additional courses of paclitaxel as described above. It is unlikely that cytokine support would be required for this patient unless there already was evidence of cumulative bone marrow damage.
   c. Altretamine. This is an important agent which is underutilized in ovarian cancer management because it almost always was incorporated in first-line treatment programs and not used as a single agent with dose-intensive courses. Altretamine has been reported to induce objected responses in 15 to 30% of patients who have received prior cisplatin-containing regimens. More importantly, its use has been associated with prolonged survival durations in patients who have clinical complete responses following primary therapy. Thus, it would be a rational choice for treatment in this patient.
   d. Topotecan. This drug received FDA approval in June, 1996, for the salvage therapy of ovarian cancer. In a phase III study, the time to progression of recurrent disease was significantly longer with topotecan (23 weeks) than with paclitaxel administered at 175 mg/m^2 over 3 hours (14 weeks) (2). Topotecan is for more myelosuppressive than paclitaxel, but the bone marrow toxicity does not appear cumulative.
2. Standard FDA-approved drugs for other indications.
   a. Intraperitoneal cisplatin. This drug is FDA-approved to be administered by the intravenous route at doses of 50 to 100 mg/m2 for

patients with advanced ovarian cancer. It has not been approved for administration by the intraperitoneal route. In a recent presentation of an Intergroup study (Intergroup 0051 or SWOG-8501/GOG-104) at the 1995 American Society of Clinical Oncology meeting in Los Angeles (3). I reported that intraperitoneal cisplatin was superior to intravenous cisplatin administered at the same dose level (i.e., 100 mg/m^2 every 3 weeks for six courses when combined with intravenous cyclophosphamide 600 mg/m^2) with respect to patient survival duration and the degree and frequency of clinical hearing loss and neutropenia. This pivotal trial for the intraperitoneal efficacy of cisplatin was performed in previously untreated patients with < 2 cm residual intraperitoneal tumor. Intraperitoneal cisplatin has proven active in the salvage treatment of patients who have minimal residual (in this case, microscopic) disease after second-look surgery. Several studies have documented high objective response rates and prolonged survivals to intraperitoneal cisplatin (100 to 200 mg/m^2) in previously treated patients. Thus, it remains a potential treatment of choice in this category of patient.

b. Tamoxifen. Several studies have documented response rates of 10 to 20% to standard-dose tamoxifen (10 mg twice daily) in patients with advanced, drug-refractory ovarian cancer. Tamoxifen is considered to be safe, especially in women. This drug has virtually no severe toxicities, but requires > 2 months to express its anticancer activity.

c. Oral or intravenous etoposide. Various studies have documented 0 to 25% objective response rates to etoposide when used as a second-line drug in patients who have had prior cisplatin-containing therapy. In a recently reported Gynecologic Oncology Group phase II study, prolonged (i.e. 21 day), low dose (i.e. 50 mg/m^2/day) oral etoposide was associated with a 27% response rate in patients with platinum refractory cancers.

d. Intraperitoneal FUDR. In a recently completed SWOG phase II randomized study, high-dose intraperitoneal FUDR appeared superior to intraperitoneal mitoxantrone. Data analyses showed that patients treated with intraperitoneal FUDR lived for a prolonged period.

3. Experimental Treatments

a. Intraperitoneal paclitaxel. When administered intraperitoneally, paclitaxel has an extremely prolonged half-time and extremely large intraperitoneal AUC. Whether it will prove as active as intraperitoneal cisplatin remains to be documented by an ongoing phase II trial in GOG.

b. Intraperitoneal alpha-interferon. This biological agent has proven active in patients with minimal intraperitoneal residual disease during phase I and II trials at a few different institutions.

If this patient had been referred to me for further treatment decisions, I would probably have placed her on at least six additional cycles of paclitaxel, 175 mg/m^2 over 3 hr or 135 mg/m^2 over 24 hr every 3 weeks. I believe that this approach would have the greatest chance of success. Since the patient had shown an excellent prior response to paclitaxel/carboplatin, there is strong reason to believe that her cancer may continue to be sensitive to both of these drugs. A strong alternative in a patient who desires treatment with an oral agent would be the use of dose-intensive altretamine for up to six courses of therapy. Additionally, topotecan could be used for consolidation therapy.

References

1. Calvert AH, et al. Carboplatin dosage: Prospective evaluation of a simple formula based on renal function. *J Clin Oncol.* 1989; 7(11):1748–1756.
2. Carmichael J, et al. Topotecan, a new active drug, vs paclitaxel in advanced epithelial ovarian carcinoma; international topotecan study group trial. Proc Amer Soc Clin Oncol 1996; 15:283 (Abs. 765).
3. Alberts DS, et al. Phase III study of intraperitoneal (IP) cisplatin (CDDP)/intravenous (IV) cyclophosphamide (CPA) vs IV CDDP/IV CPA in patients (Pts) with optimal disease stage III ovarian cancer. Proc Amer Soc Clin Oncol 1995; 14:273 (Abs. 760).

PHYSICIAN'S RESPONSE

MARCUS E. RANDALL

Surgical reassessment (SRA) following primary chemotherapy documents residual disease in the majority of patients with stages III and IV ovarian carcinoma. In the Gynecologic Oncology Group (GOG) experience, only 30 of 483 suboptimal stage III patients undergoing SRA had negative findings; of these, 18 subsequently relapsed (1). Although emerging data suggest higher rates of negative SRA and longer median survivals with platinum/paclitaxel regimens, the problem presented in this case remains common.

In view of the demonstrated curative potential of radiotherapy (RT) in certain subsets of patients with ovarian carcinoma, many investigators have evaluated this modality following primary chemotherapy in a consolidation or salvage setting. Published series have been reviewed by various authors. (2,3)

Two approaches have been used. Intraperitoneal chromic phosphate (^{32}P) has been advocated for high-risk patients with negative SRA and in those with microscopic or very small tumor deposits restricted to the peritoneal surface. In patients with negative SRA, retrospective analyses have given conflicting results. A clearer picture of the benefit, if any, should emerge from an ongoing GOG trials. Data are similarly conflicting in patients with microscopic or minimal residual disease. Rigorous analysis of the data is complicated by the various selection factors employed in these retrospective series and the fact that other therapies (e.g., second-line chemotherapy) have also been administered. However, in view of the favorable experience reported by Rogers et al., the relatively small risk or acute of late morbidity, and the lack of adequate second-line chemotherapy, administration of intraperitoneal ^{32}P is a reasonable treatment approach in the patient described (4).

The second RT approach that has been used in patients with positive SRAs is external RT directed to the whole abdomen (WAR). Clearly, significant benefit is lacking in patients with significant residual disease. Results are quite variable in patients with microscopic or minimal residual disease. The weight of the data, both prospective and retrospective, suggests no significant treatment effect in patients with residual disease, particularly in patients with "suboptimal" disease after initial surgical cytoreduction. Although it is possible that different sequencing and/or intensities of WAR and chemotherapy or altered radiation fractionation schemes will prove more effective, the use of WAR in the patient presented is unlikely to be helpful and would generally not be recommended outside of a clinical protocol.

In summary, my recommendation would be for intraperitoneal ^{32}P, assuming adequate isotope distribution can be achieved. Otherwise, the patient is a candidate for phase I clinical trials or close follow-up and subsequent treatment as appropriate.

References

1. Omura GA, Brady MF, Homesley HD, et al. Long-term follow-up and prognostic factor analysis in advance ovarian carcinoma: The Gynecologic Oncology Group experience. J Clin Oncol 1991; 9:1138–1150.
2. Lanciano RM, Randall ME. Update on the role of radiotherapy in ovarian cancer. Semin Oncol 1991; 18:233–247.
3. Thomas GM. Is there a role for consolidation or salvage radiotherapy after chemotherapy in advanced epithelial ovarian cancer? Gynecol Oncol 1993; 51:97–103.
4. Rogers L, Varia M, Halle J. et al. P-32 following second-look laparotomy for epithelial ovarian cancer. Int J Oncol Biol Phys 1990; 19:167–168.

PHYSICIAN'S RESPONSE

BONNIE S. REICHMAN

This case clearly demonstrates that a clinical complete remission is not synonymous with a pathological complete remission. Of patients who have clinical complete remission—resolution of symptoms, disappearance of radiographic abnormalities, and normalization of CA-125—approximately 60% will have residual disease at second look laparotomy (SLL). Among the patients who are pathologically free of disease at SLL, 30 to 50% will eventually recur and die of disease. The role of SLL remains controversial, since there is a lack of evidence that it significantly improves survival. Second-look laparotomy is the most sensitive means of diagnosing persistent disease in patients who appear to be clinically free of disease. Secondary cytoreduction at SLL might be beneficial for a small subset of patients. As per the 1994 National Institutes of Health Consensus Development Conference on the treatment of ovarian cancer, "Second-look laparotomy should be done only for patients on clinical trials or for those patients in whom the surgery will affect clinical decision making and clinical course. It should not be employed as routine care for all patients" (1).

This patient's tumor is chemosensitive to both platinum and paclitaxel. However, it is unusual for responders to first-line intravenous chemotherapy with residual disease at second-look surgery to convert to complete responders after more of the same intravenous chemotherapy. Continuing intravenous chemotherapy with carboplatin and paclitaxel would be of minimal benefit. Since the tumor appears to be sensitive to these agents, overcoming relative resistance by increasing dose intensity via intraperitoneal chemotherapy administration or high-dose treatment intravenously with bone marrow support could be considered on an investigational protocol. The long-term benefit of these investigational regimens is not known, but they appear to benefit a small subset of patients. This patient would be an appropriate candidate for investigational second-line chemotherapy. The doses and side effects of the patient's prior chemotherapy should be reviewed in detail before further treatment could be recommended.

Prior to consideration of intraperitoneal chemotherapy, the status of the peritoneal cavity regarding adhesions needs to be clarified. The presence of significant adhesions would interfere with drug distribution. For selected patients with microscopic residual disease, there appears to be a survival benefit to intraperitoneal platinum-based treatment and/or intraperitoneal paclitaxel. However, there are no randomized studies to establish a clear benefit.

Clearly, without further treatment, this young patient will ultimately die of disease. Salvage intravenous chemotherapy regimens are palliative at best, with responses in the range of 10 to 20% of short duration. Since, this patient does not have clinically measurable or evaluable disease, it would be difficult to monitor the response to any treatment without further surgical intervention. Since the patient is asymptomatic at present, an argument could be made to monitor the patient until evaluable or measurable disease recurs. Alternatively, in theory cancer treatment is most effective in the setting of minimal tumor burden. Moreover, one feels compelled to continue treatment, especially in the setting of prior response, young age, and excellent performance status. Unfortunately, there is not standard treatment in this scenario. This patient should be encouraged to participate in an investigational protocol.

Reference

1. National Institutes of Health Consensus Development Conference Statement. Ovarian Cancer: Screening, treatment, and follow-up. Gynecol Oncol 1994; (suppl):4–14.

41

Stage I Mixed Mesodermal Cancer of the Uterus

CASE

A 62-year-old woman who was previously in excellent health notes a 3-month history of mild, crampy lower abdominal pain. On physical examination her uterus is found to be enlarged. At surgery the mass is found to be a mixed mesodermal tumor of the endometrium. There is no evidence of spread outside the uterus. Pelvic and periaortic lymph nodes demonstrate no evidence of cancer. Postoperative computed tomography (CT) scans of the abdomen, pelvis, and chest are unremarkable.

(*Note*: A cousin of your patient is a gynecologist in another city who asks you whether chemotherapy and/or radiation therapy are indicated in this clinical setting.)

PHYSICIAN'S RESPONSE

THOMAS MONTAG

This 62-year-old woman has apparent surgical stage I malignant mixed mesodermal tumor (MMMT) of the endometrium. Additional information will be valuable in making a recommendation for adjuvant postoperative therapy. As you would intuitively expect, the extent of disease discovered at the time of surgery has implications with regard to recurrence. Extensive myometrial invasion and serosal involvement by tumor are recognized as poor prognostic factors. The presence of malignant cells in peritoneal washings usually correlates with a clinical course similar to that of patients with visible extrauterine disease. Prior pelvic irradiation

327

is considered by some to predict a poor outcome. Knowledge of these factors may influence decision making, since the benefit of adjuvant therapy for surgical stage I MMMT remains controversial.

This type of tumor, MMMT of the uterus (endometrium), has traditionally been associated with aggressive behavior and poor prognosis. Although surgical therapy may be curative in some patients with early disease, reported 5-year survival rates in stage I disease rarely exceeds 50%. Despite such poor survival rates, the role of adjuvant therapy remains unsettled. If available, I would recommend participation in a multi-institutional study investigating adjuvant therapy.

Off study, a strong recommendation for postoperative external whole pelvic radiotherapy can be made. Data suggest a pelvic recurrence rate in MMMT of approximately 30 to 50% and a similar rate of distant recurrences. In the Gynecologic Oncology Group (GOG) study of adjuvant postoperative radiation therapy for stage I/II uterine sarcomas (1), 54% of initial recurrences were pelvic in the group not receiving radiation versus 23% in the group receiving whole pelvic irradiation postoperatively. There is additional literature supporting a reduction in the local recurrence rate following adjuvant whole pelvic radiotherapy. However, the effect of radiation on overall survival remains unclear due to the high incidence of distant metastases.

The high recurrence rate of MMMT and the propensity to recur at distant sites demonstrate the need for effective chemotherapy. Studies show that ifosfamide and cisplatin are the most active agents identified to date. It remains speculative whether adjuvant chemotherapy for MMMT is effective. A GOG study (2) that required 11 years to accrue an adequate number of patients randomized stage I MMMT patients to receive eight course of doxorubicin (Adriamycin) or no further therapy. In the no-treatment arm, the number of distant metastases was greater, the recurrence rate higher, and the survival rate worse. These differences were *not* statistically significant. However this study provides supportive evidence for adjuvant chemotherapy. Should this patient have poor prognostic factors, it is recommended that she receive adjuvant chemotherapy with cisplatin and ifosfamide.

References

1. Hornback NB, Omura G, Major FJ. Observations on the use of adjuvant radiation therapy in patients with stage I and II uterine sarcoma. Int J Radiat Oncol Biol Phys 1986; 12:2127.

2. Omura GA, Blessing JA, Lifshitz S, et al: A randomized clinical trial of adjuvant Adriamycin in uterine sarcomas: A Gynecological Oncology Group Study. J Clin Oncol 1985; 3:1240.

PHYSICIAN'S RESPONSE

MURRAY JOSEPH CASEY

Although there are no large randomized studies to prove a survival advantage for patients treated with postoperative radiotherapy for mixed mesodermal tumors confined to the uterus, retrospective analyses in several substantial series have documented decreased pelvic recurrences among patients treated with surgical removal and pelvic irradiation compared with those who were treated with surgery alone. One series reported fewer pelvic recurrences and improved survival rates in the patients treated with combined external pelvic irradiation plus brachytherapy compared with those who received lower pelvic doses or no radiotherapy at all. Others have noticed fewer central recurrences when higher doses of pelvic irradiation were given. However, some authors have found neither improved central control nor increased survival rates in patients who received pelvic radiotherapy for mixed mesodermal tumors.

Adjuvant cytotoxic chemotherapy has not been convincingly demonstrated to enhance survival or diminish either central recurrences or metastatic disease in patients who are treated with complete removal of uterine mixed müllerian tumors and radiation therapy. On the other hand, both ifosfamide and high-dose cisplatin as single agents have induced objective responses in measurable persistent and metastatic mixed mesodermal tumors, giving results that have surpassed those previously obtained with more toxic multiple drug regimens.

Currently, the best advice for treating stage I mixed müllerian tumors following hysterectomy and bilateral salpingo-oophorectomy seems to be the addition of high-energy photon external irradiation to wide-field whole pelvic ports designed to encompass the entire iliac lymphatic systems and upper vagina, delivering a total tumor dose of at least 5000 cGy to the lymphatic systems and upper vagina over 5 to 6 weeks. A four-field box technique with cut corners or rotational therapy may have some bowel-sparing effect. For those patients in whom the vagina is found to be free of adherent small bowel on roentgenographic contrast studies, brachytherapy may be used to supplement the mucosal surface dose at the vault to a total of 8000 cGy, including external therapy, with little danger of significant untoward effects. If the patient is in otherwise good health and she is interested in trying to maximize her outcome, introduction to a collaborative, controlled prospective phase III trial that includes randomization to a promising cytotoxic regimen may be considered.

References

Hornback NB, Omura G, Major FJ. Observations on the use of adjuvant radiation therapy in patients with stage I and II uterine sarcoma. Int J Radiat Oncol Biol Phys 1986; 12:2127–2130.

Larson B, Silfverswärd C, Nilsson B, Pettersson F. Mixed müllerian tumors of the uterus—Prognostic factors: a clinical and histopathologic study of 147 cases. Radiother Oncol 1990; 17:123–132.

PHYSICIAN'S RESPONSE

J. SAXTON

It is not clear from the history whether the lymph nodes were negative by inspection or pathologically. Although no benefit in survival has been demonstrated by selective lymphadenectomy, it may have prognostic value. Although the lesion was described as limited to the uterus, the degree of myometrial involvement was not described.

The use of postoperative radiation therapy in the treatment of malignant mixed mesodermal tumors (MMMT) is very controversial. Previous reports have shown conflicting data in the benefit of local regional control and no benefit to overall survival. Some authors have reported a 15 to 16% incidence of pelvic nodal involvement. Perez has recommended preoperative intracavitary radiation therapy for stage I disease and postoperative external-beam radiation for stage II disease, suggesting a trend toward improvement and survival (1). The numbers of patients have been small in a nonrandomized series; however, these data have been supported by other clinical studies. Spanos showed a high local regional recurrence rate in spite of postoperative radiation therapy (2).

The overwhelming factor leading to the poor prognosis is hematogenous spread. Studies by the Gynecologic Oncology Group have shown response in advanced disease with doxorubicin alone and with decarbazine (DTIC) but no significant improvement in survival with stage I and stage II disease. Cisplatin and ifosfamide have more recently shown activity in advanced and recurrent MMMT of the uterus. A present study was recently closed to accrual in stage I and II surgically resected disease. Lymph node sampling was not required; data are pending.

In a clinical setting where the prognosis is poor and the management is equivocal, patient choice should play an important role in the treatment decision. Armed with what current information is available, the patient can become the determining factor of the final treatment decision.

Ideally, I would recommend this patient to a clinical trial to evaluate the benefits of systemic management. Eventually, with better systemic control, pelvic radiation may play an important role in improving local regional control and ultimately quality of life.

References

1. Perez CA, Askin F, et al. Effects of irradiation on mixed muellerian tumors of the uterus. Cancer 1979; 43:1274–1284.

2. Spanos WJ, Wharton JT, et al. Malignant mixed muellerian tumors of the uterus. Cancer 1984; 53:311–316.

PHYSICIANS' RESPONSE

JUDY CHENG
WILLIAM J. MANN

Uterine sarcoma accounts for 1 to 3% of all uterine cancers, and less than half of these are malignant mixed mesodermal tumors (MMMT). Since first reported in 1899, MMMT, a rapid-growing, aggressive, lethal tumor, remains a clinical frustration for gynecological oncologists, with a 5-year survival rate of less than 38%. Vaginal bleeding followed by abdominal pain and weight loss are the most common symptoms. The mean age of patients is 63 years, which is similar to that for endometrial carcinoma (62 years of age). Obesity, hypertension, and prior pelvic irradiation are associated risk factors. This lesion is further classified as homologous, consisting of elements such as leiomyosarcoma and stromal sarcoma, and MMMT with heterologous mesenchymal cells such as rhabdomyosarcoma, osteosarcoma, and chondrosarcoma. There is no significant difference in survival between the two groups.

Oncologists disagree on the histological identification, behaviors, prognostic factors, spread, and management of MMMT. There are theories that these biphasic tumors arise from transformation of a single epithelial clone with metaplasia into the sarcomatous component or that the transformation occurs independently from separate epithelial and mesenchymal populations. The behavior of MMMT resembles that of papillary serous carcinoma or other high-grade carcinomas of the endometrium. The carcinomatous elements influence the prognosis of MMMT. The more aggressive the carcinomatous components, the higher the frequency of metastases. Features of the stromal component such as the grade, mitotic index, and heterologous elements have no prognostic value. Tumor extension at diagnosis is the main prognosticator for survival. Patients with stage I disease have a 5-year survival of 30 to 50%, while stages II and IV disease have been grouped together, with a 5-year survival of 7 to 12%. Measurement of DNA content using flow cytometry and image analysis has been done to predict prognosis. Patients with diploid tumors have 5-year survivals of 72% while patients with hyperdiploid and hypodiploid tumors have median survival of 18 and 12 months. A study has reported that pedunculated tumors with a 5-year survival of 53% have a significantly better prognosis than broad-based tumors (< 30% 5 year survival). Debates over whether age, tumor size, depth of myometrial invasion, or lymphovascular involvement predict the prognosis are still unresolved. Initial metastases in MMMT often involve the pelvic and paraaortic nodes. Pulmonary metastasis usually occurs later in the course of disease, as in aggressive endometrial cancer. In addition, the extrauterine metastases of MMMT are most commonly carcinoma or a combination of carcinoma and sarcoma. Pure sarcomatous metastases are very rare.

This patient has apparent stage I disease. We agree with total abdominal hysterectomy/bilateral salpingo-oophorectomy and sampling of pelvic and para-aortic nodes as initial therapy. We favor adjunctive pelvic radiation, which improves local tumor control but not long-term survival.

The role of chemotherapy is still controversial, and we reserve it for recurrence or metastatic disease. Doxorubicin has traditionally been used as a single agent or in combination with vincristine, cytoxan, or cisplatin. However, with a response rate of < 10%, there was no evidence of benefit when doxorubicin was used in early-stage MMMT. Cisplatin and ifosfamide, with response rates exceeding 15%, are promising chemotherapeutic agents for MMMT. Serum CA-125 levels can be used to follow response to therapy or progression of disease.

References

Salazar OM, Bonfiglio TA, Patten ST, et al. Uterine sarcomas: Analysis of failures with special emphasis on the use of adjuvant radiation therapy. Cancer 1978; 42:1161–1170.

Silverberg SG, Major FJ, Blessing JA, et al. Carcinosarcoma (malignant mixed mesodermal tumor) of the uterus: A Gynecological Oncology Group pathologic study of 203 cases. Int J Gynecol Pathol 1990; 9:1–19.

42

Stage I Endometrial Cancer with Positive Washings

CASE

A 59-year-old woman with diet-controlled diabetes is found to have adenocarcinoma of the endometrium on dilatation and curettage (D&C) performed to evaluate postmenopausal bleeding. A total abdominal hysterectomy/bilateral salpingo-oophorectomy (TAH/BSO) was performed and the patient appeared to have a stage IB endometrial cancer. The procedure was concluded before any other staging could be completed due to unexplained intraoperative hypotension. However, no gross disease was observed outside the uterus. Pathology review revealed a grade 2 adenocarcinoma of the endometrium with just under 50% myometrial invasion. Unfortunately, peritoneal washings contain adenocarcinoma cells.

PHYSICIAN'S RESPONSE

HENRY KEYS

The intrauterine findings in this case place the patient in a good-prognosis group with some uncertainty as to whether there would be any benefit from the addition of adjuvant postoperative treatment. If that were the whole story and there had been full operative staging, including negative pelvic and paraaortic lymph node staging, the patient would fit the eligibility criteria for randomization onto Gynecologic Oncology Group (GOG) protocol #99, which compares postoperative pelvic radiation therapy to observation for patients with low/intermediate-risk disease.

333

However, there are two factors complicating the picture in this specific case. First, intraoperative staging could not be done, and thus the pathologic status of the lymph nodes is unknown. The risk of lymph node involvement for Fédération International de Gynécologie et d'Obstétrique (FIGO) grade 2 lesions is 9% and that for paraaortic nodes is 5%, while the figures for grade 1 lesions are 3 and 2% respectively (1). The FIGO staging system divides stage I patients into A, B, and C subcategories based on there being either no myometrial invasion, less than 50% invasion, or greater than 50% invasion. When the lymph node positivity rate is studied as a function of which third of the myometrial thickness is invaded, there is very little difference between the inner third and the middle third (5 and 6%, respectively, for pelvic nodes, and 3 and 1%, respectively, for paraaortic nodes). Another pathological factor that is an important prognostic variable is the presence or absence of invasion of endothelium-lined space within the myometrium. The presence of capillarylike space involvement quadruples the risk of lymph node involvement in the pelvis (from 7 to 27%), and doubles the paraaortic nodal involvement (from 9 to 19%). There is no comment about this element in this case description, which could mean that it was not present, but it could also mean that it was not looked for.

The second confounding factor here is the presence of adenocarcinoma cells in the peritoneal fluid. The significance of positive peritoneal washings is generally believed to be determined by the other pathological prognostic factors associated with the positive cytology. Thus, in the absence of any other evidence of extrauterine involvement, positive peritoneal cytology has little if any significance, while findings of parametrial, omental, or lymph node involvement give positive peritoneal cytology a much more ominous significance. Pelvic and paraaortic lymph node involvement is much more likely to be present when the cytology is positive than when it is negative (25 versus 7% for pelvic nodes and 19 versus 4% for paraaortic nodes). Once again the absence of node sampling makes determination of the clinical significance of this finding problematic.

A rational discussion of postoperative treatment options for this patient could consider all of the following:

1. Observation
2. Adjuvant progestational treatment
3. Adjuvant systemic chemotherapy
4. Adjuvant pelvic irradiation
5. Adjuvant vaginal irradiation
6. Intraperitoneal chromic phosphate (^{32}P)
7. Adjuvant whole abdominal/pelvic irradiation

Progestational and systemic chemotherapy is of no proven benefit in the adjuvant setting, and would not be my recommendation. If the patient had *negative* peritoneal cytology and negative lymph node sampling, I would consider vaginal irradiation as a viable treatment option, with pelvic irradiation as the other choice. Others might choose observation as a viable option. However, the absence of nodal pathological evaluation and the presence of positive cytology makes these options less attractive in this case.

The use of intraperitoneal instillation of ^{32}P provides another method of treating the entire peritoneal surface. This approach has been used for patients who are considered at higher risk of intraperitoneal relapse without having a heightened risk of pelvic relapse or lymph node failure. In this case, with the uncertainty about the actual extent and distribution of disease, treating the peritoneal surface without including deeper structures and lymph nodes would not seem desirable.

The appropriate role for whole abdominal irradiation in endometrial cancer is not well defined at the present time. It is clearly well tolerated by most patients while having more acute side effects than pelvic treatment. In GOG protocol #94, whole abdominal treatment was delivered to 205 patients with generally well-tolerated side effects. Of the 77 patients with stage III/IV typical endometrial adenocarcinoma histology, 55 (71.4%) have died and 47 (61%) are known to have relapsed (2). Thus, if we take the worst-case scenario and assume that a more thorough intraoperative evaluation would have discovered stage III/IV disease, then the use of whole abdominal treatment would be a reasonable but only moderately effective treatment choice.

This would be my recommendation: 3000 cGy to the whole abdomen in 20 treatment fractions of 150 cGy each, delivered through anterior and posterior fields with full kidney shielding from the posterior direction, to be followed by 1980 cGy to the pelvis in 11 fractions of 180 cGy each, delivered through a four-field pelvic technique.

References

1. Creasman W, et al. Cancer 1987; 60:2035.
2. Axelrod J. Personal communication, March 1995.

PHYSICIANS' RESPONSE

M.S. PIVER
J. GOLDBERG

In most instances, surgical staging is necessary in endometrial cancer to determine appropriate therapy. However, not every patient needs to undergo every step of a staging procedure. Fortunately, there are risk factors for extrauterine spread of endometrial cancer that are well quantified. Creasman et al. have reported, in a large Gynecologic Oncology Group study, that of 231 patients with grade 2 endometrial adenocarcinoma not invading the outer third of the myometrium, only 14 (6%) had metastasis to the pelvic nodes and only 6 (3%) had metastasis to the paraaortic nodes. Therefore, in the absence of any grossly enlarged lymph nodes noted at surgery, the chances of this patient having significant extrauterine disease are small. Conversely, to use postoperative pelvic radiation at a standard dose rate of 5040 cGy in $5^1/_2$ weeks for 100% of patients with similar grade 2 superficially invasive stage I endometrial adenocarcinoma for the 6% at risk of pelvic lymph node metastasis would result in excessive morbidity for the 94% not at risk. Brachytherapy to the vaginal cuff, to reduce the risk of vaginal cuff recurrence, should complete the major part of this patient's therapy. In such a setting, brachytherapy has resulted in a 0% vaginal recurrence rate.

The significance of peritoneal cytology is less clear. Numerous studies have reported that the presence of malignant cells in peritoneal washings is an independent negative prognostic factor. However, in patients whose only extra-uterine disease is positive peritoneal cytology, recurrence of gross disease can easily be prevented in most cases. Creasman et al. reported the reduction of recurrence in patients with disease confined to the uterus except for positive peritoneal cytology from 46% (6/13) to 10% (2/20) using intraperitoneal chromic phosphate (^{32}P). At Roswell Park Cancer Institute, we have reported on 45 such patients entered into a protocol utilizing oral megestrol 160 mg daily or intramus-cular medroxyprogesterone 1.0 g IM weekly for 1 year. Of 36 patients who consented to second-look laparoscopy, 34 had no evidence of disease. Two patients with persistent positive peritoneal cytology received an additional year of progesterone therapy and subsequently had negative third-look laparoscopies. None of the 45 patients have had a recurrence of their cancer. These results with such minimal therapy would tend to question the prognostic significance of positive peritoneal washings.

Despite the presence of positive peritoneal cytology and the lack of patho-logical confirmation of the absence of nodal metastases, the patient can be reassured that her prognosis is quite good. We have reported on 92 patients treated at our institution for grade 1 or 2 endometrial carcinoma limited to superficial myometrial invasion and adjuvant brachytherapy to the vaginal cuff. None of the patients have had a recurrence, and the estimated 5-year disease-free survival is 99%. Given such an excellent outcome, there is really no role for any further therapy beyond adjuvant radiation to the vaginal cuff and 1 year of progesterone, followed by second-look laparoscopy and repeat cytological washings.

References

Creasman WT, DiSaia PJ, Blessing J, et al. Prognostic significance of peritoneal cytology in patients with endometrial cancer and preliminary data concerning therapy with intraperitoneal radiopharmaceuticals. Am J Obstet Gynecol 1981; 141:921–929.

Creasman WT, Morrow CP, Bundy BN, et al. Surgical pathological spread patterns of endometrial cancer. Cancer 1987; 60:2035–2041.

Piver, MS, Hempling RE. A prospective trial of postoperative vaginal radium/cesium for grade 1-2 less than 50% myometrial invasion and pelvic radiation for grade 3 or deep myometrial invasion in surgical stage I endometrial adenocarcinoma. Cancer 1990; 66: 1133–1138.

Piver MS, Recio FO, Baker TR, and Hempling RE. A prospective trial of progesterone therapy for malignant peritoneal cytology in patients with endometrial carcinoma. Gynecol Oncol 1992; 47:373–376.

PHYSICIAN'S RESPONSE

ERNEST KOHORN

Positive cytology for endometrial carcinoma cells in an endometrioid endometrial carcinoma without other high-risk factors has been recognized as a significant prognostic factor. If there are extrauterine metastases, particularly in lymph nodes, on the peritoneal surface, in the omentum, or at other intraabdominal sites, it is doubtful whether the finding of positive cytology adds significantly to an already grave prognosis. The problem arises with grade 1 or 2 histology when positive cytology is the only factor and pelvic and paraaortic nodes have been examined and are negative. With extrauterine or nodal disease, adjuvant treatment is clearly indicated. The question is whether adjuvant treatment is required if there is positive cytology in the absence of extrauterine disease in patients with grade 1 or 2 tumors. Creasman and Rutledge (1) had reported 13 from a group of 26 patients with positive cytology where there was no disease outside the uterus. Six of these patients (46%) died of carcinomatosis. DiSaia and Creasman (2) in their textbook state that "when malignant cells are present in peritoneal fluid this tends to neutralize the good prognostic factors and cytologic findings become a predominantly important consideration." Sutton (3) confirmed that positive peritoneal cytology remained an independent significant risk factor. Grimshaw et al. (4) showed that although 24 of 381 patients with positive cytology had a significantly worse prognosis, there was no statistical difference with positive cytology among patients with surgical stage I disease. There is thus disagreement in the literature.

The Oncology Group at Duke University has utilized chromic phosphate (^{32}P) to treat patients with malignant cytology (5). It was shown 53 of 65 patients with clinical stage I disease had an 89% disease-free survival, 94% in surgical stage I cases. These data suggests that it is better to treat such patients with ^{32}P than not to treat them. The dilemma is that a patient with diabetes, arteriosclerotic heart disease, and hypertension who presumably also has peripheral vascular disease may develop morbidity from external-beam irradiation. The Duke University Group found very little morbidity with ^{32}P if no additional external-beam radiation therapy was given. The Yale practice has been to give external-beam irradiation with myometrial invasion greater than 50% and with grade 3 tumors (neither of these factors applied in this case) and also to offer whole abdominal radiation for positive cytology.

This patient with diabetes and apparent vascular disease who has a grade 3 tumor with less than 50% myometrial invasion but does have positive cytology should have adjuvant therapy. The therapy should be dependent on the experience of the institution. If this is with intraperitoneal ^{32}P, this will produce the least side effects. In the absence of such experience, carefully administered external-beam radiation therapy should be given, preferably to the whole abdomen, with pelvic boost.

References

1. Creasman WT, Rutledge FN. The prognostic value of peritoneal cytology in gynecologic malignant disease. Am J Obstet Gynecol 1971; 110:773.
2. DiSaia PJ, Creasman WT. Clinical Gynecological Oncology, 4th ed. St. Louis, Mosby-Year Book, 1993:170.
3. Sutton GP. The significance of positive peritoneal cytology in endometrial cancer. Oncology 1990; 4:21.
4. Grimshaw RN, et al. Prognostic value of peritoneal cytology in endometrial carcinoma. Gynecol Oncol 1990; 36:97.
5. Soper J, et al. Intraperitoneal chromic phosphate P-32 suspension therapy in malignant peritoneal cytology and endometrial cancer. Am J Obstet Gynecol 1985; 153:191.

PHYSICIANS' RESPONSE

ROBERT A. BURGER
ALBERTO MANETTA

For patients with clinically early-stage adenocarcinoma of the endometrium, accepted prognostic surgical-pathological variables include tumor grade, depth of myometrial invasion, vascular space invasion, cervical spread, status of pelvic peritoneal cytology, and histological type. In the absence of medical contraindications, patients with grade 2 tumors displaying myometrial invasion but grossly confined to the uterus should undergo complete surgical staging, including bilateral pelvic and paraaortic lymph node sampling, in order to facilitate the most appropriate postoperative management decision. Assuming that this patient's tumor is not of the high-risk histological type, i.e. serous papillary or clear cell, based on uterine factors alone, she would be considered at intermediate risk of recurrence (approximately 20% at 5 years), with no prospective data to support the routine application of adjunctive pelvic radiotherapy. Unfortunately, the absence of lymph node data, the finding of positive peritoneal cytology, and the increased morbidity of restaging, given previous intraoperative medical problems, complicate this patient's plan of management.

The incidence of positive peritoneal cytology in patients with clinical stage I disease is approximately 15%. It is clear that positive cytology is found most commonly in the setting of other adverse prognostic features such as high grade, deep myometrial invasion, adnexal spread, or nodal metastasis. For example, in the highly quoted GOG surgicopathological study of 621 patients with clinical stage I endometrial cancer, Creasman and colleagues reported that 25 and 19% of patients with positive cytology had pelvic and paraaortic lymph node metastases, respectively, and 48% had metastasis to other extrauterine sites. Nevertheless, many studies have also documented positive cytology in the absence of other evidence of extrauterine spread. According to a recent metaanalysis of 242 patients with isolated positive peritoneal cytology, the predicted risk of recurrence is on the order of 23%. Furthermore, a recent multivariate analysis of 858 patients with clinical stage I disease identified positive peritoneal cytology as independently prognostic for both pelvic and distant failure.

A number of adjunctive modalities have been investigated in patients with isolated positive peritoneal cytology. These include intraperitoneal chromic phosphate (^{32}P) pelvic or whole abdominal radiation (WART), hormonal therapy, and cytotoxic chemotherapy. In the absence of placebo-controlled randomized studies to demonstrate reduction in recurrence risk with any of these adjuvant therapies, theoretical benefits of their implementation outside a research protocol must be weighed against known risks. Nevertheless, based on this patient's risk for both pelvic and distant recurrence, in the absence of a suitable clinical trial, she should be offered some form of adjuvant therapy off protocol.

Intraperitoneal ^{32}P, although previously shown to be feasible for patients with isolated positive peritoneal cytology, would not be a reasonable choice of treatment for this patient with a statistically high risk of retroperitoneal disease. One should first discuss with the patient the options of WART with a pelvic boost versus whole pelvic radiotherapy combined with either doxorubicin/cisplatin chemotherapy or progestin therapy. With positive peritoneal cytology as her only evidence of extrauterine spread, the excessive morbidity associated with WART and a low 30% objective response rate documented for doxorubicin/cisplatin in advanced clinically measurable endometrial cancer would, however, make the use of either modality in this setting controversial.

For doses no higher than 50 Gy, adjuvant whole pelvic radiation has been found to carry a 5-year severe complication rate on the order of only 2% in patients younger than age 65 who have not undergone lymph node dissection at the time of TAH/BSO. Since patients with positive peritoneal cytology have a 25% risk of pelvic node metastasis at the time of diagnosis and since pelvic radiotherapy has been shown to reduce the risk of pelvic failure for patients with pelvic nodal spread, the potential benefits of pelvic radiation as an adjuvant greatly outweigh the risks of the known morbidity rate. Because patients with paraaortic node metastases have been cured with extended-field radiation, it would also be recommended that she undergo CT examination of the abdomen, with extended-field radiation prescribed in the event of CT-guided, biopsy-proven paraaortic node involvement. In considering a low-risk systemic therapy, one should note a recent study reported by Piver and colleagues, in which 1 year of adjuvant progestin therapy (+/– pelvic irradiation depending on tumor grade and depth of invasion) given to 45 patients with endometrial carcinoma confined to the corpus except for positive peritoneal cytology was associated with a recurrence rate of 0% and an estimated 5-year survival of 89%. In this study, approximately 33% had either grade 3 tumors or outer-half myometrial invasion.

With all the above considerations, given the nearly equivalent risk of distant and pelvic relapse in patients with positive cytology, it would be recommended that this patient receive 50 Gy adjuvant pelvic radiation with the addition of at least 1 year of continuous oral progestin.

References

Creasman WT, Morrow CP, Bundy BN, et al. Surgical pathologic spread patterns of endometrial cancer: A Gynecologic Oncology Group study. Cancer 1987; 60:2035–2041.

Piver MS, Recio FO, Baker TR, Hempling RE. A prospective trial of progesterone therapy for malignant peritoneal cytology in patients with endometrial carcinoma. Gynecol Oncol 1992; 47:373–376.

PHYSICIAN'S RESPONSE

F. MONTZ

In this case, it is next to impossible to offer a learned consultation without obtaining much more information. I would like to know the following:

1. What is the patient's body habitus and what has been done in an attempt to identify the cause of the intraoperative hypotension?
2. The following information from the pathologic review is needed:
   a. Size of the lesion
   b. Presence of extension to the cervix/isthmus
   c. Adnexal involvement
   d. Presence of lymphovascular space involvement
   e. Hormone receptor status
   f. Quantification of the nature of the positivity of the washings

This information is critical, as it would help to determine the risk for nodal spread and recurrence of disease.

3. Was a perioperative CA-125 determination performed, and if so, what was the result?

I would *strongly* encourage that the patient undergo re-exploration, potentially via laparoscopy, so as to complete adequate surgical staging, emphasizing lymph node sampling. Until such staging is completed, she is not a candidate for a GOG protocol.

If I were forced to give a consultation based only on the information offered in the case (something I would adamantly resist), my recommendations would be as follows:

1. Obtain a chest x-ray and a CT scan of the abdomen prior to instituting therapy.
2. Obtain a CA-125 determination if not already completed.
3. Treat the patient with whole-pelvis external-beam radiation to a dose of 4500 cGy using a four-field technique.
4. Institute progestogen therapy, using either oral dosing [e.g., megestrol (Megace) 320 mg/day in divided doses] or intramuscular progestogen (e.g., Depo-Provera 400 mg IM weekly for 3 months and then every 2 weeks).
5. Follow the patient with quarterly physical examinations and CA-125 determinations with chest x-rays and CT scans twice yearly for a period of 3 years. Thereafter, she should be followed on a twice-yearly basis.

References

Morrow CP, Bundy BN, Kurman RJ, et al. Relationship between surgical-pathological risk factors and outcome in clinical stage I and II carcinoma of the endometrium: A Gynecologic Oncology Group Study. Gynecol Oncol 1991; 40:55.

Turner DA, Gershenson DM, Atkinson N, et al. The prognostic significance of peritoneal cytology for stage I endometrial cancer. Obstet Gynecol 1988; 74:775.

43

Papillary Serous Adenocarcinoma in an Endometrial Polyp

CASE

A 57-year-old (5 ft 8 in, 120 lb) woman develops postmenopausal bleeding. Evaluation reveals an endometrial polyp that is found to contain papillary serous adenocarcinoma. At hysterectomy, the patient is found to have no palpable lymph nodes and the upper abdomen reveals no gross disease. An omental biopsy is negative and there is no residual disease in the uterus. Cytologies from peritoneal washings reveal no cancer.

PHYSICIANS' RESPONSE

BABAK EDRAKI
SETSUKO K. CHAMBERS

Endometrial carcinoma is the most common gynecological malignancy in the United States. It is blessed with the early symptom of postmenopausal bleeding; therefore the majority of cases are diagnosed in the early stages. Factors that have been shown to influence survival are histology, grade, depth of invasion, presence of lymphovascular space invasion, peritoneal cytology, and extrauterine disease. The tumor volume is also an important prognosticator. Uterine papillary serous carcinoma was first described by Hendrickson et al. in 1982 as a highly malignant form of endometrial carcinoma (1). Histologically, this tumor resembles papillary serous carcinomas of the ovary and often demonstrates the presence of psammoma bodies. The majority of patients with stage I disease have myometrial invasion and approximately three-quarters have lymphatic space invasion. Fifty percent of all patients with clinical stage I uterine papillary serous carcinoma have evidence of extrauterine disease at surgery. Fifty to sixty percent of the cases are understaged. A third of patients who are thought to have the tumor confined to the uterus have lymph node metastases, underscoring the importance of a thorough surgical evaluation in patients with this subtype of endometrial carcinoma. Reports of local/regional and distant recurrence in patients with favorable prognostic indicators are not uncommon. Indeed, Carcangiu and Chambers (2) demonstrated that patients with stage I disease and no residual tumor or tumor confined to an endometrial polyp or endometrial mucosa without lymphovascular space invasion had a survival not statistically different from those with stage I disease but with myometrial and/or vascular invasion. This patient had an appropriate initial workup of her postmenopausal bleeding, which led to the diagnosis of uterine papillary serous carcinoma; however, once this diagnosis was made, it would have been more appropriate that the patient undergo extensive surgical staging by a gynecological oncologist, at which time a total abdominal hysterectomy and bilateral salpingo-oophorectomy, as well as periaortic and bilateral pelvic lymph node sampling and full omentectomy, would have been performed. At the present time, it is unclear whether this patient has micrometastases to the omentum or retroperitoneal lymph nodes. This staging, therefore, is considered inadequate. Open and laparoscopic restaging procedures have been proposed and are being performed in a number of centers in the United States. However, for such procedures to be cost-effective, the information gained should be significant enough to change management strategies. In this particular case, given the aggressive behavior of this subtype of endometrial carcinoma, the risk of recurrence is still present even with the absence of nodal or omental metastases. Therefore a restaging procedure will not change the management of this patient. Currently at our institution, all patients with uterine papillary serous carcinomas receive adjuvant therapy. Because of the mode of spread and frequency of distant metastases, the treatment of choice should not be localized to the pelvis alone. Whole abdominal radiation has been employed extensively in the United States. However, Frank et al. (3) reported a 66% recurrence rate in patients with uterine papillary serous carcinoma treated with whole abdominal radiation, with median time to recurrence of only 7.5 months. This type of therapy also carries a high rate of morbidity. Price et al. (4) have reported reasonable efficacy with cyclophosphamide, doxorubicin, and platinum (CAP) chemotherapy in patients without metastatic or only microscopic extrauterine disease. Our recommendations in the management of this particular patient would be to obtain a pretreatment CT scan of the abdomen and pelvis as well as a CA-125 level followed by six cycles of CAP chemotherapy. After the completion of this regimen, the patient should be followed routinely.

References

1. Hendrickson M, Ross J, Eifel P, et al. Uterine papillary serous carcinoma: A highly malignant form of endometrial adenocarcinoma. Am J Surg Pathol 1982; 6:93–108.
2. Carcangiu ML, Chambers JT. Uterine papillary serous carcinoma: A study of 108 cases with emphasis on the prognostic significance of associated endometrioid carcinoma, absence of invasion, and concomitant ovarian carcinoma. Gynecol Oncol 1992; 47:298–305.
3. Frank AH, Tseng PC, Haffty BG, et al. Adjuvant whole-abdominal radiation therapy in uterine papillary serous carcinoma. Cancer 1991; 68:1516–1519.
4. Price FV, Chambers SK, Carcangiu ML, et al. Intravenous cisplatin, doxorubicin and cyclophosphamide in the treatment of uterine papillary serous carcinoma. Gynecol Oncol 1993; 51:383–389.

PHYSICIANS' RESPONSE

N. NIKRUI
R. SAINZ DE LA CUESTA

Uterine papillary serous carcinoma (UPSC) is a rare (3 to 4%) but aggressive type of endometrial carcinoma that resembles ovarian serous adenocarcinoma in its morphology as well as its clinical behavior. It frequently presents with extrauterine disease and has a high recurrence rate even in early stages, where it is confined to the uterus. Because of this progressive behavior, a complete surgical staging is recommended. This should include peritoneal cytology, total hysterectomy, bilateral salpingo-oophorectomy, lymph node sampling, and omentectomy. Even though myometrial invasion is a well-known independent prognostic factor for typical endometrioid-type adenocarcinoma of the endometrium, it seems to play a little role in the overall prognosis of patients with UPSC. At initial laparotomy, this cancer presents with a high rate of intraperitoneal metastasis (70%). In addition, positive peritoneal cytology is found in 44% of the cases, lymph node metastases in 46%, and lymphovascular space involvement (LVSI) in 40% (1). In this particular case, we lack information of lymph node status, as lymph node palpation can be inaccurate in 15% of the cases. Another important piece of histological information is knowing if there was LVSI within the polyp. The presence of LVSI by the tumor has been associated with poor prognosis. In this case and given no LVSI, restaging laparotomy or laparoscopy is probably not necessary, because positive lymph nodes in the absence of extrauterine disease and no myometrial invasion is a rare event. In the largest series of UPSC arising from an endometrial polyp, Sherman et al. (2) reported 9 cases, out of which 4 had no myometrial invasion. However, the majority had extrauterine disease at the time of presentation, and all those patients died of the disease. Based on this and other studies, some authors advocate adjuvant chemotherapy or radiation therapy for all patients with UPSC. However other authors have reported a few cases, similar to this one, with an excellent survival rate. In our case, where there is no myometrial invasion and no evidence of extrauterine disease, we believe that adjuvant therapy should not be necessary. We would, however, recommend close follow-up for evidence of recurrent disease because of the tendency of this tumor to recur intraabdominally. A tumor marker such as OC-125 may be useful for this patient's follow-up case. A complete physical exam with an OC-125 should be performed every 3 months for 1 year, then every 4 months for 1 year, and finally every 6 months for 3 more years, and yearly from then onward.

References

1. Goff et al. Uterine papillary serous carcinoma: Patterns of metastatic spread. Gynecol Oncol 1994; 54:264–268.
2. Sherman et al. Uterine serous carcinoma: A morphologically diverse neoplasm with unifying clinicopathologic features. Am J Surg Pathol 1992; 16:600–610.

PHYSICIAN'S RESPONSE

THOMAS F. ROCERETO

Papillary serous adenocarcinoma of the endometrium is an aggressive disease with a poor prognosis. It accounts for approximately 5% of all endometrial carcinomas and has a cure rate of only 25%. These tumors tend to deeply invade the myometrium. Pelvic and/or paraaortic lymph nodes are involved in 25% of the cases; in close to 50%, there is extrauterine involvement. The natural course of this disease more resembles that of tubal and ovarian carcinomas.

The findings at the time of surgery in patients with serous adenocarcinoma of the endometrium usually show that the tumor is more advanced than thought clinically. The recommended surgery for patients with adenocarcinoma of the endometrium consists of a total abdominal hysterectomy and bilateral salpingo-oophorectomy with sampling of the lymph nodes, depending on tumor grade and depth of myometrial invasion. This is not adequate surgical evaluation for the patient with a serous adenocarcinoma. These patients should have the same operative procedure normally used in patients with ovarian carcinoma. This surgery includes a total abdominal hysterectomy, bilateral salpingo-oophorectomy, sampling of the para-aortic and pelvic lymph nodes, infracolic omentectomy, and multiple abdominal and pelvic peritoneal biopsies. The depth of penetration of the tumor into the myometrium should not influence the extent of surgery. Peritoneal washings should include the entire abdominal cavity, not just the pelvic cavity.

Over 50% of patients grossly free of tumor at the end of surgery will recur. Recurrence is common in the upper abdomen and along the peritoneal surfaces.

There is no standard postsurgical treatment. Pelvic irradiation increases the rate of local control only. Whole abdominal radiation (WAR) has been used in experimental protocols, but the overall results with respect to cure are not known as yet; however, WAR may improve the survival of some patients with only microscopic disease at the end of surgery. Even though the technique for WAR has been improved upon, the side effects may not warrant its general use in this disease. Multiple chemotherapeutic regimens have been studied, including those used for ovarian carcinomas; however, the results are not promising.

As in most cases, the patient in this case was known to have a papillary serous adenocarcinoma of the endometrium prior to surgery. She has had inadequate surgery with respect to the proper evaluation for the extent of tumor involvement. There is no myometrial invasion and, in fact, there is no residual tumor in the endometrium. Patients with no myometrial involvement have done well without any further treatment. This patient's tumor was isolated in an endometrial polyp. Chances are very small that further surgery will uncover tumor outside the uterus. No further treatment is recommended in this case. Good follow-up is most important.

References

Jeffrey JF, Krepart GV, Lotocki RJ. Papillary serous adenocarcinoma of the endometrium. Obstet Gynecol 1986; 67:670–674.

Ramirez-Gonzalez CE, et al. Papillary adenocarcinoma of the endometrium. Obstet Gynecol 1987; 70:212–215.

Sutton GP, et al. Malignant papillary lesions of the endometrium. Gynecol Oncol 1987; 27:294–304.

Ward BG, Wright RG, Free K. Papillary carcinomas of the endometrium. Gynecol Oncol 1990; 39:347–351.

PHYSICIANS' RESPONSE

EDWARD KAPLAN
DATTA NORI

This 57-year-old woman was found to have uterine papillary serous carcinoma (UPSC) in an endometrial polyp on endometrial biopsy after she presented with postmenopausal bleeding. No residual disease was identified in the hysterectomy specimen, nor was there any evidence of extrauterine disease at exploratory laparotomy. Lymph nodes were not taken, although intraoperatively no suspicious adenopathy was seen. This patient has stage IA endometrial UPSC limited to a polyp.

Initially described in 1982, UPSC is a histological variant of endometroid adenocarcinoma and represents the most common of the unfavorable histologies.

The others include clear-cell, undifferentiated, and squamous carcinoma, which together represent less than 10% of all endometrial tumors. There is a general consensus that UPSC is a high-grade tumor, but definitive therapy remains controversial. This case is especially interesting because the tumor was confined to a polyp.

Consistent evidence drawn from several small series indicates that the typical prognostic factors used to assess ordinary adenocarcinoma of the endometrium— such as depth of myometrial invasion, histological grade, lymphovascular invasion, and absence of extrauterine disease—do not apply to UPSC. It is a virulent tumor and must be dealt with aggressively, including the unusual polypoid presentation.

One series from a single institution parallels our patient's presentation (1). Ten cases with clinical stage I disease presenting as UPSC confined to endometrial polyps were identified among all patients treated at the M.D. Anderson Cancer Center from 1985 to 1990. The polyps ranged in size from 1 by 1 cm to 4 by 2.5 cm, and only one showed any myometrial invasion, which was less than 1 mm. Two patients were found to have positive pelvic washings; two had microscopic foci of disease on an ovary and fallopian tube, respectively; two had other superficial foci of UPSC in the endometrium; and three patients had lymphvascular invasion (LVI). Surgical stage was not provided, and it is not certain which cases had which pathological findings. Nevertheless, 6 of the 10 patients developed recurrences in the peritoneum. One was salvaged with external-beam radiotherapy (EBRT) and is NED at 12 months, while no patient was salvaged with chemotherapy. The two patients who received preoperative intracavitary implants remain NED, while the one who was given EBRT failed. Since only three patients had LVI, it was postulated that this was not an important route of spread. Beyond that, however, no conclusions were drawn except to say that these patients were at high risk for failure. Tumor volume was not evaluated, but the proportion of polyp involved was mentioned as a potential prognostic factor.

In a similar study from Johns Hopkins (2), 9 patients among 41 cases had UPSC limited to a polyp. Four of the nine polyps showed no myometrial invasion, and the deepest was 3 mm. Five patients had extrauterine disease found at surgery. All four patients with noninvasive UPSC in polyps died and only one patient remains NED. Overall, survival was no better in patients with polyps than in other patients with myometrial invasion and/or LVI. Five of the nine polyp patients received adjuvant irradiation, but it is not known whether they were among the survivors.

In summary, review of the few reports in the literature offers compelling evidence that the classic prognostic factors for endometrial carcinoma are not applicable to UPSC and that all clinical stage I UPSCs deserve adjuvant treatment. This tumor is so lethal that even disease limited to a polyp can behave unpredictably, as shown above, where three-quarters of the patients failed. Some investigators believe that papillary serous carcinoma may be inherently multicentric, similar to the field cancerization effect in the aerodigestive tract. Our recommendation in this case is for postoperative whole pelvic irradiation to 45 Gy, followed by three fractions of intravaginal brachytherapy, much the same as we would administer for patients with grade 2 or 3 endometrial adenocarcinoma or for any patient with more than one-third myometrial invasion. We would reserve abdominal irradiation for salvage, since it carries a significant risk of morbidity and is of uncertain benefit.

References

1. Silva EG, Jenkins R. Serous carcinoma in endometrial polyps. Mod Pathol 1990; 3:120–128.
2. Sherman ME, Bitterman P, Rosenshein NB, et al. Uterine serous carcinoma. Am J Surg Pathol 1992; 16:600–610.

44

Uterine Cancer, Stage IC, Grade 3

CASE

A 71-year-old woman, gravida I, para I, who experienced 1 week of postmeno-pausal bleeding and came to her doctor's office. An endometrial biopsy revealed a grade 3 adenocarcinoma of the endometrium. Abdominal pelvic computed tomography (CT) and a chest x-ray were negative preoperatively, as were all standard chemistries and a complete blood count (CBC). The patient is diabetic, controlled by diet; she has mild hypertension that is currently being managed without medication. She underwent an exploratory laparotomy, total abdominal hysterectomy/bilateral salpingo-oophorectomy (TAH/BSO), and bilateral pelvic as well as paraaortic lymph node sampling. Approximately 10 lymph nodes were removed from each side of the pelvis and 4 to 6 nodes on first the left and then the right para aortic regions respectively. Final pathology showed a grade III adenocarcinoma with 75% myometrial invasion, negative peritoneal washings, and negative pelvic and paraaortic lymph nodes. The patient developed some shortness of breath on her third postoperative day and a ventilation/perfusion scan was highly suspicious for multiple pulmonary emboli. The patient was im-mediately placed on heparin and then, over the next 5 days, converted to warfarin (Coumadin). No source was found by Doppler exam in her lower extremities. The patient was discharged home on warfarin on her eighth postoperative day.

PHYSICIAN'S RESPONSE

HANS KREBS

The patient described in this case has a stage IC, grade 3 adenocarcinoma of the endometrium based upon 75% myometrial invasion of a grade 3 adenocarcinoma without cervical involvement, positive peritoneal cytology, or spread to lymph nodes or other organs. Although there is no mention of vascular space involvement or other prognostic factors, the presence of a poorly differentiated adenocarcinoma with deep myometrial invasion in an elderly woman over 70 years old projects a high risk for treatment failure, reported in the literature to be as high as 75%. It has been thought in the past that this group of women may benefit the most from adjuvant therapy. The medical problems listed (diabetes mellitus, deep vein thrombosis with pulmonary embolus) are considered incidental and should not interfere with the treatment decision.

Unfortunately, the treatment of high-grade endometrial carcinoma with deep myometrial invasion has never been studied in a controlled, randomized fashion. Even the data presented in retrospective reviews are scant. For example, a recent comparatively large Gynecologic Oncology Group (GOG) study of 895 women contains only 12 patients with a grade 3 tumor invading to the outer third of the myometrium without other risk factors such as lymph nodes, adnexal involvement, capillary space invasion, extension to the uterine isthmus/cervix, cytology, or gross disease outside the uterus (1). All patients in that study received external radiation to the pelvis postoperatively. The fact that only 1 of the 12 women developed a recurrence suggests that adjuvant radiation therapy is beneficial.

The strongest support in favor of radiation therapy in the given situation comes from the fact that 37.5% of women in the GOG study with grade 3 lesions invasive to the inner or middle third of the myometrium developed recurrences when treated by surgery only compared to 18.2% when external radiation therapy was given postoperatively (1).

This view, however, is not shared unanimously. For one thing, the number of women in the high-risk groups in the GOG study was small. In addition, Chen prospectively studied 18 patients with stage IC, grade 3 endometrial carcinomas. None of the patients who received only primary surgical treatment without postoperative irradiation showed evidence of disease in follow-up of 5 to 13 years. Chen concluded that patients with stage I endometrial carcinoma may not require postoperative irradiation even when poor prognostic factors of deep myometrial invasion and/or grade 3 tumor are present (2).

It is of interest that women with similar lesions in the GOG study suffered no recurrences when vaginal cuff instead of whole pelvic irradiation was given. This suggests that vaginal cuff irradiation may be preferable to whole pelvic irradiation should adjuvant radiation therapy be considered (1).

In conclusion, we must await the arrival of firm data derived from prospective, randomized studies before firm recommendations in regard to adjuvant radiation can be given. In the meantime I would err on the side of postoperative therapy either in the form of a vaginal cylinder or whole pelvis irradiation.

References

1. Morrow P, Bundy BN, Jurman R, et al. Relationship between surgical-pathological risk factors and outcome in clinical stage I and II carcinoma of the endometrium: A Gynecologic Oncology Group study. Gynecol Oncol 1991; 40:55–65.
2. Chen S. Operative treatment in stage I endometrial carcinoma with deep myometrial invasion and/or grade 3 tumor limited to the corpus luetem: No recurrence with only primary surgery. Cancer 1989; 63:1843–1845.

PHYSICIAN'S RESPONSE

JOHN CURRIE

Following appropriate surgical therapy, this 71-year-old woman experienced a promptly diagnosed and treated pulmonary embolus. It is presumed she had been exposed to prophylactic intermittent pneumatic compression stockings and/or heparin perioperatively; if so, her development of thromboembolic phenomena is worrisome for systemic hypercoagulation (Trousseau's syndrome), and the possibility of extant tumor should be entertained. A baseline CT scan of the lungs should be obtained to document tiny metastasis or serve as a benchmark for future imaging. If such prophylaxis was not ordered and executed, the provider should include current prevention techniques in subsequent patients with planned pelvic surgery. If recurrent emboli are documented, a vena cava filter device should be inserted, and anticoagulation should be maintain at upper levels of therapeutic values for 6 months, with consideration of lower levels for life.

If randomized clinical trials are available in the institution where this patient is being treated, she should be considered for entry into a trial randomizing her to pelvic radiation therapy or no further treatment. Trials combining radiation therapy with chemotherapy are available in some centers and could also be considered. The results of such studies are eagerly sought by all providers rendering care for this group of patients. While this patient has several risk factors for recurrence, most notably grade 3 disease and deep (75%) myometrial invasion, there are no randomized data available that would confirm a survival benefit from the addition of adjunctive radiation or other treatment in this patient. At the same time, the known potential complications of radiation therapy in this diabetic patient would suggest withholding such treatment in the absence of a proven benefit. In addition, lymphedema, which often results when patients who have undergone lymphadenectomy receive external-beam therapy, would cloud the monitoring of possible subsequent lower extremity thromboembolic disease.

Thus, if randomized clinical trials were unavailable to this patient or if she refused entry into such, only close follow-up should be offered after informing the patient of the available options. There is no indication for progestational therapy; not only is it unlikely to be of benefit even in the case of occult extant disease (poorly differentiated tumors rarely respond to such treatment), but the known thromboembolic risks of such therapy would contraindicate its use prophylactically.

Close follow-up would entail pelvic exams and Pap smears every 3 months for 2 years, every 6 months for 3 years, and yearly for life. The benefit of periodic chest imaging is not established; the cost/benefit ratio should be carefully considered in the asymptomatic patient.

PHYSICIAN'S RESPONSE

A. ROBERT KAGAN

Most of our management regimens for adenocarcinoma of the endometrium are from investigations of patients who have *not* had adequate removal of bilateral pelvic and paraaortic nodes to be histologically examined. There is universal agreement on TAH/BSO being the corner-stone of treatment, but whether the additional treatment of pre- or postoperative irradiation, external irradiation, intrauterine/intravaginal curietherapy, or transvaginal roentgen therapy is also needed has been a source of debate fueled by the fervor of the debaters rather than by the logic of definitive studies.

The pathological stage is IC, grade 3, with negative nodes, and I would recommend external pelvic irradiation to 5000 cGy with intravaginal irradiation, 2100 cGy in three fractions if a high dose rate is used or 2500 gamma rads if a low dose rate is given in one application to the lateral vaginal surface, maintaining the anterior rectal dose below 1600 cGy. Knowing that the pelvic/paraaortic nodes are negative and the patient was obese might influence me to forgo the pelvic irradiation, but my belief is that in patients with grade 3 and greater than 50% myometrial involvement, the vaginal and pelvic recurrence rate is 20%, and this can be reduced to less than 5% with external beam irradiation plus or minus intravaginal irradiation.

I would be more likely to forgo external-beam irradiation in an obese patient or one with a history of diverticulitis if the grade of the tumor were 1 or 2 or if the grade 3 tumor infiltrated the myometrium by *less* than 50%. I have never understood how the cancer can recur in the vagina with a negative lower uterine segment, hence my "faith" in external-beam irradiation. Perhaps in the future, I will become convinced that the knowledge that the nodes are negative can allow me to safely eliminate external-beam irradiation.

PHYSICIAN'S RESPONSE

MICHAEL HOPKINS

The current method for staging uterine malignancy is through surgery. Postoperatively, the patient would be classified as stage IC, grade 3. Prior to the staging trials conducted in the 1970s and early 1980s, virtually all patients with endometrial cancer received some form of radiotherapy either pre- or postoperatively. Now that we are doing extensive lymphadenectomy or lymph node sampling, we obtain information that is of prognostic benefit but not always used for planning postoperative therapy. This patient presents such a dilemma. All the lymph nodes are negative and the question now is whether radiotherapy would add any benefit to her treatment. The two most common sites of recurrence are at the vaginal cuff and in the lungs. Clearly, pelvic radiotherapy is a localized treatment and can only prevent localized recurrence. If small emboli have already traveled to the lungs, pelvic radiotherapy at this point will not help. If the lymphadenectomy has been thorough and all nodal tissue has been removed, I believe there is little benefit to pelvic radiotherapy beyond preventing a recurrence at the vaginal cuff. I would consider this patient to be a candidate for observation or cuff radiotherapy only.

The fact that this patient had a pulmonary embolism postoperatively is consistent with the high risks faced by these patients, who are usually older and overweight. The pulmonary embolism would not alter my decision making.

PHYSICIAN'S RESPONSE

MARK D. ADELSON

Many patients with endometrial cancer are obese, diabetic, and hypertensive. These diseases often result in vascular, cardiac, and renal compromise; therefore these patients may not be optimal surgical candidates. The state-of-the-art approach to endometrial cancer is operative laparoscopy (1), which is accompanied by a lower morbidity and shorter recovery compared to laparotomy. This patient had risk factors for thromboembolic disease such as cancer, diabetes, and hypertension. You should be commended for promptly evaluating this patient's shortness of breath to rule out pulmonary embolism, since the mortality from a promptly diagnosed pulmonary embolism is 10%, versus 30% if diagnosis is delayed. Patients with thromboemboli causing cardiorespiratory embarrassment can initially be given fibrinolytic therapy to rapidly remove the clot prior to anticoagulation. Since pelvic thrombosis is uncommon in the non-pregnant state, it is likely that this patient's source was her lower extremities, even with a negative Doppler.

Postoperative adjunctive therapy is problematic. The lack of clear evidence showing a survival advantage for adjunctive therapy, especially with grade 3 disease, mandates that we completely discuss the material risks and benefits of the different types of treatment versus nontreatment. Pelvic radiation is often considered the standard of care. Radiation does appear to reduce the risk of pelvic recurrence, but it does not appear to reduce the overall risk of recurrence (2). Pelvic radiation therapy would have no impact on disease outside the pelvis. Grade 3 cancers generally do not contain estrogen or progesterone receptors and so are generally not responsive to hormonal manipulation, which has not been shown to be helpful in the adjunctive setting. It is possible that progesterone and tamoxifen would increase the risk of repeat thromboembolic disease. Chemotherapy could be given even though the patient is anticoagulated. The risk of bleeding secondary to thrombocytopenia (from chemotherapy) plus anticoagulation is increased. Chemotherapy does not appear to influence survival in this setting.

I follow these patients postoperatively every 3 months with a general and pelvic examination and a Pap smear. I generally do not obtain radiographic studies in the absence of specific symptoms. I advise pelvic radiation if the patient wishes to take advantage of the "standard" therapy, realizing that there is always a chance it would help, and the risk of serious complications is low. If the patient does not wish to receive any treatment that is not of proven benefit and therefore does not wish to experience any unnecessary treatment and risk, she might wish to be followed without further therapy.

References

1. Childers JM, Brzechffa PR, Hatch KD, Surwit EA. Laparoscopically assisted surgical staging (LASS) of endometrial cancer. Gynecol Oncol 1993; 51:33–38.
2. Aalders J, Abeler V, Kolstad P, et al. Postoperative external irradiation and prognostic parameters in stage I endometrial carcinoma. Obstet Gynecol 1980; 56:419.

45

Uterine Cancer: Adenocarcinoma Stage II

CASE

A 58-year-old woman, gravida II, para II, presents to your office with postmeno-pausal bleeding of 6 months' duration. She has otherwise been in good health and is on no medication. At 5 ft, 3 in in height and 180 lb in weight, she is a bit overweight. On examination there are no palpable supraclavicular nodes. The chest is clear. The heart shows a regular rate and rhythm. No breast or abdominal masses are noted. There are no suspicious palpable inguinal nodes, and no vulvar or vaginal lesions are present. The cervix seems somewhat irregular, although it is only a couple centimeters in diameter and not particularly firm. The uterus is approximately 8 weeks in size and mobile. No adnexal masses are noted. Rectovaginal exam confirms this and there is no cul-de-sac nodularity. A punch biopsy is done of the cervix as well as a pipelle of the endometrium. The biopsies show a grade 2 adenocarcinoma of the endometrium with some areas of atypical adenomatous hyperplasia. In addition, there is a similar nonmucinous adenocar-cinoma, endometrioid in type, involving the cervix.

The patient underwent abdominal pelvic computed tomography (CT) using oral IV rectal contrast as well as a vaginal tampon, and the study was interpreted as negative.

PHYSICIAN'S RESPONSE

PEYTON T. TAYLOR

The patient described could either have a primary endocervical adenocarcinoma (stage IB) or endometrial adenocarcinoma (clinically occult stage II). The distinction between the two is difficult to make on the basis of either the physical examination or biopsies alone. Endometrioid adenocarcinoma in the cervix and uterus, especially when the endometrial biopsy is admixed with adenomatous hyperplasia, most likely represents an endometrial primary involving the cervix (clinically occult stage II). Most primary endocervical adenocarcinomas are of the mucinous or endocervical epithelial type.

I would not advise hysteroscopic examination as an aid in establishing the anatomic "epicenter" of malignancy in this patient for concern that efflux of malignant cells out the tubal ostia into the peritoneal cavity could have adverse significance. Except for a chest radiogram and serum CA-125, I would not advise any additional preoperative diagnostic studies and would not have ordered the abdominal-pelvic CT scan based on the information presented.

Two less traditional alternatives were considered but neither was advised: primary radiation therapy and radical hysterectomy. Radiation therapy alone utilizing four-field whole pelvic radiation (4500 to 5000 cGy) followed by cesium brachytherapy (approximately 3500 cGy to point A) would be a reasonable and effective plan, especially if the patient was a poor surgical candidate. Radical hysterectomy and lymphadenectomy would also be effective, regardless of whether the tumor is endocervical or endometrial in origin, and may be as effective as the more conventional combined surgery plus radiation schemes.

I favor primary surgical staging of this patient, followed by integrated and specific postoperative therapy based on the extent of disease. In addition to abdominal hysterectomy and adnexectomy, this includes assessment of the pelvic and paraaortic nodes, peritoneal washings, and assessment of the general abdominal cavity. I believe that staging lymphadenectomy can be performed in many if not most patients efficiently and with little added risk to the basic procedure (1). Some advise nodal sampling in only selected patients, basing their decision on intraoperative frozen-section analysis of grade and depth of myometrial invasion (2). Others question the value of lymphadenectomy and recommend no or minimal nodal sampling coupled with complex algorithms for postoperative therapy based on the statistical likelyhood of occult nodal metastasis (3,4).

The staging data obtained will allow the patient to be placed into one of the following risk groups: (a) those with metastatic disease, (b) those at high or intermediate risk for subsequent recurrent or metastatic disease (occult invasion of cervical stroma; $\geq 1/2$ myometrial wall invasion; lymphovascular space invasion) and (c) those at low risk for subsequent relapse (for whom no additional therapy is usually advised). Because the cervical punch biopsy (not just a positive endocervical curettage) revealed invasive adenocarcinoma, this patient will actually have metastatic disease or will remain at high to intermediate risk. She will, therefore, likely benefit from participation in one of the prospective clinical trials comparing adjuvant postoperative treatments now being conducted by the Gynecologic Oncology Group (GOG).

Patients with metastatic disease are at high risk of developing progressive and fatal disease and need additional treatment; unfortunately, the "best" treatment is not known. If this is the case, I would advise her to enter a prospective GOG trial comparing two schemes of systemic chemotherapy or whole abdominal-pelvic radiation versus systemic chemotherapy. Those with intermediate-risk disease are the most problematic because there is an observation arm; i.e., additional pelvic radiation has not been shown to improve the long-term survival of these patients and therefore is the subject of current investigation.

References

1. Orr JW, Jr, Holloway RW, Orr PF, Hoilman JL. Surgical staging of uterine cancer: An analysis of perioperative morbidity. Gynecol Oncol 1991; 42:209.
2. Goff BA, Rice LW. Assessment of depth of myometrial invasion in endometrial adenocarcinoma. Gynecol Oncol 1990; 38:46.
3. Belinson JL, Lee KR, Badget GJ, et al. Clinical stage I adenocarcinoma of the endometrium: Analysis of recurrences and the potential benefit of staging lymphadenectomy. Gynecol Oncol 1992; 44:17.
4. Kim YB and Niloff JM. Endometrial carcinoma: Analysis of recurrence in patients treated with a strategy minimizing lymph node sampling and radiation therapy. Obstet Gynecol 1993; 82:175.

PHYSICIANS' RESPONSE

RICHARD REID
GARTH D. PHIBBS

The diagnosis in this patient is adenocarcinoma arising in a background of atypical adenomatous hyperplasia and showing apparent clinical extension to the cervix. Using positive endocervical curettage as the sole criterion, cervical involvement is falsely suspected in 40 to 50% of cases. Since November 1988, endometrial cancer has been a surgically staged disease; however, a positive punch biopsy from an abnormally firm cervix clearly suggests that this is a Fédération Internationale de Gynécologie et d'Obstétrique (FIGO) stage II tumor. Differentiation from primary adenocarcinoma of the cervix can also be difficult, but positive uterine curettings from a bulky uterus in a postmenopausal patient plus the endometrioid histological pattern indicates that this is an endometrial carcinoma. Associated workup to date, including a comprehensive abdominal/pelvic CT with contrast, does not indicate any evidence of extrauterine disease. Given the observed tumor distribution and lack of associated symptomatology, endoscopic evaluation of the bladder and rectum is unlikely to yield positive findings.

In light of the small number of stage II cases in the reported endometrial cancer series, together with the lack of prospective randomized studies, it is difficult to be dogmatic about the optimal therapy for this patient. The basic principles, however, are clear. Optimal local control requires uterine removal. Given the 35% incidence of positive pelvic nodes in this group of patients, any treatment protocol must also include treatment of these lymph nodes. Hence, unless absolutely medically contraindicated, all stage II endometrial cancers should be treated with some form of hysterectomy.

There are two specific options available to this patient. One is radical hysterectomy, bilateral salpingo-oophorectomy, and bilateral pelvic lymphadenectomy. The other is combined therapy using preoperative external pelvic irradiation and intracavitary radium or cesium, followed by a total extrafascial abdominal hysterectomy and bilateral salpingo-oophorectomy. Theoretically, preoperative external irradiation should optimize the geometry of the intracavity insertion with less resultant risk of fixed (and thus easily injured) bowel within the pelvis. Nonetheless, most papers on combined therapy have reported significant intestinal morbidity, with up to 30% of patients experiencing a bowel complication severe enough to require surgical correction (1,2). Hence, our preference in medically fit patients with no clinical evidence of parametrial invasion is primary laparotomy with surgical staging. This permits adherence to the principle of wide local excision of the primary cancer along with the attendant sites of primary extension yet minimizes postoperative morbidity.

At surgery, pelvic and abdominal peritoneal washings are collected for cytological assessment. The peritoneal cavity is explored and any suspicious areas are biopsied. The omentum should also be sampled. The uterus is then removed for thorough histological assessment by extended or modified radical (type 2) hysterectomy, with bilateral salpingo-oophorectomy. Additional staging includes thorough pelvic lymphadenectomy, resection of the lower periaortic lymph nodes, and removal of any other grossly enlarged periaortic lymph nodes. Recently, Partridge et al. have stressed the possible therapeutic benefit of thorough lymphadenectomy in this high-risk group of patients (3).

As in most gynecological malignancies, goals of therapy are to individualize treatment, maximizing resultant cure, but also minimize resultant morbidity so as to focusing upon improved quality (rather than quantity) of life.

If all resected lymph nodes prove to be negative, we would recommend vaginal vault cesium without external beam therapy. Conversely, if either a grossly positive pelvic node or multiple microscopically positive pelvic lymph nodes are found, we would recommend extended-field teletherapy without added vault cesium. In the unlikely event that this patient should be found to have intraabdominal disease, a concerted attempt would be made to complete resection, with consideration given to whole abdominal irradiation therapy or possibly systemic chemotherapy, although the benefits of systemic therapy at this advanced stage are not firmly established. Because this appears to be a biologically aggressive lesion with apparent cervical extension, a tumor sample would also be sent for estrogen and progesterone receptor analysis to help guide subsequent systemic therapy.

Despite the obvious importance of clinical stage, histological grade remains the prognostic indicator of paramount importance. This patient, with a low-grade stage II tumor, has a better prognosis than she would if she had a stage IC, grade 3 lesion (4).

References

1. Larson DM, Copeland LJ, Gallagher HS, et al. Stage II endometrial carcinoma: Results and complications of a combined radiotherapeutic/surgical approach. Cancer 1988; 61:15–28.
2. Kinsella TJ, Bloomer WD, Lavin PT, Knapp RC. Stage II endometrial carcinoma: Ten year follow-up of combined radiation and surgical treatment. Gynecol Oncol 1980; 10:290.
3. Boente MP, Orandi YA, Yordan EL, Miller A, et al. Recurrence patterns and complications in endometrial adenocarcinoma with cervical involvement. Ann Surg Oncol 1995; 2:138–144.
4. The annual report on the results of treatment of gynecologic cancer, Table B1VA. 1992; 21:140.

PHYSICIAN'S RESPONSE

GEORGE W. MORLEY

It is interesting to note that this 58-year-old woman who had postmenopausal bleeding for a period of 6 months apparently had not sought medical attention any sooner. In this day and age it should be pretty well recognized that abnormal uterine bleeding after the menopause is serious until proven otherwise, and certainly such patients should be thoroughly investigated at the earliest possible moment. This patient is apparently in good health, but it would be interesting to know if she has been treated for hypertension or diabetes mellitus in addition to her obesity. Also, was she on hormone replacement therapy—either unopposed estrogen or a combination estrogen/progesterone medication—and if she had a previous Pap smear, what the findings were.

On review of this case history there is no known clinical extension of her disease beyond the endometrium and cervix. This lesion is therefore classified as stage II, grade 2; however, there is no mention as to whether the cervical component involves only the endocervical glands or whether there is cervical stromal invasion. Actually this glandular component of the cervix could be considered a contaminant of the endocervix rather than involvement in this area, and this should be rereviewed with the pathologist. If so, this patient should be treated as if she had stage I disease (1,2).

The differential diagnosis here would be between stages IIA and IIB. Even though this patient has had a CT scan that was interpreted as negative, I would personally want a lymphangiogram, especially in the presence of an adenocarcinoma involving both areas of the uterus. If this report is suspicious or positive for metastatic disease, then a fine needle aspiration should follow. Given that this pathology report revealed metastatic disease to either the pelvic or paraaortic lymph nodes, this might alter the therapeutic approach, or at least its sequence, since this lesion is now considered stage IIIC. If, however, the fine needle aspiration is negative for metastatic disease, the final surgical staging will be deferred until more definitive therapy has been carried out and the results from the pathologist have been reported, thus more accurately staging the disease. The FIGO staging for carcinoma of the endometrium has certainly been a step forward, since it not only increases the accuracy of the diagnosis but also improves the uniformity of reporting survival rates, etc., in the future.

In this case, with the CT scanning being negative, it must be assumed that no regional lymphadenopathy was detected on this examination. For the purpose of this discussion, one must then consider this lesion to be a stage II, grade 2 adenocarcinoma of the endometrium. Last, before therapy is initiated, one must review the slides with the pathologist, since it is possible that this is an adenocarcinoma of the endocervix with endometrial extension and thus would be treated as a stage I carcinoma of the cervix. Still more remotely, this could be a double primary lesion, but again one would need the entire specimen to rule in or out this possibility.

Given that this patient has a stage II, grade 2 adenocarcinoma of the endometrium, currently most investigators would treat her with full-course preoperative radiation therapy to a dose of 4500 to 5000 rads to the whole pelvis followed in approximately 4 weeks with an extrafascial total abdominal hysterectomy, bilateral salpingo-oophorectomy, and paraaortic selective lymphadenectomy. Peritoneal cytology should be obtained on all patients. The significance of positive peritoneal cytology without extrauterine disease remains unclear, but basically it is thought to be part and parcel to the current surgical staging and does not alter this staging in either direction. The paraaortic lymph node sampling is necessary, since the radiotherapy given this patient would not include this area of nodal distribution. If other unusual findings were encountered, these areas would be treated accordingly. If, following surgery, the paraaortic nodes were reported positive for metastatic disease, this area would receive additional radiation therapy. In addition, most physicians would add high-dose megestrol (Megace) as adjunctive hormone treatment. Chemotherapy as adjunctive treatment for patients with endometrial carcinoma is still evolving and several single agents or combination regimens have been used, but all of these are considered palliative at this time.

There are a number of variations to the treatment outlined above; these include the following: (a) radical hysterectomy and bilateral pelvic and paraaortic lymphadenectomy with adjunctive x-ray therapy and/or progestin hormone treatment, being considered on an individual basis depending on the final report from the pathologist; (b) extrafascial total abdominal hysterectomy and bilateral salpingo-oophorectomy with a pelvic and paraaortic selective lymphadenectomy, to be followed by at least a vaginal cylinder of brachytherapy; and (c) an initial extrafascial hysterectomy and pelvic and paraaortic selective lymphadenectomy followed by postoperative radiation therapy depending on the pathology report. However, if, in the latter situation a grossly involved cervix were detected preoperatively, the treatment would be reversed, with preoperative whole-pelvis irradiation carried out initially. Given that the final surgical diagnosis was carcinoma of the endometrium stage IIIC, the patient would receive paraaortic irradiation and megestrol hormone therapy.

On review of the literature, the survival rates for stage I carcinoma of the endometrium are approximately 85 to 90% overall, whereas when stage II endometrial carcinoma is the diagnosis, the consensus is that there is a 5-year survival of 75%, although there are some reports giving 5-year survival rates even lower, in the 50 to 60% range.

Finally, what about postoperative estrogen? Given stage II disease, it seems reasonably safe to institute estrogen as prophylaxis against menopausal symptoms, osteoporosis, and heart disease in 3 to 5 years if there has been no evidence of recurrence. In the more advanced situation where megestrol is already used, this drug can be continued for 5 years, following which estrogen can be given, depending on physician preference. Whether or not combination hormone replacement therapy is used rather than unopposed estrogen is a moot point.

Again, the earlier the diagnosis, the better the survival. It would be interesting to have investigated this patient at 6 weeks rather than 6 months following the onset of symptoms, since 75% of all carcinomas of the endometrium when diagnosed are confined to the uterine corpus only.

References

1. Morrow CP, Curtin JP, Townsend DU. Synopsis of Gynecologic Oncology. New York: Churchill Livingstone, 1993.

2. DiSaia PJ, Creasman WT. Clinical gynecologic oncology. St Louis: Mosby, 1989.

PHYSICIAN'S RESPONSE

ROBERT C. WALLACH

There are two different management situations for this patient, depending on the nature of involvement of the cervix. The endometrioid carcinoma in the cervix is assumed to be extension of the disease arising in the corpus. It may either be an extension along the mucosal surface or may involve the stroma of the cervix.

Assuming that the cervical extension of disease is only on the mucosal surface, I would recommend extrafascial total abdominal hysterectomy, bilateral salpingo-oophorectomy, sampling of paraaortic nodes, and sampling of any enlarged pelvic nodes (1). If the sampled nodes and peritoneal washings were negative for tumor, I would recommend whole pelvic external radiation on the basis of extension of disease into the cervix and the potential for occult lymphatic spread. Depth of myometrial invasion would not be a consideration. Dependent on the dose distribution, the use of a remote after-loading iridium source to the vaginal vault could be added at the end of external treatment to the whole pelvis. If paraaortic nodes were involved, extension of the radiation field to include the paraaortic regions would be appropriate. With positive pelvic nodes but negative paraaortic nodes, I would recommend, if possible, an increased dose aimed at the pelvic side walls, where the possibility of failure is greater, and with subtraction of the intravaginal radiation. I would not change these recommendations on the basis of positive peritoneal cytology but would add a progestogen if the cytology were positive.

If the extension of carcinoma to the cervix is into the stroma of the cervix, I would recommend (because of the potential difficulty in delivering a tumor-cidal dose to any residual disease in the pelvis) a radical abdominal hysterectomy, bilateral salpingo-oophorectomy, pelvic lymphadenectomy, and sampling of the paraaortic nodes. If the depth of invasion of the cervix or corpus were greater than 10%, I would also recommend whole-pelvis external radiation, with the under standing that the morbidity related to leg swelling might be appreciable. I would also recommend extended-field radiation if the paraaortic tissue yielded positive tumor.

Although an endometrial carcinoma with atypical adenomatous hyperplasia present in an obese woman might suggest one of the less aggressive varieties of this neoplasm, I believe the extension to the cervix as well as advanced grade indicate that this is a potentially lethal disease and merits the aggressive treatment program outlined above. In the absence of any dependable chemotherapeutic agents for endometrial carcinoma, I would not offer chemotherapy this time.

Reference

1. Belinson JL, Lee KR, Badger GJ, et al. Clinical stage I adenocarcinoma of the endometrium: Analysis of recurrences and potential benefits of staging lymphadenectomy. Gynecol Oncol 1992; 44:1723.

PHYSICIAN'S RESPONSE

PETER FLEMING

This patient is staged $T_2N_0M_0$, according to the American Joint Committee on Cancer, wherein T_2 indicates that tumor invades the cervix but does not extend beyond the uterus. The T_2 category is further broken down to T_{2a} (endocervical glandular involvement only) and T_{2b} (cervical stromal invasion). The corresponding classification in the FIGO system is stages IIA and IIB, respectively.

The rationale for treatment of this disease is based upon the perceived risk for regional lymph node metastasis. Homesley et al. determined that the incidence of lymph node metastasis was similar in the case of overt and occult spread of disease to the cervix, i.e., 25 and 21%, respectively (1). Morrow et al., reporting on a Gynecologic Oncology Group Study of 136 stage II cases, found the 5-year recurrence-free interval for patients with involvement of the isthmus/cervix to be 70% (2). Cervical involvement is more often associated with poor tumor differentiation and deep myometrial invasion as opposed to cases without cervical invasion, both factors being predictive for metastatic disease. Larson et al. investigated the prognostic significance of the variants of cervical involvement (3). In a study of 58 stage II patients, 10 patients were found to have gross cervical involvement, 25 patients had occult stromal invasion, and 23 patients had no evidence of stromal invasion. There was no difference in survival among the three groups, 70, 65, and 64%.

For the above reasons, recommended definitive therapy for known stage II disease involves either definitive radical hysterectomy and pelvic lymph node dissection or combined external-beam radiation therapy and intracavitary brachytherapy followed by an extrafascial total abdominal hysterectomy and bilateral salpingo-oophorectomy. The algorithm is as follows:

1. External beam radiotherapy, 39.6 Gy, 1.8 Gy/fx, 22 fx, APPA or four-field pelvic portal technique, 4.5 weeks elapsed treatment time, megavoltage treatment machine.
2. Rest interval of 1 to 2 weeks.
3. Fletcher-Suit Tandem and Ovoids application, delivering 30 Gy, 50 cGy/hr, to point A (or equivalent HDR therapy).
4. Rest interval of 4 to 6 weeks.
5. Extrafascial TAH/BSO.

Extrafascial TAH/BSO for clinical stage I (but surgical stage II) may be followed by whole-pelvis irradiation, i.e., 45 to 50.4 Gy, 1.7 Gy/fx.

References

1. Homesley, HD, et al. Stage II endometrial adenocarcinoma. Obstet Gynecol 1977; 49:604–608.
2. Morrow CP, et al. Relationship between surgical-pathological risk factors and outcome in clinical stage I and II carcinoma of the endometrium: A gynecologic oncology group study. Gynecol Oncol 1991; 40:55–65.
3. Larson DM, et al. Nature of cervical involvement in endometrial carcinoma, Cancer 1987; 59:959–962.

46

Uterine Cancer, Stage IV, Grade 3 Adenocarcinoma of the Endometrium

CASE

A 60-year-old woman presents with a 9-month history of postmenopausal bleeding. She has noticed no change in bowel function, but she has had some recent urinary frequency with no dysuria. Her appetite is good. She has had no weight loss, no abdominal swelling. She has no pain or swelling in her extremities. Family history is negative. Past medical history: no previous operations. She is currently on no medications except for a daily vitamin. She has never taken hormone replacement therapy since she stopped having menses 10 years prior.

There are no palpable supraclavicular nodes. The chest is clear; the heart shows a regular rate and rhythm. No breast or abdominal masses are noted. There are no palpable suspicious inguinal nodes. No vulvar lesions are present. On examination of the vagina, there is a 1 cm suburethral nodule in the distal third of the vagina. The cervix is without lesions. There is a small amount of blood coming from the os. The uterus is 12 weeks in size and mobile. There are no separate adnexal masses nor is any cul-de-sac nodularity noted. Workup includes a biopsy of the suburethral nodule as well as an endometrial biopsy both of which show grade 3 adenocarcinomas. A chest x-ray shows a 1-cm nodule in the right lower lobe of the lung.

PHYSICIANS' RESPONSE

TIMOTHY O. WILSON
IVY A. PETERSEN
KARL PODRATZ

This patient has evidence consistent with stage IIIB or IV high-grade endometrial carcinoma, depending upon the result of computed tomography (CT) of the chest and probable thoracoscopy or thoracotomy with excision of the right-lower-lobe pulmonary nodule. If this is found to be a solitary lung metastasis, a benign lung lesion, or a surgically curable primary lung cancer, we would initiate systemic chemotherapy with MVAC (1) beginning approximately 2 to 3 weeks after the thoracic procedure and continuing for three to four cycles before further pelvic surgery. Prior to definitive surgery, reassessment by chest, abdominal, and pelvic CT scanning would be done; if no recurrent or progressive disease existed, wide local excision of the previous metastatic vaginal wall site and type II radical hysterectomy with pelvic and paraaortic lymph node samplings would be recommended. If all disease could be excised, pelvic irradiation would most likely be added postoperatively.

Reference

1. Long HJ, Langdon RM Jr, Cha SS, et al. Phase II trial of methotrexate, vinblastine, doxorubicin, and cisplatin in advanced recurrent endometrial carcinoma. Gynecol Oncol, 1995. In press.

PHYSICIAN'S RESPONSE

JOHN KAVANAGH

The patient represents the problem of having an endometrial carcinoma that is grade III in histology by endometrial biopsy as well a metastatic suburethral nodule. A chest x-ray shows a 1-cm nodule in the right lower lung.

    The case should be viewed from the aspects of controlling both pelvic and metastatic disease. Further information will be necessary in order to make the appropriate decisions. First and foremost, an old chest x-ray should be obtained. If a lesion has been present and unchanged on a previous x-ray at least 1 year old, we would assume it represents a benign lesion of the lung and is unrelated to the endometrial carcinoma. If no previous chest x-ray is available, a CT scan of the chest should be done to determine if there are multiple lesions. A screening mammogram should be ordered considering the relationships of the two malignancies and the presence of a possible metastatic pulmonary lesion. In addition, it would be warranted to do a cystoscopy to determine extent of urethral involvement and whether there is any bladder extension. The purpose of the cystoscopy would be to consider the feasibility of either a local excision or radiotherapy consolidation with implants or boosts to the urethral lesion. A CT scan of the abdomen and pelvis should also be done. If, as stated before, comparisons of the chest x-rays or CT of the chest show lesions that are consistent with a growing metastasis and/or the CT scan of the abdomen shows extensive spread in terms of lymphadenopathy, ascites, or liver metastasis, the systemic approach to therapy would be most reasonable. This could represent a single-agent carboplatin therapy or the more traditional use of a platinum/anthracycline combination. My preference would be single-agent carboplatin therapy. If the patient has an excellent response to therapy with complete remission of the lung lesion and resolution of disease on CT scan, an abbreviated course of radiotherapy to the pelvis might be considered. This would be particularly useful in terms of controlling future uterine bleeding. If the patient develops progressive systemic metastatic disease in a generalized sense, salvage therapy with paclitaxel (Taxol) may be considered. However, the data on the use of paclitaxel in endometrial cancer are limited. If progression continues on these regimens, then palliative care utilizing a progestational agent and local irradiation as needed is most reasonable. The response rate to hormones in undifferentiated and poorly differentiated tumors is lower than in well or moderately differentiated tumors. In addition, the patient should be treated symptomatically as various problems develop. Radiotherapy would again be in order if the patient begins to develop urethral obstruction and bleeding or significant symptomatology such as bleeding, discharge, or pain from the primary uterine lesion. The radiotherapy could consist of external beam with a boost to the involved lesions or intrauterine radiotherapy devices. Hospice care would eventually be in order.

If the patient, on metastatic evaluation, has only the chest lesion and there are no previous chest x-rays for comparison, then a biopsy of the lung lesion should be considered. If the biopsy is positive, systemic therapy should be administered. If it is negative or chemotherapy is considered contraindicated, one should proceed with curative intent. The chest lesion may then be followed by serial chest x-rays. If the patient has no evidence of disease other than what has been stated in the known information, with a negative cystoscopy and CT scans of the chest, abdomen, and pelvis (i.e., a positive endometrial biopsy and a suburethral nodule), consideration should be given to a modified radical hysterectomy with excision of the urethral nodule. This would be followed by radiotherapy with particular attention to the suburethral area. Adjuvant chemotherapy is not recommended.

Reference

1. Kudelka AP, Gonzalez de Leon C, Edwards CL, Kavanagh JJ: Tumors of the uterine corpus. In: Pazdur R, ed. Medical Oncology: A Comprehensive Review. Huntington, NY: PRR, Inc. 1993/1994: 21:271–280.

PHYSICIANS' RESPONSE

BOB TAYLOR
ROBERT PARK

This 60 year old postmenopausal patient presents with what we fear will most likely be a stage IVB endometrial carcinoma. The endometrial biopsy reveals a poorly differentiated endometrioid adenocarcinoma, and a biopsy of a noncontiguous distal vaginal lesion is consistent with metastatic disease. We would argue that although she may qualify to be clinically stage III, the presence of a noncontiguous, distal vaginal lesion having an anatomically different venous and lymphatic drainage suggests that she is stage IV via hematogenous spread. This suspicion is strengthened by the finding of a pulmonary nodule and the knowledge that the lung is a favorite trophic site for endometrial carcinoma metastasis and recurrence.

We would expand her metastatic survey to include chest and abdominopelvic tomography. Given no additional sites suspicious for metastatic disease, we believe that her treatment involves the precise knowledge of the pulmonary nodule's pathology. Transbroncheal or CT-guided needle biopsy of this lesion would further guide management options. If the biopsy was positive for metastatic endometrial carcinoma, she would be stage IVB and her prognosis would be considered dismal. In this case, nontoxic hormonal therapy with progestational agents or the antiestrogen tamoxifen would be offered, to be followed by cytotoxic chemotherapy for progression of disease (1). Alternatively, she may be eligible for phase II cytotoxic chemotherapy trials. Hysterectomy and bilateral salpingoopherectomy or perhaps intracavitary radiotherapy would be considered only for unmanageable uterine bleeding.

If the pulmonary lesion was negative for malignancy, we would consider this patient to have locally advanced endometrial adenocarcinoma and surgical staging would be recommended, including excision of the suburethral nodule. Should she have disease limited to the pelvis (no diseased paraaortic lymph nodes), whole-pelvis radiotherapy would be recommended. We would disfavor exenterative procedures based on the assumption that the suburethral metastasis represents hematogenous spread and subclinical disease likely exists elsewhere.

Reference

1. Thigpen JT, Blessing J, DiSaia P. Oral medroxyprogesterone acetate in advanced or recurrent endometrial carincoma: Results of therapy and correlation with estrogen and progesterone levels: the Gynecologic Oncology Group experience. In: Baulieu EE, Slacobelli S, McGuire WL, eds. Endocrinology of Malignancy. Park Ridge, NJ: Parthenon, 1986:446.

PHYSICIAN'S RESPONSE

WILLIAM CREASMAN

This patient presents with what appeared to be a clinical stage III, poorly differentiated adenocarcinoma of the endometrium. Metastases to the periurethral area without any disease between the cervix and the urethral nodule are seen not uncommonly. The unresolved question at presentation is whether or not the 1-cm nodule in the chest is metastasis. Knowledge concerning this nodule is important, because it may very well determine definitive therapy. Therefore it is reasonable to proceed with a fine needle aspirate (FNA) of the lung nodule. A 1-cm nodule in the lower lobe should be easily accessible by the interventional radiologist. If the lung nodule is metastatic, there may be several therapeutic options. One would be to explore the patient, do a full surgical staging, and determine the possibility of extrauterine disease within the pelvis and abdomen. In a clinical stage IG3 lesion, over 20% of these patients will have metastasis to the pelvic or paraaortic lymph nodes. An additional 4 to 5% will have intraperitoneal disease. Approximately 12 to 15% will have positive peritoneal cytology. With at least a stage III cancer, the incidence of extrauterine (intra- or retroperitoneal) disease increases even more. This would determine true extent of disease and allow one to direct therapy pending upon true disease status. If, for instance, there is gross or even microscopic intraperitoneal disease, one may very well consider palliative therapy. Instead of using external radiation, systemic therapy in either the form of chemotherapy or hormone therapy would be indicated. If, however, there is no evidence of intraperitoneal disease, radiation therapy could be given to the pelvis, including the paraurethral nodule, with the intent of local control of tumor, and use systemic therapy in order to take care of the lung lesion. Although long-term survival in this group of patients is small, nevertheless, some patients with this extent of disease do have long-term survival. Obviously if there is retroperitoneal disease in either the pelvic or paraaortic nodes, radiation therapy can be directed to this area. If the patient is a surgical candidate, then primary surgical staging would be this investigator's choice of action. At 60 years of age, one would expect that she could withstand thorough surgical evaluation with hopes of long-term survival or at least good palliation.

The other approach would be to proceed with pelvic irradiation without surgery. This would need to cover not only the uterus and pelvic node area but also the periurethral area. Since the uterus is 12 weeks in size, the pelvic port would have to be increased in order to cover the uterus and extend down to cover the periurethral area. With a large radiation port, complications could be increased. Chemotherapy, either in the way of cytotoxic agents or hormones, could be used. If the nonsurgical approach is used, this suggests that the decision has been made not to be aggressive; therefore hormonal therapy is probably indicated as first line.

If, in fact, after fine needle aspirate, the lung nodule is negative for adenocarcinoma cells, then the primary surgical approach as noted above would be indicated in this investigator's opinion. The exact extent of the disease can be identified and radiation therapy can then be specifically directed to the areas of known disease. Since extrauterine disease can be quite common in this situation, it is important to know where the disease might be located; otherwise metastasis to the paraaortic nodes, for instance, could be overlooked and the patient inappropriately treated. Patients with known pelvic or paraaortic metastasis treated with radiation therapy may have a long-term survival of 50% or greater. If palliation only is feasible, then radiation to cover the uterus as well as the periurethral area should be performed. Periurethral nodules do respond very well to external radiation and in most instances do not require local interstitial impants.

References

Behbakht K, Yordon EL, Casey C, et al. Prognostic indicators of survival in advanced endometrial cancer. Gynecol Oncol 1994; 55:363–367.
Pliskow S, Penalver NL, Averette HE. Stage III and stage IV endometrial carcinoma: A review of 41 cases. Gynecol Oncol 1990; 38:210–215.

PHYSICIANS' RESPONSE

M. J. SCHMITZ
C. T. MACRI

Endometrial cancer is the most common female pelvic malignancy, ranking fourth in cancer frequency behind breast, bowel, and lung cancers. Of an anticipated 32,800 cancers of the uterus projected for 1995, some 5900 women will die from their disease. Success of therapy is largely attributed to diagnosis at an early stage, despite the fact that there is no effective screening method. Seventy-five percent of cases occur after menopause at a mean age of 60, when the finding of vaginal bleeding or discharge, the most common symptom expressed, usually alerts women to seek medical care. The diagnosis is then made on endometrial biopsy or dilation and curettage (D&C). The vast majority of patients present when the tumor is confined to the uterus. Only 10% present with stage III or IV disease and have a considerably worse prognosis. Risk factors for the development of endometrial cancer include endometrial hyperplasia, particularly complex atypical hyperplasia, hypertension, obesity, nulliparity, diabetes, and unopposed estrogen.

For endometrioid adenocarcinomas, grade is the most sensitive predictor of tumor spread. Other cell types such as clear-cell carcinoma and serious endometrial cancers portend a poor prognosis regardless of grade. Up to 50% of grade 3 tumors invade the outer half of the endometrium. Metastasis to the pelvic lymph nodes occurs in 30% and to the paraaortic lymph nodes in 20% of cases.

Histological grade determined from biopsy and D&C specimens is found to be at least one grade lower than the grade found in the hysterectomy specimen in 15 to 20% of patients.

In the case presented, both the endometrial and vaginal biopsies reveal grade 3 adenocarcinomas, most likely indicating metastasis of an endometrial cancer to the suburethral area, a common metastatic site in the vagina. Primary vaginal adenocarcinoma is considered "one of the rarest malignant processes in the body." Ninety percent of primary vaginal cancers are squamous in origin, with adeno-carcinomas comprising only 1 to 2%. The most common tumor of the vagina is metastatic, originating from endometrium, ovary, urethra, bladder, rectum, and trophoblast. The nodule noted on chest x-ray should be evaluated either by biopsy or excision. Disease outside the abdomen and pelvis would not respond to local therapeutic modalities, leaving systemic chemotherapy or hormonal therapy as the available options for treatment.

Interpretation of the results of traditional therapy for endometrial cancer is hampered by inaccurate clinical staging. Frequently, treatment was begun with preoperative radiation therapy, followed by hysterectomy. In 1988, the Fédération Internationale de Gynécologie et d'Obstétrique (FIGO) adopted a surgical staging system that consists of cytologic washings, simple hysterectomy, bilateral sal-pingo-oophorectomy, and, in most patients, bilateral pelvic and paraaortic lymph node sampling. Since hysterectomy is not curative in advanced-stage endometrial cancer and neither depth of myometrial invasion nor grade is additive in terms of prognosis, its role is controversial in this patient. Surgery in patients with ad-vanced-stage endometrial cancer can relieve the problem of vaginal bleeding, confirm location of tumor metastases, and assess the status of pelvic and para-aortic lymph nodes. Extrapolating from data in ovarian cancer, it is possible that removing large tumor masses would increase the effectiveness of chemotherapy, but there are no prospective studies to substantiate this. Each patient must be evaluated individually, with surgical staging performed in the majority of patients, particularly with clinically early-stage disease. Low-volume intraperitoneal dis-ease or disease confined to paraaortic or pelvic lymph nodes may be accessible to radiotherapy, including whole-pelvis irradiation and whole abdominal radiation with or without brachytherapy as well as radioactive isotopes instilled intra-peritoneally.

Chemotherapy or hormonal therapy is the treatment of choice for patients with stage III or IV disease not limited to the pelvis and/or abdomen. Endometrial cancer has a low response rate to chemotherapy. Of systemic chemotherapy options, doxorubicin has been shown to have the most activity in endometrial cancer, with response rates of 30 to 40% in prospective clinical trials of the Gynecologic Oncology Group. Cisplatin has also been found to have activity as single-agent, first-line chemotherapy in advanced or recurrent endometrial can-cers. Multiple combinations of cytotoxic agents with or without hormonal therapy have been tried but have yielded response rates similar to that of doxorubicin alone. Some early data reported that circadian-timed chemotherapy has a response rate of up to 60% with reduced toxicity in advanced-stage endometrial cancer, a concept currently being studied by the Gynecologic Oncology Group in a prospective, randomized fashion.

Hormonal therapy has been investigated in the setting of disseminated disease or recurrence after initial surgical and adjuvant radiation therapy. Response rates of 15 to 30% have been reported, with well-differentiated tumors responding better than their more poorly differentiated counterparts. Estrogen and progesterone receptor status may help identify the rare patient with a grade 3 tumor who may benefit from hormonal therapy. Specific hormonal regimens that have been studied include high dose medroxy-progesterone acetate, tamoxifen 20 mg twice daily, and megestrol acetate 160 to 320 mg daily. Remissions lasting 6 months to several years with overall survival of approximately 1 year were reported.

References

DiSaia PJ, Creasman WT. Adenocarcinoma of the uterus. In: Clinical Gynecologic Oncology, 4th ed. St Louis: Mosby-Year Book, 1993.

Grigsby PW, Perex CA, Kuske RR, et al. Results of therapy, analysis of failures, and prognostic factors so clinical and pathologic stage III adenocarcinoma of the endometrium. Gynecol Oncol 1987; 27:44–57.

Huang SJ, Berek JS, Fu YS. Pathology of endometrial carcinoma. In: Malcolm Coppleson, ed. Gynecologic Oncology, 2d ed. New York: Churchill Livingstone, 1992.

Kadar N, Malfetano J, Homesley H. Determinants of survival of surgically staged patients with endometrial carcinoma histologically confined to the uterus: Implications for therapy. Obstet Gynecol 1992; 80:655–659.

Kurman RJ, Zaino RJ, Norris HJ. Endometrial carcinoma. In: Robert Kurman, ed. Blaustein's Pathology of the Female Genital Tract. 4th ed. New York: Springer-Verlag, 1994.

Morrow CP, Curtain JP, Townsend DE. Tumors of the endometrium. In: Synopsis of Gynecologic Oncology, 4th ed. New York: Churchill Livingstone, 1993.

Piver MS, Hempling RE. A prospective trail of postoperative vaginal radium/cesium for grade 1–2 less than 50% myometrial invasion in surgical stage I endometrial adenocarcinoma. Cancer 1990; 66:1133–1138.

Thigpen JT, Blessing JA, Lagasse LD, et al. Phase II trial of cisplatin as second-line chemotherapy in patients with advanced or recurrent endometrial carcinoma. Am J Clin Oncol 1984; 7:253–256.

Thigpen JT, Blessing JA, Monesley HD, et al. Phase II trial of cisplatin as first-line chemotherapy in patients with advanced or recurrent endometrial carcinoma: A Gynecologic Oncology Group study. Gynecol Oncol 1989; 33:68–70.

47

Solitary Lung Lesion 9 Months After the Diagnosis of Endometrial Cancer

CASE

A 58-year-old woman is found to have a solitary lung nodule (1 by 1 cm) on a routine chest x-ray obtained 9 months after she underwent surgery for a grade 2 adenocarcinoma of the endometrium. The endometrial surgery was performed by a gynecological oncologist and there was no evidence of disease outside the uterus. The patient's past medical history is significant for a 1/2-pack-per-day smoking history for 30 years. A CT scan of the chest reveals only a solitary lung lesion. Unfortunately, a chest x-ray had not been taken at the time of the patient's previous surgery, and her last x-ray was over 4 years ago.

PHYSICIAN'S RESPONSE

PETER ROSE

Additional information should be obtained from the radiologist. Is the nodule calcified? This would suggest an indolent process. The old chest x-ray report and films should be obtained if the study was not completely normal. The operative and pathology reports and pathology slides must be obtained, since evaluation of the patient's original disease extent is an essential step in trying to determine if this is recurrent disease or a second primary. Were poor prognostic pathological features such as deep myometrial invasion, vascular or lymphatic invasion, cervical extension, or adnexal extension present? Was a nodal dissection performed at the original operation? In a surgically staged patient, the presence of nodal metastasis is highly prognostic of the possibility of recurrent disease (1). Did the patient receive any postoperative therapy? If the patient had poor prognostic pathological features originally present, it is more likely that this is recurrent disease. In this case, an abdominal pelvic computed tomography (CT) scan should be obtained. If disease is found in the abdomen or pelvis, this would favor recurrent disease and not a second primary. Alternatively, if the patient had no poor prognostic pathological features originally present, a second primary is more likely. Additionally, a family history of other malignancies should be obtained from the patient. The second malignant solid tumors (and relative risks) after endometrial cancer are kidney (2.1), thyroid (2.0), bladder (1.7), rectum (1.6), colon (1.4), lung (1.4), and breast (1.3) (2). A careful physical exam with stool guaiac and CT scan of the abdomen and pelvis will aid in this evaluation. The mass should then be biopsied by CT guided fine needle aspiration or bronchoscopy. A comparison of the histology of the pulmonary mass and the original endometrial tumor is essential. If the mass cannot be biopsied, if the previous chest x-ray was normal, the patient has no poor prognostic pathological features in her original tumor, and there is no evidence of metastatic disease on her abdominal/pelvic CT scan, consult thoracic surgery for a surgical resection.

References

1. Morrow CP, Bundy BN, Kumar RJ, et al. Relationship between surgical-pathologic risk factors and outcome in clinical stage I and II carcinoma of the endometrium: A Gynecologic Oncology Group study. Gynecol Oncol 1991; 40:55–65.
2. Curtis RE, Hoover RN, Kleinerman RA, Harvey EB. Second cancer following cancer of the female genital tract in Connecticut, 1935–1982. Natl Cancer Inst Monogr 1985; 68:113–137.

PHYSICIANS' RESPONSE

GINI FLEMING
PHILIP HOFFMAN

We will assume that this is a noncalcified nodule. Almost all calcified nodules are benign and could be followed up with a repeat chest x-ray in 6 months. If it is available, it would be worthwhile to review an earlier chest x-ray even if over 4 years old, since any lesion present and unchanging for over 4 years is quite unlikely to be malignant. In general, the probability that an asymptomatic solitary nodule is malignant increases with the age of the patient and with a prior smoking history or prior cancer history. The question is whether this lesion is a metastasis from the known endometrial cancer, for which the value of pulmonary resection is not well established, or a new 1-cm primary carcinoma of the lung, in which case a lobectomy should yield a 5-year survival in the range of 80% (assuming there is no nodal involvement, as no lymph nodes over 1 cm appear to have been identified on CT scan).

This patient should have a complete physical exam, including a pelvic exam to look for any obvious local recurrence of her endometrial cancer. A CT scan of the abdomen and pelvis should also be obtained. If these prove within normal limits, she should have the nodule resected. The overall probability that a stage I (confined to the corpus) endometrial carcinoma would recur is only in the range of 10% at 5 years; grade and depth of myometrial invasion are the most important factors in predicting recurrence. Her risk would be significantly greater if she had invasion of the outer third of the myometrium.

Attempts to obtain a preoperative histological diagnosis of a small, solitary, noncalcified pulmonary nodule will probably not be helpful unless this nodule is central and accessible to bronchoscopy. Needle aspiration for diagnosis of a lesion this size may be difficult. Moreover, a diagnosis of adenocarcinoma will likely not distinguish a primary lung cancer from a metastatic lesion, and the chances of a definitive benign diagnosis are small. It may not be possible, even on final pathology, to distinguish an endometrial metastasis from a primary lung cancer if the histological diagnosis proves to be adenocarcinoma.

If the lesion is an isolated pulmonary metastasis from endometrial cancer, resection is a reasonable treatment approach, since neither chemotherapy nor hormonal therapy has any curative potential. Five-year survival following resection averages 30 to 40% for solitary lung metastases from a wide variety of primary cancers. Little is published about resection of solitary metastases from endometrial cancer. One large series of resection of pulmonary metastases included 9 patients with endometrial cancer and reported a 5-year survival of 53.3% in this group (1).

If the patient is in good health and has adequate pulmonary function, resection of the nodule should have an operative mortality of less than 1%. Because lobectomy is considered to be the operation of choice for an early-stage lung cancer, with lesser resections reserved for patients with marginal pulmonary function, removal of the nodule alone is appropriate only if, after seeing the frozen section, the pathologist's level of certainty is very high that the lesion is a metastasis from the endometrial cancer. Otherwise a formal lobectomy should be performed.

Reference

1. Mountain CF, McMurtrey MJ, Hermes KE. Surgery for pulmonary metastasis: A 20-year experience. Ann Thorac Surg 1984; 38:323–329.

PHYSICIANS' RESPONSE

BABAK EDRAKI
JOSEPH T. CHAMBERS

The main issue in this case is to determine whether the 1-cm nodule on the chest x-ray so soon after initial therapy represents a metastatic lesion from the patient's endometrial carcinoma or a secondary benign or malignant lesion. It is unusual that a preoperative chest x-ray was not performed in a woman with a known malignancy (as part of the metastatic workup), especially in a smoker, who is thus at risk of developing intra- and postoperative pulmonary complications. The presence of the lung lesion pre-operatively would have prompted a diagnostic workup that might have affected the patient's management. We have found a preoperative CA-125 level evaluation helpful in that approximately 80% of patients with an elevated level have extrauterine disease.

In looking back at the case, we have to ascertain whether the patient has risk factors that increase the chance of recurrence. According to the GOG data, an appropriate surgical staging is of paramount importance in evaluation of a patient's prognosis. Risk factors that were found to be important for recurrence include the status of pelvic and periaortic lymph nodes, peritoneal washings, histology of the tumor, grade, depth of myometrial invasion as well as presence of lymphatic space invasion, and cervical involvement. Since the surgery was performed by a gynecological oncologist, we assume that a proper staging was done and revealed no evidence of extrauterine disease. It is widely accepted that papillary serous, clear-cell, high-grade endometrioid and mixed müllerian histology bode a poor prognosis and that local/regional and distant recurrences, even in the absence of high-risk factors, do occur. Thus we would review the initial pathology for any suggestion of these high-risk features.

Assessment of the patient's current status is quite important to detect any other evidence of disease. On physical examination, particular attention should be paid to the suburethral as well as the vaginal cuff areas. A CT scan of the abdomen and pelvis is indicated to rule out widespread disease. In the absence of aggressive endometrial histology and extra-uterine spread, a pulmonary metastasis is unusual and other etiologies must be considered. A breast examination along with a mammogram should be performed. However, the cornerstone of our approach to this patient involves obtaining tissue diagnosis of the lung lesion via a CT-guided biopsy. If the biopsy reveals a primary lung process or a lesion related to another process such as breast carcinoma, then appropriate referrals and treatments can be initiated. If, however, the nodule is consistent with metastasis from the prior endometrial carcinoma, further therapy should be based on the patient's tumor burden and symptomatology. Treatment must be individualized and consideration may be given to either systemic cytotoxic chemotherapy or progestational agents.

References

1. Morrow CP, Bundy BN, Kurman RJ, et al. Relationship between surgical-pathological risk factors and outcome in clinical stage I and II carcinoma of the endometrium: A Gynecologic Oncology Group study. Gynecol Oncol 1991; 40:55–65.
2. Chambers SK, Kapp DS, Peschel RE, et al. Prognostic factors and sites of failure in FIGO stage I, grade 3 endometrial carcinoma. Gynecol Oncol 1987; 27:180–188.

PHYSICIAN'S RESPONSE

JOE YON

Although this patient was operated upon by a gynecological oncologist, a chest x-ray was not done as part of her exclusion workup, and one wonders why not. However, we must accept that we do not have that information. It is also noted that there was no disease outside of the uterus, but we were not told the stage of the disease, what the patient's risk factors were, whether she had adjunctive therapy, whether she was at high risk for recurrence, and so on. Therefore it would be useful to know the final stage of her endometrial cancer.

However, with a smoking history and a lung nodule confirmed by CT scan as being solitary, the patient needs to be worked up for that lesion. One might consider a CT of the abdomen or pelvis looking for recurrent endometrial cancer, and one might possibly consider a CA-125 level in that this may be elevated in patients with metastatic endometrial cancer, but if the patient has received adjunctive radiation therapy, this can give a false elevation of the CA-125, so we need more information in that regard.

Once the patient's abdominal evaluation, which, of course, should include a pelvic examination, has been done and if this is normal or negative, the patient needs to have pulmonary function studies, possibly a bronchoscopy (although the yield will be low). Then, if this is negative, the patient will have to undergo a thoracotomy. If the solitary lesion should prove to be an endometrial cancer, the patient should have the lesion resected if at all possible. This could confer as high as a 40% 5-year disease-free interval from that disease alone. If the patient proves to have a primary lung cancer, she needs to be treated accordingly.

To summarize then, we need more information about the patient's endometrial disease, the actual treatment applied, and further evaluation of abdomen and pelvis at this time. Then aggressive diagnostic steps need to be taken to evaluate the chest lesion with a view to resecting either a primary or a solitary metastatic lesion.

PHYSICIAN'S RESPONSE

WIM TEN BOKKEL HUININK

This case evokes many questions regarding the differential diagnosis. One should certainly try to find the patient's last x-ray, since it seems highly probable that this lung nodule has been documented previously. This means that a long-standing lung tuberculosis scar and other infectious diseases should be excluded as well, as should histoplasmosis, coccidiomycosis, and so on.

Only after diagnostic procedures have excluded infectious diseases as the origin of the lung nodule should neoplastic diseases be considered. In their overview of 379 patients suffering from a relapsed endometrial cancer, investigators of the University of Gröningen found lung metastases in only 10% of them. Since this patient has a grade II adenocarcinoma of the endometrium (of which further definitions are lacking, it may be stage IA or IB), the chance of a relapse within 1 year is very small. Only 10% of patients such as this have a relapse after 5 years. Of these, 50% of the cases are related to a grade III and 50% to a grade II lesion. If one calculates the chance that a relapse in grade IA or IB can be documented before 1 year of follow-up, the chance is only 1%. The chances that this woman, who has been smoking more than 1/2 pack per day for 30 years, now suffers from a secondary tumor, that is, lung cancer, seem to be far higher.

Therefore, diagnostic procedures to exclude infectious diseases and lung cancer should be performed. If serological tests exclude fungal diseases and staging procedures indeed show only a solitary lung lesion excluding abdominal recurrences, suggested by the case history, surgical removal of the mass should be performed. In case of a secondary lung tumor, appropriate measures should be taken.

48

Cervical Cancer, Stage IIB, Squamous Cell

CASE

A 28-year-old woman initially presented $1^1/_2$ years ago with a stage IIB squamous cell carcinoma of the cervix. She was treated with radiation therapy and within 8 months had a recurrent mass in the central pelvis. In addition, a chest x-ray showed two pulmonary nodules. She was treated with platinum/ifosfamide and initially had some response, but now, with two additional nodules, she has a 10-cm painful mass occupying the central pelvis. By computed tomography (CT), her left ureter is obstructed, but the mass does not appear to involve either pelvic side walls. The CT scan shows a couple of nodes measuring 2 cm in size that are suspicious for metastatic diseases in the right paraaortic area, but there is no evidence of liver metastasis. The patient requires two oxycodone/acetaminophen (Percocet) tablets plus 600 mg of ibuprofen (Motrin) every 4 hours for pain. She is bothered by severe urinary spasms and pain with urination.

PHYSICIANS' RESPONSE

PATRICK S. ANDERSON
CAROLYN D. RUNOWICZ

It is estimated that approximately 35% of all patients with invasive cervical cancer will have recurrent or persistent disease following therapy. Autopsy series have revealed that the location of these recurrences includes the central pelvis (33%), pelvic side wall (43%) and distant areas (24%). Following radiation

379

therapy, the 5-year survival rate for patients with stage IIB disease is approximately 60 to 65%. This patient has both central and distant recurrence following treatment with pelvic radiation and chemotherapy.

Due to widely metastatic disease, this patient is not a candidate for a surgical intervention, such as a pelvic exenteration. At our institution, the patient would be offered experimental therapy with alpha-interferon and *trans*-retinoic acid. Interferon has cytotoxic, antiproliferative, and antiviral activity. *Trans*-retinoic acid (tRA) is a metabolite of vitamin A. Retinoids have long been known to play an important role in a variety of biological processes including growth, differentiation, and stimulation of immune function. Thus, there is a good biological rationale to test this combination of therapies in this clinical setting.

In addition to experimental therapy, the patient's symptoms should be palliated. The severe urinary spasms are probably related to an obstructed ureter. Although, in a patient with recurrent cervical cancer, we prefer not to place ureteral stents or percutaneous nephrostomies, in this particular patient it may be necessary for pain control. Pain control can be optimized by switching from a weak opioid (Percocet) to a stronger opiate narcotic that includes drugs such as meperidine, morphine, hydromorphone, methadone, and fentanyl. The new sustained-release morphine preparations (MS Contin and Roxanol SR) are readily available and provide analgesia for up to 8 to 12 hr. A supplemental immediate-release medication such as morphine or Dilaudid can be added to treat breakthrough pain. The patient will require stool softeners and laxatives to prevent constipation and stool impaction. She should be instructed on their use and the need to supplement her diet with fiber and roughage.

If the patient is sedated from the medications, the narcotic dose can be adjusted and central nervous system stimulants can be added to the regimen (Ritalin 5 mg tid). Tricyclic anti-depressants (amitriptyline 50 to 75 mg PO hs) will improve sleep and potentiate the effect of the narcotic analgesics. Corticosteroids can also enhance analgesia and may, in addition, stimulate appetite and mood.

The patient and her family should be counseled as to the aggressive nature of her disease and be prepard for hospice care and dealing with her demise. The issue of advance directives and power of attorney should be discussed, and the patient should express her wishes in writing to the physician and the family regarding resuscitation and terminal care.

References

Cherry NI, Portenoy R. Cancer pain management—Current strategy. Cancer 1993; 72:3393.

Greer DS, Mor V, Morris JN, et al. An alternate in terminal care: Results of the National Hospice Study. J Chronic Dis 1986; 39:9–26.

PHYSICIAN'S RESPONSE

JAVIER MAGRINA

This patient, a 28-year-old woman, presented with recurrent and metastatic lesions in the pelvis and lungs, respectively, 8 months after completing pelvic irradiation for squamous cell carcinoma of the cervix stage IIB. After completing therapy with platinum and ifosfamide, her chief complaints are pain, pain with urination, and severe urinary spasms. Evaluation demonstrates:

1. A persistent pelvic mass
2. A left ureteral obstruction, presumably secondary to metastatic pelvic nodes, since the pelvic mass does not reach the left pelvic side wall
3. Persistent and increased metastases to the lung (four nodules)
4. Metastases to the right periaortic nodes

The goals of the treatment are three:

1. Evaluation of the cause of the pain and urinary symptoms
2. Symptomatic treatment based on the results from the evaluation
3. Treatment of the disease if the patient desires

Evaluation and palliation would include the following:

1. A UA and urine culture are indicated to rule out urinary tract infection. A superimposed urinary tract infection would worsen the symptomatology of an already existing radiation cystitis.
2. A cystoscopy would be helpful to determine whether any intravesical treatments could be beneficial to alleviate bladder symptomatology.
3. A left retrograde urography would be useful to delineate the nature and level of obstruction of the left ureter.
4. Systemic urinary antispasmodics, and antibiotics if indicated, could be beneficial.
5. A CT scan would be helpful to ascertain the nature of the pelvic mass. A hydrometra or pyometra secondary to cervical stenosis can result in severe pelvic pain. If appropriate, cervical dilatation and probing of the uterus under anesthesia would rule out this possibility.
6. Adnexal pathology, acute or chronic, must also be considered in the differential diagnosis of the pelvic mass.
7. A fine needle aspirate would demonstrate whether the large central pelvic mass is a recurrent cervical carcinoma.
8. Should there be no symptomatic benefit from local measures or systemic therapy, urinary diversion must be considered. In this patient with a dismal prognosis and an obstructed left ureter, a right cutaneous ureterostomy would be the preferred choice to divert the urine; a right

nephrostomy with right ureteral ligation (to prevent the passage of urine to the bladder) would be an alternative. It must be emphasized that urinary diversion does not guarantee complete disappearance of the urinary symptoms.

9. In the presence of residual pain, escalating doses of oral morphine should be used.

As to treatment of the disease, in our experience, the use of M-VAC—methotrexate, vinblastine, doxorubicin (Adriamycin), and cisplatin—has resulted in a response rate, partial and total, of about 60% in patients with recurrent cervical carcinoma. Even in the absence of an objective response, significant improvement of the pain can be obtained. Because this patient has already received a first-line chemotherapy, I would expect a lower chance of response with a second line.

PHYSICIAN'S RESPONSE

JAMES NELSON

This 28-year-old woman with stage IIB squamous cell carcinoma of the cervix has central recurrence, unilateral ureteral obstruction, and presumed distant metastases after initial radiation therapy and later platinum chemotherapy; she has severe central pelvic and urinary pain requiring constant oral analgesia. Prognosis in this patient is poor and the treatment goal should be palliation.

Attempt at surgical cure of previously irradiated recurrent cervical cancer through pelvic exenteration is limited to central pelvic recurrence; the presence of distant metastases precludes surgical cure and is a contraindication to radical pelvic surgery. It is, therefore, important to obtain histological confirmation of tumor via fine needle aspirate cytology of pulmonary nodules found on radiological exam. Lung metastases occur in 1 to 2% of advanced cases of cervical cancer. If a lung nodule is the sole evidence of recurrence, surgical resection is an option; in this case, central pelvic recurrence precludes resection of metastatic lung disease.

Reirradiation of recurrent cervical cancer is controversial. The bladder is very sensitive to radiation injury, and this patient's urinary symptoms can be attributed to chronic radiation damage including vasculitis and fibrosis. If her symptoms were due to tumor growth in the bladder, this would prohibit cure with further irradiation. The bladder pain may be treated with antispasmodics. Ureteral obstruction is due to recurrent carcinoma in 95% of instances; however, if CT-guided cytological evaluation of periureteral tissue causing obstruction reveals radiation fibrosis rather than tumor, ureterolysis may be attempted to relieve obstruction and spamodic pain.

In previously irradiated recurrent and/or metastatic cervical carcinoma, chemotherapy is palliative only, not curative. Palliative chemotherapy is reserved for those cases not curable by surgery or irradiation. This pessimistic outlook is adopted for two main reasons: (a) of all tumors, the squamous cell histologic variety has had the least response to any type of chemotherapeutic agent, and (b) tumor cells in previously irradiated areas are encased with fibrosis, making attainment of adequate blood and tissue levels of drug difficult.

Many trials with a variety of chemotherapeutic agents show response rates varying from 8 to 45%. Park and Thigpen reviewed activity of single and combination cytotoxic chemotherapeutic regimens and found that no regimen for advanced or recurrent carcinoma of the cervix is more effective than single-agent cisplatin. New agents and combinations need to be found to offer greater antitumor activity.

This unfortunate patient needs to have these facts, options, and alternatives explained to her so that she can understand her situation and contribute to decision regarding making her treatment. If the lung lesions are metastatic by biopsy and the pelvic mass also, we would not be aggressive surgically unless all detectable pulmonary disease was unilateral and could be removed completely. The patient is very young and should be given every chance to control her disease. One should not attempt surgical resection of the pelvic mass unless the lung disease is resectable and the paraaortic nodes are checked for histologic evidence of carcinoma or lack thereof. Only then should the decision be made to attempt resection of the pelvic mass. This would almost certainly require a pelvic exenteration. If this can be done, a continent urinary conduit should be made available to the patient. In addition, every attempt should be made to restore continuity of the colon by a low anterior bowel resection and transrectal stapling of the colon.

References

Park RC, Thigpen JT. Chemotherapy in advanced and recurrent cervical cancer: A review. Cancer 1993; 71:1446.
Vermorken JB. The role of chemotherapy in squamous cell carcinoma of the uterine cervix: A review. Int J Gynecol Cancer 1993; 3:129.

PHYSICIANS' RESPONSE

JOHN L. LOVECCHIO
DAVID GAL

This unfortunate 28-year-old woman possesses a diagnosis of recurrent, progressive stage IIB squamous cell carcinoma of the cervix, characterized by both persistent regional and radiographically documented distant metastatic disease to the paraaortic nodes and multiple pulmonary sites. It is clear that despite therapeutic measures, consisting of radiation therapy and systemic cytotoxic chemotherapy, this malignancy is refractory to treatment. At present, the patient has pelvic pain, urinary spasms, and dysuria. Objectively, prospects for survival are negligible and interventions of any dimension are to be considered palliative in nature.

If further chemotherapy is contemplated, one must be cognizant of the fact that this patient possesses radiographic evidence of a unilateral obstructive uropathy. Ureteral stenting is suggested only if additional chemotherapy is pursued. This may provide a suitable uremia-free interval so that the potential effect of chemotherapy can be assessed. Stenting is not indicated if no further treatment is contemplated, whereupon death from uremia will likely ensue. Additionally, consideration might be given to instituting selective intraarterial pelvic chemotherapy in an attempt to control pelvic disease and provide relief of pelvic pain.

Exenterative surgery in this clinical setting is not an acceptable option. Surgery of this nature is reserved for curative intent. If vesicovaginal or rectovaginal fistulas become apparent, then diverting nephrostomies and/or colostomy would be warranted. Although this is an imperfect solution, a reasonable degree of perineal hygiene can thus be secured.

In the absence of profound uremia or hypercalcemia, it becomes predictable that this patient will suffer from progressive pelvic pain as well as possible bone pain. It is incumbent upon the treating physician to be responsive to this development with escalating doses of narcotic analgesics and, as indicated, by periodic consultation with experts in cancer pain management. Providing pain relief, emotional support, maintaining hygiene, and responding to disease-related complications is instrumental in preserving human dignity for patients in this catastrophic clinical setting.

PHYSICIANS' RESPONSE

MANUEL A. PENALVER
ADRIANA SUAREZ

The factors to be considered in this case are that (a) the patient has recurrent pelvic disease refractory to radiotherapy; (b) the metastatic pulmonary nodes, were only initially responsive to the platinum/ifosfamide combination; (c) there are suspicious periaortic nodes; and (d) the left ureter is obstructed. The presence of pulmonary metastases and questionable paraaortic nodes precludes a surgical option in this patient. Therefore, a total pelvic exenteration with urinary diversion, which is done in order to provide a possible cure, is not indicated in this patient.

The major goal of management in cases with obvious metastasis to distant organs refractive to both radiotherapy and/or surgical treatment is palliation. Palliation is achieved with systemic therapy producing (a) an objective remission of disease, thereby relieving symptoms, and (b) a reduction in the rate at which the locally advanced disease is progressing.

Factors to consider in the chemotherapeutic management of recurrent or advanced cervical cancer are staging, histological grade, renal status, and prior radiotherapy. Squamous cell carcinomas represent approximately 80% of cervical cancers and are therefore the histological type upon which most chemotherapeutic regimens are based.

Prior radiotherapy may adversely affect systemic treatment by decreasing the vascularization of tumor area, including cellular resistance to alkylating agents and impaired marrow reserve. Renal status must be considered in dealing with chemotherapy, since excretion of the drugs may be affected by ureteral obstruction and nephrotoxicity, especially in the case of compounds such as cisplatin.

The approach for additional chemotherapy in this patient is first to decide whether to use a single agent or a combination treatment regimen. Out of the 48 single agents tested in the past 20 years in squamous cell carcinoma of the cervix, cisplatin has been the most extensively studied. Cisplatin is a heavy metal complex and has the most consistent objective response rates of greater than 20%. However, it has been shown that cisplatin is more effective in patients who have not received prior chemotherapy. Another heavy metal complex showing a greater than 15% response is carboplatin, which can be substituted for cisplatin.

Alkylating agents showing promise are ifosfamide and dibromodulcitol, both of which have response rates of greater than 20%. Doxorubicin and epirubicin represent the anthracyclines, from among the antitumor antibiotics, with response rates greater than 15% and greater than 20% respectively. Other agents with antitumor activities include the vinca alkaloids, 5-fluorouracil, 5-floxuridine, folic acid antagonists, CPT-11, ICRF-159, and hexamethylmelamine. The single agents mentioned previously have response rates ranging from 15 to 35%, yet palliation from single-agent therapies is relatively brief, with a 4- to 9-month response rate.

Studies of combination chemotherapy are also numerous, yet no effective controlled studies showing conclusive data has offered any evidence that combination therapy is superior to that of single agents. To date, combinations that have shown some patient improvement are platinum drugs combined with either 5-fluorouracil, ifosfamide, dibromodulcitol, and doxorubicin. Yet all these combinations showed decreased response rates, shorter response duration, and shorter survival after prior radiotherapy. A recent combination of interest that has already undergone two phase II clinical trials is that of 13-*cis*-retinoic acid (13-c-RA), 1 mg/kg orally daily, plus interferon-alpha (IFN-alpha), 6 million units subcutaneously every day. The combination demonstrates the synergistic antiproliferative actions of IFN-alpha with the differentiating effects of 13-c-RA.

Combination chemotherapy and radiotherapy is another modality that is being considered and investigated. Yet subjecting this patient to more radiotherapy poses more chance for radiotherapy complications and is therefore contraindicated.

Although this 28-year-old woman initially responded to a cisplatin-based combination regimen, she later relapased, indicating the possibility of using another chemotherapeutic regimen. The only form of management besides placing a urostomy for urinary symptomatic relief, is to offer her palliative chemotherapy, most likely with agents that are still experimental. The option of participating in an experimental chemotherapeutic regimen or not to receive any palliative treatment should ultimately be offered to the patient.

49

Locally Advanced Cervical Cancer in a Young Woman

CASE

A 32-year-old woman is found to have a clinical stage IIIB carcinoma of the cervix. Both she and her family have asked you to be aggresive in her management as she "wants to live." She is willing to try experimental treatments if you think this might help. She has heard about radiosensitizers, neoadjuvant chemotherapy, and biological treatments and wants to know your opinion of these strategies in the management of her disease. The patient has normal renal function and a CT scan reveals the kidneys to be unobstructed.

PHYSICIANS' RESPONSE

BRADLEY J. MONK
ALBERTO MANETTA

Patients with advanced cervical carcinoma are generally treated with a combination of external and intracavitary irradiation. Using this combination, approximately 9000 and 6000 cGy are delivered to points A and B, respectively. According to the patterns-of-care study, patients with unilateral or bilateral side-wall involvement have a 4-year survival rate of 44 and 34%, respectively. The majority of these deaths are associated with infield failures. In an attempt to improve infield control and survival, investigators have studied radiosensitizers, neoadjuvant chemotherapy, biological therapies, radiation dose intensification, and surgical staging.

The use of systemic chemotherapy as a radiosensitizer remains controversial. The current phase III Gynecologic Oncology Group (GOG) Trial (No. 120) for patients with advanced cervical cancer randomizes patients between one of three chemotherapy regimens in combination with standard radiotherapeutic techniques. Regimen I is weekly intravenous cisplatin at 40 mg/m^2. Regimen II includes two administrations of intravenous cisplatin at 50 mg/m^2 on days 1 and 29, followed by two 4-day infusions of 1000 mg/m^2 per day of systemic 5-fluorouracil (5-FU) from days 2 to 5 and days 30 to 33 and hydroxyurea, 2 g/m^2, twice weekly during external-beam irradiation. The final regimen, regimen III, includes hydroxyurea alone at 3 g/m^2 twice weekly during external-beam irradiation. It has been our practice to routinely include patients with negative periaortic lymph nodes in this multicenter, randomized national protocol.

Another novel approach in the treatment of advanced cervical cancer includes the use of chemotherapy prior to irradiation or radical surgery. Although the feasibility of this multimodality therapy has been demonstrated, few studies have demonstrated substantial benefit in local control and survival. Patients should be treated with such neoadjuvant chemotherapy protocols only in a research setting.

The least studied medical therapy in advanced cervical cancer is the use of biological response modifiers. Perhaps the most widely studied agents include *cis*-retinoic acid, alpha-interferon, and bacille Calmette-Guérin (BCG). Once again, none of these agents have demonstrated increased efficacy either alone or in an adjuvant setting. Consequently, their use can be recommended only as part of a research protocol.

Since the mainstay of therapy in advanced cervical cancer is radiation, clinicians have studied methods of increasing parametrial dosimetry to overcome the inadequacies of standard external-beam and intracavitary techniques. Indeed, the patterns-of-care study demonstrated a dose-response relationship for infield pelvic control among stage III patients, with the highest rate of pelvic control being associated with paracentral doses to point A of more than 8500 cGy. In addition, the only treatment factor associated with improved pelvic control in multivariate analysis was the use of intracavitary brachytherapy. Two methods have been proposed to improve parametrial dosimetry. The first is multiple daily fraction irradiation. This treatment modality, piloted by the GOG in combination with either hydroxyurea or cisplatin/5-FU as a sensitizer, was found to be feasible, with acceptable morbidity. Nevertheless, this methodology has yet to be tested among large groups of patients. Second, Syed and colleagues have investigated the transperineal interstitial-intracavitary "Syed-Neblett" applicator in the treatment of advanced cervical carcinoma. In comparing a 42-day accelerated fraction regimen with a 48-day interstitial irradiation regimen, the effective dose delivered to point B is approximately one-third higher with the interstitial technique, providing a theoretical basis for the superiority of dose intensification with interstitial brachytherapy as compared to hyperfractionated techniques. This explains the improved local control reported by Syed and colleagues among patients with stage IIIB lesions. Interstitial irradiation achieved durable remissions among 13 (50%) of 26 patients. Among the 13 patients who expired, 7 were noted to be disease-free in the pelvis at the time of death. Thus, the overall infield control was over 75% when interstitial irradiation was used together with an intracavitary tandem and external irradiation. Therefore, I would counsel this patient concerning our single institutional experience and, if she were not interested in participating in the current GOG study, would recommend that she receive interstitial irradiation as described above.

Patients eligible for the current GOG study must have negative periaortic lymph nodes. We are currently studying the use of the laparoscope in performing retroperitoneal periaortic lymphadenectomy. The therapeutic benefit of surgical staging is yet to be demonstrated. Assuming that 30% of patients with stage III cervical cancers have periaortic metastases and only 15 to 25% of these patients are salvageable with extended-field irradiation, then approximately only 5% of patients would benefit from this operative intervention. In addition, bulky periaortic metastases may be detected with CT scanning, making the incidence of periaortic nodal metastases and the benefit from this operation much less. Thus, surgical staging in advanced cervical cancer can be recommended only in a research setting.

References

Syed AM, Nisar P, Ajmel A, et al. Transperineal interstitial-intracavitary "Syed-Neblett" applicator in the treatment of carcinoma of the uterine cervix. Endocuriether/Hypertherm Oncol 1986; 2:1–13.

Bloss D, Lucci JA III, DiSaia PJ, et al. A phase II trial of neoadjuvant chemotherapy prior to radical hysterectomy and/or radiation therapy in the management of advanced carcinoma of the uterine cervix (abstr). Society of Gynecologic Oncologists, San Francisco, February 1995.

PHYSICIANS' RESPONSE

EDWARD KAPLAN
DATTA NORI

The vast majority of cervical carcinomas are squamous cell tumors, which is the most likely histology in this case. The standard of care for all locally advanced lesions starting with stage IIB is radiotherapy alone. Certainly, this is true for our patient with stage IIIB disease. Given the fact that 50 to 75% of patients with her stage perish by 5 years, it is understandable that the patient and her family wish to follow an aggressive therapeutic approach, including investigational protocols.

A brief overview of past and current efforts to enhance local control and survival in this disease is instructive.

During the past decade, there have been dozens of phase II and several phase III chemotherapy trials aimed at defining any potential role for chemotherapy in the management of cervical cancer. Though initial responses are sometimes dramatic, they are inconsistent and virtually never durable. Cisplatin has been shown to have the highest degree of activity as a single agent. Other active agents include ifosfamide, doxorubicin (Adriamycin), and mitolactol. A randomized trial has never confirmed the efficacy of single-agent or combination chemotherapy, including studies of neoadjuvant chemotherapy from Brazil (BOMP) and France (CDDP/MTX/chloramb/VCR) or concomitant chemotherapy (CDDP/5-FU) tested by the GOG (protocol #85). Further, in early disease subjected to radical hysterectomy with the subsequent finding of positive pelvic nodes, a phase III trial of adjuvant chemotherapy (CDDP/VCR/BLM) did not improve survival. One GOG study (protocol #4) is sometimes represented as a positive trial in support of concomitant radiotherapy and hydroxyurea, but these data are highly criticized and not convincing. Thus, there is absolutely no evidence at this time to support offering this woman chemoradiation in any form.

Interesting work has been done in the area of biological therapy, again without encouraging results. The combination of 13-*cis*-retinoic acid and alpha-interferon was tried on 32 previously untreated patients with locally advanced disease in a phase II format; half the patients attained an objective response, which was short-lived. In a phase III study by the GOG (protocol #24), *Coryne-bacterium parvum* did not improve the response over radiotherapy alone.

Efforts to modulate radiation therapy technique have similarly not resulted in improvements in local control or survival. The GOG (protocol #56) showed that misonidazole, a hypoxic cell sensitizer, does not increase survival over radiotherapy/hydroxyurea controls. RTOG 8805, a phase I/II study of hyper-fractionated irradiation, now has a minimum follow-up of 4 years and has shown no benefit from 1.2 Gy bid versus historical controls treated on a conventional schedule. Two GOG trials that also looked at hyperfractionated radiation therapy (RT) have closed and their data are maturing. The first (protocol #8801) combined hydroxyurea with 1.2 Gy bid and the second used 5-FU/CDDP with the same RT regimen. No results have been published so far.

Our recommendation at this time is for this patient to proceed with conventional definitive RT, adhering to the caveats and guidelines derived from the patterns-of-care studies. First, total treatment time should be limited to 8 weeks if possible, and 10 at the most, in order to maximize local control and survival (1). Second, intracavitary radiation must be used to achieve local control and improve survival, although it is sometimes more practical to use interstitial radiation. The point A (paracentral) dose should reach 85 Gy to take advantage of the dose-response effect shown for stage III disease (2), bearing in mind that late complications are most apt to occur at this dose level. Finally, if this patient desires enrollment in a randomized trial, she may be a candidate for GOG protocol #120, which is a three-arm trial for locally advanced disease comparing radiotherapy with concomitant hydroxyurea or cisplatin or hydroxyurea/cisplatin/ 5-FU. In order to be eligible for this study, she would have to submit to an extraperitoneal paraaortic node sampling and would be randomized if her nodes were negative.

References

1. Lanciano RM, Pajak TF, Martz K, Hanks GE. The influence of treatment time on outcome for squamous cell cancer of the uterine cervix treated with radiation: A patterns-of-care study. IJROBP 1993; 25:391–397.
2. Lanciano RM, Won M, Coia LR, Hanks GE. Pretreatment and treatment factors associated with improved outcome in squamous cell carcinoma of the uterine cervix: A final report of the 1973 and 1978 patterns-of-care studies. IJROBP 1991; 20:667–676.

PHYSICIAN'S RESPONSE

MURRAY JOSEPH CASEY

The patient is a 32-year-old woman with squamous cell carcinoma of the cervix, stage IIIB. Conventional methods of management by radiation therapy directed to the primary tumor and confined to pelvic fields will predictably provide only 36% prognosis for long-term survival. Reasons for treatment failures are local and pelvic recurrences and distant metastasis beyond the pelvic field of irradiation. Squamous cell carcinoma of the cervix is believed to be a disease that generally advances from the primary site to pelvic and thence paraaortic lymph nodes before becoming more widely disseminated. Patients who are surgically explored for stage III cervical carcinomas have been found to have positive pelvic lymph nodes in 46 to 66% of cases, and some 29% are found to have positive paraaortic nodes (range, 19 to 46%). Nonetheless, aggressive combinations of radiation brachytherapy and external irradiation to the pelvis will successfully control pelvic tumor in 49 to 64% of patients with stage III tumors, while some 20% of cases so treated will develop distant metastasis.

Efforts to improve survival rates for patients with stage III cervical cancers have been designed to decrease local and pelvic recurrences and prevent metastatic dissemination. Because of the hypothesized stepwise progression of cervical cancer from pelvic to paraaortic nodes, studies were aimed at control of paraaortic metastasis through surgical lymph node resection and extension of radiation fields beyond the pelvis to encompass paraaortic abdominal fields. These approaches have been disappointing. Although occasional individual reports have indicated marginal improvement in survival rates for patients who have undergone paraaortic node dissection followed by external irradiation in instances of positive nodes, the bulk of available evidence demonstrates no significant survival advantage with these approaches; often, there is a considerably increased incidence of surgical and radiation-induced complications. Attempts to avoid the enhanced comorbidities of surgery and radiotherapy led some to advocate paraaortic irradiation for patients shown to harbor nodal metastasis by current widely available scanning modalities, such as computed tomography (CT) and magnetic resonance imaging (MRI). However, this approach overlooks the relatively low 66 to 75% sensitivity of these scanning techniques and the surprisingly high occurrence of scalene node metastases, which have been reported in several series of advanced cervical cancers. The rationale of controlling microscopic metastasis by the extension of external radiation to paraaortic fields without prior surgical exploration and regardless of scanning results is improved control of tumor within the irradiated fields. One prospective randomized study also demonstrated a significantly higher survival rate when radiotherapy was extended to paraaortic fields in patients with large central tumors confined to the cervix and parametria. But another randomized study, which included patients with stage III cervical cancers, found that similar regimens conveyed no significant survival advantages, and virtually all reports indicate that paraaortic irradiation increased the incidence of serious radiation complications, particularly to the small bowel. So, while extended radiotherapy can be shown to be effective in controlling clinically detectable and preclinical deposits of cancer in the paraaortic regions, the prognosis for survival of patients with stage III cervical cancers has not been improved by these methods.

To overcome the problem of occult metastatic disease and improve the effectiveness of local and regional radiotherapy, many studies have been undertaken that employ various antineoplastic chemotherapeutic agents in conjunction with irradiation or subsequent extirpative radical surgery in resectable cases. The literature is replete with anecdotal reports and nonrandomized series documenting complete and partial objective responses with such approaches. Improved radioresponsiveness and surgical resectability have been claimed with the use of such neoadjuvant chemotherapy with numerous cytotoxic agents, including especially cisplatin, 5-fluorouracil, methotrexate, mitomycin-C, vincristine, bleomycin, and the alkylating agents chlorambucil, melphalan, ifosfamide, and dibromodulcitol alone or in several combinations. However, there is no convincing evidence through randomized prospective studies that neoadjuvant chemotherapy actually decreases local and pelvic recurrences or improves survival rates, particularly in bulkier, more advanced tumors. Furthermore, a critical analysis of three prospective randomized controlled studies of neoadjuvant cisplatin containing chemotherapy followed by radiation therapy versus primary radiotherapy for advanced cervical cancers has raised the caveat that local recurrences may be enhanced and survival diminished for those who receive neoadjuvant therapy, possibly because of delays in the initiation of potentially curative radiation regimens and the biological selection of more aggressive tumor clones through action of the chemotherapy.

Although currently there are no proven advantages to be gained through the use of debulking surgery, extended-field irradiation or neoadjuvant cytotoxic chemotherapy in patients with locally advanced cervical squamous cell tumors, some of the observations made in the course of clinical trials remain encouraging. If this young woman with stage IIIB cervical carcinoma wishes to attempt to improve her chances for survival beyond that which may be available through standard regimens of radiotherapy, she is well advised to submit to one of the controlled, well-supervised prospective studies operating under the aegis of reputable scientific groups. Randomized trials are open testing paraaortic irradiation and neoadjuvant therapy with several regimens known to contain agents effective against squamous cell cervical carcinoma. Emerging drugs and biological response modifiers undoubtedly will find their way into such trials in the future.

References

1. Jones WB. New approaches to high-risk cervical cancer: Advanced cervical cancer. Cancer 1993; 71(4 suppl):1451–1459.
2. Perez CA, Kurman RJ, Stehman FB, Thigpen JT. Uterine cervix. In: Hoskins WJ, Perez CA, Younge RC, eds. Principles and Practice of Gynecologic Oncology. Philadelphia Lippincott, 1992:591–662.
3. Potish RA, Twiggs LB. On the lack of demonstrated clinical benefit of neoadjuvant cis-platinum therapy for cervical cancer. Int J Radiat Oncol Biol PHys 1993; 27:975–979.

PHYSICIAN'S RESPONSE

JONATHAN BEREK

Clinical stage IIIB squamous cell carcinoma of the cervix is still a curable disease. While optimal therapy is evolving, it appears that the use of a radiosensitizer— i.e., either 5-fluorouracil (5-FU) and cisplatin or hydroxyurea—is useful when given concurrently with radiation therapy to the pelvis (1).

Because the standard radiation field is to the pelvis only and not extended to the periaortic area, some have recommended the use of a staging laparotomy in young stage IIIB patients to maximize the probability of success (2). With a normal CT scan, there still is a 20 or 30% chance that the patient could have disease in the low paraaortic chain. If one identifies microscopic metastasis to the low periaortic area, the radiation field can be extended above the typical pelvic port.

If not otherwise on a research protocol, I would treat this patient with concurrent 5-FU and cisplatin with her pelvic radiation. I would follow a protocol that gives concurrent 5-FU for 4 to 5 days every 3 weeks for three to four cycles during the radiation therapy. The cisplatin can be given in a bolus every 3 weeks for the same number of cycles. She should also be treated with two cesium implantations of brachytherapy to control the central disease.

Another debatable issue is whether or not a extrafascial hysterectomy should be performed at the completion of pelvic radiation therapy. Some patients with stage IIIB cervical cancer will have small persistent central disease after the radiation, and there is some evidence that the performance of an extrafascial hysterectomy in these patients improves their prognosis. In the absence of prospective randomized data, this decision must be individualized. If the patient has a prompt response to chemoradiation therapy, has no evidence of metastatic disease to the periaortic area, and is otherwise doing well, I would consider performing such a surgery 6 to 8 weeks after completing her external-beam radiation therapy.

References

1. Thomas G, Dembo A, Fyles A, et al. Concurrent chemoradiation in advanced cervical cancer. Gynecol Oncol 1990; 38:446.
2. Weiser EB, Bundy BN, Hoskins WJ, et al. Extraperitoneal versus transperitoneal selective paraaortic lymphadenectomy in the pretreatment staging of advanced cervical cancer: A Gynecologic Oncology Group study. Gynecol Oncol 1983; 33:283.

PHYSICIAN'S RESPONSE

JOHN KAVANAGH

This case presents the problem of an individual with a stage IIIb carcinoma of the cervix who has a poor prognosis and wishes to receive aggressive therapy.

At this point, given the literature concerning randomized trials of radio-sensitizers and neoadjuvant chemotherapy, one must consider them still investigational or of very marginal benefit. Long-term follow-up of the initial trials with radiosensitizers has not shown substantial survival benefit. The relapse patterns of cervical cancer involve disease outside the radiated field in about two-thirds of cases. Therefore, to be of value, the chemotherapy should provide curative potential for subclinical metastatic disease. Considering the historical experience of available agents, this remains unproven (1,2). Although the reported single-arm trials that utilize a variety of prognostic factors are of provocative interest, this patient represents stage IIIb cervical cancer. In addition, it must be noted that one study has found perhaps an inferior result with a neoadjuvant chemotherapy program. Also the concomitant use of radiation therapy and chemotherapy, particularly if given regionally, does enhance toxicity. Long-term toxicities are yet to be elucidated but may be worse. The biological treatments particularly the combination of retinoic acid and interferon, although fascinating, are not yet proven to be of any significant long-term benefit. One should be aware that a unilateral stage IIIB carcinoma of the cervix with negative lymph nodes and small pelvic side-wall component may have a cure rate that is above 50%. This is particularly true if the patient receives an appropriately boosted form of radio-therapy with particular attention to the intracavitary system. The dosimetry of these must be carefully directed toward the involved side wall. If the patient wishes to participate in a research protocol that both the physician and patient are comfortable with, she should indeed be offered a clinical research protocol. The advantages and disadvantages should be explained to her and the informed consent obtained.

References

1. Tattersal MHN, Lorvidhaya V, Vootiprux V, et al. Randomized trial of epirubicin and cisplatin chemotherapy followed by pelvic radiation in locally advanced cervical cancer. J Clin Oncol 1995; 13:444–451.
2. Gonzalez de Leon C, Kudelka AP, Edwards CL, Kavanagh JJ. Carcinoma of the uterine cervix. In: Pazdur R, ed. Medical Oncology: A Comprehensive Review. Huntington, NY: PRR, Inc, 1993/1994: 255–270.

50

Advanced Cervical Cancer with Bilateral Ureteral Obstruction

CASE

A 38-year-old woman with advanced cervical cancer has been treated with surgery, radiation, and several chemotherapeutic regimens. Despite this extensive treatment, she has continued to maintain a reasonably good performance status. Narcotic analgesia has recently been added to the treatment program due to a significant increase in pelvic discomfort. This has been effective in improving symptoms. Computed tomography (CT) of the pelvis is obtained to evaluate the pain, and the patient is found to have bilateral ureteral obstruction with mild to moderate hydronephrosis. The tumor has also significantly increased size since the previous CT scan 3 months earlier. Renal function is mildly abnormal (serum creatinine is 2.3).

PHYSICIAN'S RESPONSE

WELDON E. CHAFE

This unfortunate young woman with pelvic progression of her cervical cancer has exhausted therapeutic options conventionally employed in managing her disease. In spite of surgery, radiation, and chemotherapy, there is now demonstrated measurable progression of disease on a CT scan of the pelvis. This is causing her significant discomfort that has necessitated the use of narcotic analgesics in her management. More alarming in the decision-making process is the CT finding of bilateral obstructive uropathy and diminishing renal function (creatinine is 2.3).

396

Most essential here is counseling of the patient and her family. They need to be apprised of the fact that her disease is relentless in its progressive end-stage nature. Clinical concerns of appropriate analgesia in palliative symptom management now become a priority in management. Her pain management must be individualized in choice of agent, route, dose, and schedule. Potential medication side effects and the handling of breakthrough pain must be discussed. The significance of obstructive uropathy needs to be explained to the patient, and one should discuss the issue of uremia as a mechanism for death. Options in her palliation at this point in time can be addressed. A patient requiring narcotic analgesics for pain control will derive no palliation from urinary diversion. Renal failure usually leads slowly and with only moderate distress to a uremic death.

Decisions should be made after discussion with the patient and her family and must be shared by the physician. Attitudes about death, comfort methods, and so on can be elicited by the physician. Counsel with regard to attending to personal matters should be given. The patient and her family must know that with diversion severe pain, cachexia, and hemorrhage tend to be the norm and that future decisions pertaining to management (i.e., transfusions for hemorrhage, cordotomy for pain management, and so on) are no easier.

The financial concerns of prolonged hospitalization, needs of nursing, and medical care with no alteration in survival need to be discussed. Treatment and management goals should be designed to avoid undue procedures and attend to the patient's comfort and personal needs at her request.

PHYSICIAN'S RESPONSE

GREG SUTTON

One must assume several facts. First, that the "several chemotherapeutic regimens" in this case included cisplatin at one point or another. Second, that "advanced cervical cancer" is squamous or adenocarcinoma and not a small-cell neuroendocrine tumor. Third, that surgical therapy and radiotherapy were definitive for the circumstances and no option for further radiotherapy or pelvic exenteration exists. Under these conditions, there is very little tumor-directed therapy available for this patient. The central issue for discussion is the presence of hydronephrosis and renal insufficiency as a result of significant tumor growth in a 3-month period of time.

This woman has recurrent cervical cancer and is in the final months or perhaps weeks of her illness. The most important aspect of care is to meet with her and her family to discuss the implications of her recent symptoms, if this has not been done already. We know that women who develop hydronephrosis after aggressive treatment for cervical cancer have a poor prognosis regardless of therapy. Decisions at this point must be rational ones and should take into consideration the end-of-life wishes of both the patient and her family. It is important to discourage heroics and to take measures that will place the patient in a home or hospice environment if at all possible. "No code" or "do not resuscitate" orders should be written for both inpatient and outpatient settings; this is simplified if discussions about a living will have been held with the patient and her family following the initial diagnosis of recurrent cervical cancer.

A painstaking discussion must be held with the patient and responsible family members regarding the implications of hydronephrosis in cervical cancer. Education of the patient and family about the natural course of renal failure and azotemic death is critical if the temptation to place indwelling ureteral stents or percutaneous nephrostomy tubes is to be avoided, as it should be. More often than not, women with terminal cervical cancer and bilateral hydronephrosis are seen by well-meaning urologists or interventional radiologists and the hydronephrosis "problem" is "solved" by one of these means. It is often easier to perform a simple interventional procedure than it is to engage the dying patient and her family in meaningful discussion that may end the need for expensive and meaningless treatments.

References

Cain J, Stacy L, Jusenius K, Figge D. The quality of dying: Financial, psychological, and ethical dilemmas. Obstet Gynecol 1990; 76:149.

Wanzer SH, Federman DD, Adelstein SJ, et al. The physician's responsibility toward hopelessly ill patients: A second look. N Engl J Med 1989; 320:844–849

Lubitz JD, Riley GF. Trends in medicare payments in the last year of life. N Engl J Med 1993; 328:1092–1096.

PHYSICIAN'S RESPONSE

HOLLY H. GALLION

This unfortunate young woman has advanced cervical cancer despite treatment with radiation, surgery, and chemotherapy. She has now developed bilateral ureteral obstruction, presumably due to extrinsic compression of the ureter by pelvic tumor. Her prognosis is extremely grave, and if the obstruction is left untreated, death due to uremia or associated complications can be expected to occur within a matter of months. The role of palliative urinary diversion in patients with recurrent cervical cancer is controversial. Urinary diversion has generally been discouraged in such patients, as death from uremia may be replaced by a potentially more painful death from local and distant disease. However, palliative urinary diversion may prolong survival and improve quality of life in carefully selected patients with recurrent cervical cancer.

In this particular patient, palliative urinary diversion may allow the administration of potentially nephrotoxic chemotherapy with the hope of obtaining at least temporary remission of disease. However, if the patient has already failed cisplatin chemotherapy, there is little hope that a response to other salvage chemotherapy will be obtained. If this is the case, the only goal of urinary diversion in this patient would be to prolong her survival and to maintain her quality of life for as long as possible. Factors that favor urinary diversion in this case include her young age and good performance status. In the series reported by Carter, the median survival following percutaneous urinary diversion for advanced pelvic malignancy was significantly increased in younger patients and in those with good performance-status scores (1). Moreover, the median survival for patients with normal pretreatment renal function was increased from 2.5 to 16 months.

Open surgical urinary diversion in patients with advanced pelvic malignancies is associated with high morbidity and mortality. For this reason, urinary diversion should be accomplished by the cystoscopic or percutaneous placement of indwelling double-J polyurethane ureteral stents. If it is not possible to place an indwelling stent, external drainage can be established by percutaneous nephrostomy. The majority of patients will require replacement or adjustment of the stents at some time. Common complications of indwelling ureteral stents include symptomatic urinary tract infections, requiring intravenous antibiotics, and also catheter obstruction. The incidence of urinary tract infections can be decreased if the catheters are changed regularly.

Obviously, the pros and cons of diversion in this patient must be carefully considered and discussed at length with the patient and her family. It should be emphasized that this is only a palliative measure. She needs to understand that although it may prolong her life by preventing renal failure, she may develop debilitating pain from recurrent tumor. Also, she needs to be informed of the complications associated with urinary stents. In my opinion, this young patient with locally advanced cervical cancer who is in otherwise reasonably good health is a good candidate for urinary diversion. Relief of her ureteral obstruction may significantly prolong her life and allow her to spend quality time at home with her family.

Reference

1. Carter J, Ramirez C, Waugh R, et al. Percutaneous urinary diversion in gynecologic oncology. Gynecol Oncol 1991; 40:248–252.

PHYSICIAN'S RESPONSE

JOHN MALFETANO

This young patient has end-stage carcinoma of the cervix. Unfortunately, she has a progressive malignancy despite all currently available treatment modalities. Her life expectancy at this point is months, probably less than 6.

There must be a family conference with the patient to discuss her disease status and grave prognosis, to answer questions, and to formulate a supportive plan of care. The discussion must stress that there are no currently available surgical or radiotherapeutic options for her and any further chemotherapeutic approach would be futile. The issues of pain control and her renal status must be addressed. The patient and family should be reassured that pain control can be obtained by various means. Besides oral narcotics, continued parenteral drugs are feasible as well as regional narcotic therapy. Her renal status is a more complex issue and a joint understanding with an informed consensus will help plan the strategy. The decision-making process should involve either attempts at temporarily improving her renal status or allowing it to deteriorate. The latter will result in uremia and inevitable death, which as a rule is pain-free. Relief of ureteral obstruction with preservation or restoration of renal function is a prerequisite if there is consideration of further antineoplastic therapy and the patient is eligible for phase I or II drugs. Otherwise, relief of obstruction may provide palliation for pain and improve quality of life. This can be accomplished by endoscopic placement of ureteral stents or percutaneous nephrostomy placement with antegrade stent placement if there was endoscopic failure. It must be understood that these attempts are only palliative and are themselves associated with a variety of problems. These include failure to place the stents endoscopically or by antegrade techniques, leaving the patient with two nephrostomy tubes. The indwelling stents are also associated with pain, infection, hematuria, and stent occlusion.

After the family conference, plans to allow for the optimal quality of the patient's remaining life and those for terminal care should be developed. I would stress repeatedly that gynecological-oncological services would continue and always be available and that our care has not stopped but rather taken a new direction. Personally, after the patient and her family have accepted the reality of her illness and its ultimate outcome, I would put the emphasis on pain-control measures rather than her renal status, since she is symptomatic.

51

Metastatic Recurrent Cervical Squamous Cell Carcinoma

CASE

A 38-year-old woman is 18 months status post initial diagnosis of a stage 3B squamous cell carcinoma of the cervix. She was treated initially with 50 Gy whole pelvic radiation using a 12-MeV linear accelerator in 35 fractions over 44 days. In addition, the patient had two interstitial implants with Syed templates. Although she had a fair amount of difficulty with acute gastrointestinal complications from the radiation therapy, her symptoms decreased. On six Lomotil tablets (diphenoxylate HCl and atropinesulfate) a day and following a low-residue diet, she has managed to do quite well. Over the past 3 to 4 months, however, her appetite has been decreasing. She has lost about 10% of her body weight and now weighs 134 pounds. She takes two Percocet tablets (oxycodone HCl and acetaminophen) every 3 hr for pain, which is mainly sciatic in nature and on the left side. She presents now with nausea and vomiting. On evaluation, the studies of note were a serum creatinine of 12.5, potassium of 6.1, albumin of 2.6, and hemoglobin of 7.8. A renal ultrasound was done, which showed bilateral severe hydronephrosis. Physical examination revealed an ill-appearing woman with dry skin, appearing quite somnolent. Pelvic exam revealed obvious tumor and vault necrosis, with marked induration of the bladder floor.

PHYSICIAN'S RESPONSE

ED PARTRIDGE

The management of this very difficult case hinges a great deal on one's philosophical approach to a patient with incurable disease. Quality of life and benefits versus burdens of therapy are of paramount interest in this case and should be the guide to further intervention.

This patient has completed standard and maximal doses of radiation therapy for an advanced-stage carcinoma of the cervix. She now presents with obvious recurrent disease which is presumed, on the basis of hydronephrosis and sciatic pain, to be unresectable. This unresectability should be confirmed by examination. Furthermore, even if deemed resectable on examination, an attempt at an exenterative procedure should not be undertaken in this patient. The presence of bilateral severe hydronephrosis is a relative contraindication to exenteration. When this is coupled with vault necrosis, weight loss, and severe pain, an exenteration is definitely not feasible in this patient.

The issue then becomes whether or not the patient should have urinary diversion. There is very little evidence that percutaneous nephrostomy is beneficial in a patient with recurrent carcinoma of the cervix following initial treatment with radiotherapy. In one study, five of six patients died within 7 months (1) and in a second (2) the median survival was only 51 days. Percutaneous nephrostomy has substantial risk for complications in this debilitated patient. These include hemorrhage and infection. If the ureteral stents cannot be internalized, a substantial management burden is placed upon the patient and her family.

This particular patient already has significant symptomatology, with severe pain and weight loss. To add the burden of percutaneous nephrostomy to prolong for a limited time what is already a miserable existence does not seem justified. The burdens of the intervention seem to clearly outweigh the benefit. Because of the ultimate futility of this intervention, one could even make the ethical argument that it should not even be offered to the patient as an option.

On the other hand, if the patient has a directed and specific reason for prolonging life a little longer (i.e., the anticipated wedding of her son in 3 weeks), then perhaps nephrostomy could be considered. Allowing her to have the option would fulfill ethical principles of autonomy or informed consent, but the utilization of this costly intervention in the face of such ultimate futility could be considered an unjust and unnecessary waste of medical resources.

A second reason for the percutaneous nephrostomies would be to allow treatment with chemotherapy such as cisplatin (Platinol). However, the response to cisplatin for recurrent squamous cell cancer in a necrotic, previously irradiated pelvis would be quite low. Again, the benefits of treatment would be minimal and the burden considerable.

Recognition that this patient is incurable should be foremost in her care. Aggressive relief of symptoms; family, clergy, and social support; and, care and comfort constitute the most logical and indeed the most humanistic approach to the young unfortunate woman.

References

1. Gadducci A, Madrigali A, Facchini V, Fioretti P. Percutaneous nephrostomy in patients with advanced or recurrent cervical cancer. Clin Exp Obstet Gynecol 1994; 21:71–73.
2. Kehoe S, Luesley MD, Budden J, Earl H. Percutaneous nephrostomies in women with cervical cancer. Br J Obstet Gynecol 1993; 100:283–284.

PHYSICIAN'S RESPONSE

LEO LAGASSE

Initially, this patient should have stabilization of her renal failure with monitoring of her electrocardiogram (ECG) and electrolytes. The next step would be to perform a pelvic and abdominal CT scan without contrast to evaluate the pelvic mass, the left pelvic side wall, and the pelvic and paraaortic lymph nodes. Examination under anesthesia to evaluate the extent and fixation of the tumor would follow as a separate procedure. The central mass should be biopsied vaginally and any nodal mass evaluated by fine needle aspiration. If nodal biopsy is positive, the patient is not a candidate for exenteration. If node biopsies are negative, the patient should be prepared for surgical exploration with possible pelvic exenteration. This might require preoperative placement of percutaneous nephrostomies to improve renal function. At abdominal exploration, paraaortic nodes are dissected and submitted for frozen section. If node biopsies are negative, the pelvic side walls are dissected and tissue from lateral margins submitted for frozen section. If these are negative, the exenteration procedure may proceed. The distal colon and ureters are transected. The pelvic organs with tumor mass are mobilized by sectioning lateral vaginal attachments. The rectum distal to the tumor is transected. Completion of the total vaginectomy is by a perineal phase, which frees the urethra and vagina from the vulva and perineum. Since the distal rectum is preserved, a sigmoid rectal stapled anastomosis is used. Vaginal reconstruction, using either myocutaneous flaps or an omental flap with split-thickness skin graft, is carried out. Urinary tract reconstruction is preferably done with an ileocolic, Indiana pouch–type continent reservoir using detubularized ascending and transverse colon for urine storage and a narrowed segment of distal ileum as the continent efferent outflow mechanism. The procedure is a total pelvic exenteration, but the patient is left with a temporary colostomy stoma and a continent urostomy as well as the potential for a functioning vagina.

If the patient is not an exenteration candidate, very careful discussions with the patient and her family are required. Decisions may require that family members or friends be authorized by a durable power of attorney or similar instrument to safeguard the wishes of the patient. Without further treatment, an early death is expected. If the decision is to prolong life, then some form of urinary diversion will be required. This will delay death but expose the patient to the likelihood of prolonged pain, vaginal bleeding, and vaginal discharge. Erosion of the tumor into the bladder and/or the rectum may later lead to the need for surgical diversion. Both systemic and regional pain management strategies can be helpful and should be pursued vigorously. It is not clear whether delaying death by relieving renal obstruction is preferable to an earlier but more comfortable demise. The decision can only be made by the patient, supported by her family and friends and compassionately advised by her gynecological oncologist.

PHYSICIANS' RESPONSE

CLAUS TROPÉ
GUNNAR KRISTENSEN

This patient has received adequate radiotherapy for stage IIIB disease. She shortly developed progressive disease and is now admitted to hospital with fulminant uremia. Her bilateral hydronephrosis with uremia justifies immediate measures to improve urinary outlet, such as stent insertion or percutaneous pyelostomy followed by appropriate supportive care. If she does not respond to supportive care, the goal for treatment will be palliation of symptoms. In case vomiting continues after normalization of urinary function, an intestinal obstruction should be ruled out. Mechanical ileus may be caused by progressive tumor and should be managed operatively in patients fit for operation so as to improve their quality of life. If the patient responds well to supportive treatment, achieves normal renal function, and has a Karnofsky index above 60, one must deal with her progressive pelvic disease.

The survival rate for patients with locally advanced cervical cancer is not satisfactory, with 5-year survival rates of about 30%. Treatment results have not improved for the last 30 years (1). Often these patients have involved lymph nodes at the time of diagnosis and die from disseminated disease. Systemic chemotherapy have been used in the primary treatment in an attempt to improve survival, but the results have been disappointing. Therefore the use of chemotherapy has mostly been limited to patients with recurrent disease not suitable for exenteration or irradiation or to patients with primary disseminated disease. Patients with recurrent cervical disease have a poor prognosis, with less than 15% surviving for 1 year. Response rates obtained by single-agent therapy have been reported in the range of 10 to 30%, cisplatin being the most effective single agent with a response rate of 20 to 30% (2). Cisplatin in combination with 5-fluorouracil

(5-FU) has been used, but even with the most aggressive cisplatin combination, the influence on overall survival is doubtful. At the Society of Gynecologic Oncologists (SGO) meeting in 1995 we presented our long-term results with the combination of cisplatin 100 mg/m^2 on day 1 and 5-FU 1000 mg/m^2 on days 1 to 5 (3). The overall response rate was as high as 54%, with 14% complete remissions. Recurrences outside irradiated areas had a higher response rate (70%) than recurrences within previously irradiated areas (30%). The study indicates that cisplatin-containing combination chemotherapy may influence long-term survival, as 25% of patients survived for more than 2 years and 10% had 5-year survival. The highest response rates were seen in patients with their primary in early stages, a relapse-free interval after primary treatment of at least 12 months, relapse in a single site outside previously irradiated area, and a good performance status before treatment of relapse.

In the present patient with progressive disease in a previously irradiated area, we would consider palliative, nonaggressive chemotherapy and our choice would be 5-FU 500 mg/m^2 followed by Rescuvolin 60 mg/m^2 on days 1 and 2 with a cycle of 14 days.

References

1. Perez CA, Kuske RR, Camel HME. Analysis of pelvic tumor control and impact on survival in carcinoma of the uterine cervix treated with radiation therapy alone. Int J Radiat Oncol Biol Phys 1988; 14:613–621.
2. Vermorken JB. The role of chemotherapy in squamous cell carcinoma of the uterine cervix: A review. Int J. Gynecol Cancer 1993; 3:129–142.
3. Kaern J, Tropé CG, Sundfoer K, Kristensen GB. Cisplatin/5-fluorouracil treatment contribute to long-term survival in patients with recurrent cervical carcinoma. Gynecol Oncol. In press.

52

Pelvic Mass Recurrence Following Surgery and Radiation for Locally Advanced Cervical Cancer

CASE

A 47-year-old woman is treated with a radical hysterectomy and pelvic lymph-adenectomy, followed by radiation, for a stage IB carcinoma of the cervix. The radiation was administered because of two positive left external iliac lymph nodes. Three years following the completion of radiation, routine physical examination reveals the presence of a pelvic side-wall mass. The mass does not appear to be fixed. Computed tomography (CT) of the abdomen and pelvis confirms the presence of the mass, but no other disease is evident on the radiographic study. A chest x-ray is normal. The patient has an excellent performance status.

PHYSICIAN'S RESPONSE

ERNEST W. FRANKLIN, III

Impression

Probable neoplastic mass arising within the ovary. Potential malignant status can be ascertained only by laparotomy and histology.

Recommendation

Exploratory laparotomy for resection of pelvic mass.

406

Discussion

This 47-year-old woman was treated with radical hysterectomy and pelvic lymph-adenectomy but evidently did not have her ovaries removed. The subsequent pelvic radiation given for the two positive lymph nodes would have ablated ovarian function unless the ovary was transposed, thus ruling out the possibility of this being a functional ovarian cyst or mass. The possibility of the mass having arisen from the gastrointestinal or genitourinary tract should have been defined by use of CT scanning with contrast performed on the abdomen and pelvis. Fortunately that study did not show evidence of other metastatic disease, nor did the chest x-ray.

Of those patients who would have a recurrence of carcinoma of the cervix subsequent to the presence of the pelvic lymph nodes, 80 to 90% would have experienced that recurrence within 2 years of the original treatment. In addition, the probability of recurrence within the pelvis following surgical resection and radiation therapy should be small, approximately 15%, but the radiation therapy might also have delayed such a recurrence beyond the usual 2 years. In addition, the probability of this being recurrent cervical cancer is diminished because of the finding that the mass does not appear to be fixed. The majority of recurrences in these circumstances would be in the parametria or along the pelvic side wall, in which case the mass would be fixed rather than mobile. It is not possible to define the size of the mass or its consistency based on the information given by the CT scan. Review of those films is recommended. The larger the proportion of solid tissue within the mass, the greater the probability of malignant neoplasia. Under any circumstance, however, it would not be possible to determine what this mass represents without resecting it. I do not feel that a laparoscopic approach would be appropriate here, given the patient's previous radical surgery and radiation therapy. In addition, the mass is probably neoplastic, whether benign or malignant, and appears to be localized. Any risk of rupture or spillage of such a mass is to be avoided. Other studies could be undertaken, including further x-rays of the gastrointestinal and genitourinary tracts, CA-125, and other markers. These will not contribute to the final determination of management. They are not recommended and surgical resection will provide the only answer regarding the character of this mass. Needle biopsy might provide some histological evidence of the character of the mass but would not rule out malignancy if benign and would not avoid surgery if malignant. Thus, surgical removal is the appropriate next step.

PHYSICIAN'S RESPONSE

PEYTON T. TAYLOR, JR.

The pelvic mass detected in this case is very likely to be either a metastatic nodal mass from the original cervical carcinoma, an ovarian mass (benign or malignant) from a retained ovary, or a lymphocyst. Histological or cytological documentation of the nature of the mass will be critical before a management plan can be devised.

The history of ovarian preservation and a more precise description of the size and location of the mass (retroperitoneal versus intraperitoneal) would narrow the differential diagnosis. If the mass cannot be further localized and characterized by history and computed tomography, a high-resolution pelvic ultrasound would be helpful. A solid or partly solid mass almost certainly represents a malignancy; a cystic mass, even with a thickened rim, is likely to represent either a benign ovarian cyst or a lymphocyst. In either case, an image-guided needle biopsy or fine needle aspiration (FNA) for cytological examination would be the next step advised to establish a diagnosis. Both core needle biopsies and aspiration cytology have been carefully investigated and both show commendable sensitivity and specificity, especially if the cellularity of the sample is high (1,2).

Pelvic side-wall masses that represent metastatic disease after radical hysterectomy are usually fixed and as such are rarely resectable. Dissection around the iliac and other pelvic vessels, especially after radical hysterectomy/lymphadenectomy *and* pelvic radiation, is technically challenging and potentially quite complicated. However, because the mass is described as not being fixed and because of the patient's age and favorable performance status, I would consider exploration and resection, even if the FNA confirms recurrent cervical cancer. In this setting, resection provides the only real hope for disease control. If the mass is not resectable, further radiation therapy would not be helpful; the intervening and adjacent viscera would thus be near biological radiation tolerance and the tumor is demonstrably radioresistant. Metastatic cervical carcinomas respond very poorly to commercially available cytotoxic therapy, especially when the recurrences are in a heavily irradiated field. An investigational program of cytotoxic therapy would be recommended over anecdotal chemotherapy, but the outlook is rather grim.

If the mass is a primary neoplasm arising in a retained ovary, full staging is indicated: resection of both ovaries, peritoneal washings, omentectomy, random peritoneal biopsies (including samples of diaphragmatic peritoneum), and para-aortic nodal biopsies. Subsequent chemotherapy, "adjuvant chemotherapy," would likely be indicated based on the histological grade, the extent of histological involvement, and the status of the washings.

Lymphocysts are difficult to manage and no convincingly successful method of management has been reported. Several anecdotal reports have each claimed some value in exploration and "unroofing" the cyst, excising the cyst, placing an omental pedicle in the floor of the cyst, or percutaneously placing drains or sclerosing agents in the cyst. I have limited personal experience with lymphocysts, and serial follow-up seems the most prudent course to follow, if the cyst is ultrasonographically unilocular without internal papillations or complex septae, *if* the cytology is both "adequate" and "negative," *if* there is no ureteric obstruction, and if the lymphocyst remains asymptomatic.

References

1. Moriarty AT, Glant MD, Stehman FB. The role of fine needle aspiration cytology in the management of gynecologic malignancies. Acta Cyto 1986; 30:59–64.
2. Andersen WA, Nichols GE, Avery SR, Taylor PT. Cytologic diagnosis of ovarian tumors: Factors influencing accuracy in previously undiagnosed cases. Am J Obstet Gynecol. In press.

PHYSICIAN'S RESPONSE

NEVILLE HACKER

This 47-year-old, healthy, asymptomatic woman had a pelvic mass detected on routine pelvic examination. It is of note that she had a radical hysterectomy, pelvic lymphadenectomy, and postoperative pelvic radiation 3 years earlier for a stage IB cervical carcinoma with two positive left external iliac lymph nodes. The presence of the mass was confirmed on CT scan, although no details are given about the scan findings. Clinically I note that the mass appears not to be fixed.

The most likely diagnosis would be an ovarian mass, although a tubal mass, sigmoid mass, or a recurrence of the cervical carcinoma on the pelvic side wall should also be considered. The latter is the least likely, as most recurrences will appear in the first 24 months, the mass is said not to be fixed, and the patient is asymptomatic.

I would obtain a pelvic ultrasound to help define the mass. Transvaginal ultrasonography with colour Doppler should help determine whether this is a tubal or an ovarian mass and whether it is benign or malignant. A preoperative serum CA-125 titer would also be helpful as a baseline, although CA-125 titers are elevated in only about 50% of stage I ovarian carcinomas. Flexible sigmoidoscopy would also be helpful to exclude intrinsic bowel pathology.

Definitive diagnosis will necessitate laparotomy or operative laparoscopy. I would recommend laparotomy through a lower midline incision so as to allow thorough exploration of the entire abdomen. If the mass is ovarian or tubal, I would recommend unilateral salpingo-oophorectomy and frozen-section diagnosis. If benign, I would recommend removal of the contralateral tube and ovary, as this is presumably nonfunctional unless it was suspended out of the pelvis prior to the pelvic radiation.

If the mass proved to be a malignant ovary or tube, I would recommend thorough palpation of all peritoneal surfaces including the small and large bowel and their mesenteries. Any suspicious nodules should be biopsied. If there was no apparent spread, I would recommend thorough surgical staging. This would include peritoneal washings for cytology; infracolic omentectomy; biopsies from the peritoneum of the pelvis, paracolic gutters, and diaphragm; ipsilateral pelvic lymphadenectomy; and sampling of paraaortic lymph nodes.

In the unlikely event that this mass proved to be a pelvic side-wall recurrence, I would recommend surgical removal of as much of the mass as possible. This could be achieved by a combination cold knife, surgical diathermy, and CUSA (Cavetron Ultrasonic Surgical Aspirator). Intraoperative radiation would be the most useful definitive treatment, but as this is infrequently available, the CORT (combined operative and therapeutic treatment) procedure could be tried (1).

If the final diagnosis proved to be stage IA or IB epithelial ovarian carcinoma, grade 1 or grade 2, I would recommend no further treatment. If it proved to be a grade 3, stage 1 ovarian or tubal carcinoma or a stage IC ovarian carcinoma, I would recommend four cycles of cisplatin (75 mg/m^2) and cyclophosphamide (75 mg/m^2), although it is unclear whether or not the additional therapy would improve the prognosis. I would follow the patient with CA-125 titers and would not plan a second-look laparotomy.

Reference

1. Hockel M, Knapstein PG. The combined operative and radiotherapeutic treatment (CORT) (abstr). Gynecol Oncol 1992; 45:79.

PHYSICIAN'S RESPONSE

HUGH M. SHINGLETON

While postoperative irradiation for positive pelvic nodes is a common form of treatment, there is actually no evidence in the literature that this prolongs survival in women with carcinoma of the cervix. The fact that this patient received postoperative pelvic irradiation has some bearing on the selection of future therapy in that the previous irradiation may limit or even preclude use of additional irradiation should recurrent cancer be proven. The appearance of a pelvic mass in a woman who has had a radical hysterectomy 3 years before certainly raises the question of recurrent cancer. Curiously however, the mass is not fixed to the pelvic wall. A fixed pelvic side-wall mass with or without evidence of distant metastases (to paraaortic nodes, lungs, or elsewhere) and/or a central pelvic mass are the usual patterns of recurrence of cervical cancer. Pelvic lymphocysts are tense structures coming off the pelvic side walls. They should not appear this long after the lymphadenectomy (3 years) and therefore this is not likely to be the explanation for the mass. It is not stated whether this woman had her ovaries removed at the time of the radical hysterectomy, but should that not be the case, one might wonder if this is an ovarian mass. If the ovaries were removed, then one should consider some other type of pelvic pathology (masses associated with inflammatory bowel disease, etc.). It is not stated whether the CT scan revealed the mass to be solid or cystic. If solid, a fine needle aspiration could be performed to determine its nature. A cystic mass would lend more credence to the idea that this is either an ovarian cyst or a noncancerous fluid-filled silent abscess or pelvic hematoma. Most likely this woman will require a laparotomy to determine the nature of the mass short of a diagnosis of recurrent cancer being made with a fine needle. Because of the previous pelvic surgery and radiation, a laparoscopy would not be recommended, since it would be associated with a greatly enhanced chance of complications. Resection of the mass may be possible; if it is malignant, a determination would have to be made intraoperatively as to whether some type of exenterative surgery is indicated. If it is malignant and unresectable, adjunctive therapy in the form of irradiation or chemotherapy could be considered (1).

Reference

1. Shingleton HM, Orr JW. Cancer of the Cervix. Philadelphia: Lippincott, 1995:260,295–317.

PHYSICIANS' RESPONSE

NICOLETTA COLOMBO
ANGELO MAGGIONI
LUCA BOCCIOLONE
SERGIO PECORELLI

Missing information on this patient includes the following: size of primary tumor, size of recurrent lesion, and histological confirmation of recurrent tumor. Distant metastases have been ruled out by CT scan. Since the mass does not appear to be fixed and radiation has already been given in an adjuvant setting, the patient is a candidate for pelvic exenteration.

Discussion

Carcinoma metastatic to regional lymph nodes is a poor prognostic indicator in patients undergoing hysterectomy for early-stage squamous cell carcinoma of the cervix. Particularly, extensive nodal metastases or metastasis to the nodes in the region of the common iliac vessels and above are poor prognostic characteristics. Overall survival in this group is stated to be 50 to 60%. The diameter of the primary cervical lesion constitutes another significant prognostic factor in patients with metastatic lymph nodes.

Several therapeutic options have been proposed to approach local/regional recurrence of cervical carcinoma after surgery and radiotherapy. The site of recurrence largely affects the choice of treatment modality and the prognosis. Commonly, a pelvic recurrence is defined as lateral if pelvic side-wall fixation is documented or central if it involves pelvic structures but no side-wall fixation. For lateral pelvic recurrence, the treatment of choice is radiotherapy. Unfortunately, this treatment modality is usually ineffective when radiation therapy has already been given as adjuvant treatment after primary surgery. Systemic chemotherapy with platinum-based regimens can achieve a 40% response rate. These results are dependent on the site of the disease, the extent of the disease, and whether the lesions are located in previously irradiated area. Even with the most aggressive chemotherapy regimens, response duration, progression-free interval, and survival are still disappointing. Intraarterial chemotherapy has considerable theoretical interest, but it has been associated with severe toxicity and its advantage over systemic chemotherapy is uncertain.

Exenterative surgery has a significant place in the management of recurrent cervical carcinoma. Most exenterations are now performed for central pelvic recurrence after radiotherapeutic treatment. In the last two decades, improvements in pre- and postoperative care and in surgical techniques have led to improved long-term survival (40 to 60%), with an associated mortality rate of 1.4 to 13.5%.

Appropriate patient selection is the most important determinant of successful outcome after exenterative surgery. A thorough search for pulmonary and liver metastases as well as for enlarged pelvic and paraaortic lymph nodes should be performed preoperatively. The absence of extrapelvic metastases should be confirmed during the first phase of the operative procedure. If tumor is found to extend to the pelvic side wall the prognosis is poor. The presence of positive pelvic lymph nodes is also known to significantly reduce long-term survival, but when the involvement of pelvic nodes is only microscopic, a 5-year survival of 23% has been reported. Despite careful patient selection, about 50% of patients explored for exenteration will be found to have extrapelvic disease or an unresectable pelvic mass. Two innovative approaches to the subgroup of patients with tumor fixed to one pelvic side wall have recently been described. The IORT (intraoperative radiation therapy) with electrons has been utilized at the Mayo Clinic in combination with maximum debulking surgery with or without external-beam therapy in patients with paraaortic or pelvic side wall recurrences. Although actuarial control within the IORT field was 80%, the distant metastasis rate at 5 years was 47%, yielding a 5-year overall survival of 33%.

The other approach to patients with tumor fixed to one pelvic side wall has been described by Hockel and Knapstein (1). The CORT (combined operative and radiotherapeutic treatment) procedure combines radical resection of sidewall disease with postoperative high-dose-rate brachytherapy to the tumor bed. With a median follow up of 24 months (range, 5 to 48 months), the authors reported 7 of 18 patients who remained free of disease. Recurrent tumor size but not relapse location was the only prognostic factor influencing survival in the multivariate analysis. Although the data are preliminary, this novel approach deserves further study.

Reference

1. Hockel M, Knapstein PG. The combined operative and radiotherapeutic treatment (CORT) (abstr). Gynecol Oncol 1992; 45:79.

53

Central Recurrence of Advanced Cervical Cancer 10 Months Following Surgery and Radiation Therapy

CASE

A 42-year-old woman is found to have a stage IB carcinoma of the cervix. She is treated with a radical hysterectomy and pelvic lymphadenectomy, followed by 5000 rads of whole-pelvis radiation therapy and two cesium implants. Ten months following treatment, a 4-cm mass is found at the apex of the vagina, fixed to the base of the bladder. Computed tomography (CT) reveals no nodal involvement and there is no evidence of metastatic disease. A chest x-ray is negative. The patient remains asymptomatic and she has an excellent performance status.

PHYSICIANS' RESPONSE

TALLY LEVY
ROBERT GIRTANNER
ALAN KAPLAN

The initial treatment of cervical cancer offers by far the best chance for cure. Surgery and radiation therapy are equally effective treatment methods. Stage IB lesions can usually be managed by radical hysterectomy; however, many recommend postoperative pelvic radiation for patients with microscopic parametrial invasion, lymph node metastases, and positive or close surgical margins. Although the benefit in terms of increased survival has not been clearly demonstrated, the local recurrence rate is probably decreased by the addition of post-

414

operative pelvic radiation. In the present case, since the pathology results from the primary surgery are not available, we need to assume that the presence of more extensive disease was the reason for the adjuvant radiotherapy.

Recurrent disease can be expected in 10 to 20% of patients with stage IB lesions. Some 50 to 60% of these will be seen in the first year following primary treatment. Early detection of local recurrence and accurate assessment of disease extent are imperative, since pelvic exenteration offers a potential cure in selected cases. In this patient, a 4-cm mass was found at the apex of the vagina 10 months following treatment. Histological evaluation of this mass is obviously the first diagnostic step, and since the mass is palpable, a manually guided biopsy using the Tru-cut needle (1) or a biopsy forceps can be done. Another option is to perform a CT- or ultrasound-guided biopsy of the mass.

Curative therapeutic options for recurrent cervical cancer following surgery and radiation are limited. Reirradiation of previously radiated patients is reserved for very selected cases with unresectable but not bulky disease that recur 5 or more years after initial therapy. Although some tissue repair has taken place over these years, previously radiated areas do not have optimal tolerance and the morbidity of this treatment is high.

Exenterative surgery is considered the standard therapy for recurrent post-radiation disease confined to the central pelvis. This radical therapy is justified because it offers cure to more than 60% of patients who fulfill the criteria for resection (2). Moreover, improvements in anesthesia, surgical techniques, and postoperative care have reduced the operative mortality to less than 5%. Immediate and long-term morbidity have also been significantly reduced; however, complications do continue to occur in approximately 40 to 50% of patients. These complications usually involve the urinary or gastrointestinal tract. In addition, major improvements in surgical techniques involving the reconstructive phase of the operation have greatly improved quality of life for these patients and have consequently greatly increased patient acceptance. There are now options regarding urinary diversion. Contingent upon the patient's preference and her ability to care for herself, we construct either a noncontinent urinary conduit or a continent urinary reservoir. The most significant benefit of a properly functioning reservoir is the avoidance of a urinary drainage appliance, resulting in better satisfaction and improved self-esteem. We prefer to use the Miami pouch method (3), in which a segment of the ascending and transverse colon and 10 cm of the distal ileum are used. Detubularization of the right colon allows construction of a large-capacity, low-pressure reservoir of nonradiated bowel, while better continence is achieved by reinforcing the ileocecal segment with three circumferential sutures and tapering the distal ileum. The EEA stapler gives us the capability of performing a low colonic anastomosis and maintaining colonic continuity rather than performing a colostomy, when it is necessary to remove the rectum but the perineal phase of the resection is not necessary. When the perineal phase is necessary and the entire vagina is removed, vaginal reconstruction is performed utilizing full-thickness musculocutaneous flaps with either the gracilis muscle from the medial thigh or the rectus abdominis muscle from the anterior abdominal wall. This technique also fills in the defect in the levator diaphragm from the surgical excision.

The present patient is a young, asymptomatic woman with an excellent performance status. The metastatic workup included a chest x-ray and abdominal and pelvic CT scan, which revealed no nodal or metastatic disease. Although the pelvic examination is important to the preoperative assessment of tumor resectability, radiation fibrosis can cause immobility, and even radiological evaluation by CT scan or magnetic resonance imaging (MRI) (4) is not reliable for distinguishing tumor invasion from radiation changes involving the pelvic side walls. Consequently, when the disease seems to be locally unresectable based on the pelvic examination, if other factors are favorable, the final decision regarding resectability should be made at the time of laparotomy. At surgery, careful exploration of the abdomen and pelvis should be done for any evidence of intraperitoneal or extrapelvic disease. The lower aortic lymph nodes should be sampled first, followed by pelvic node dissection and evaluation of tumor resectability. Pelvic exenteration has a questionable role if the pelvic nodes contain metastatic tumor, as only a few of these patients can be cured. If the lesion is deemed resectable, the operation is individualized on the basis of the distribution of the disease and the patient's desires. In this patient, unless more extensive disease is noted at laparotomy, an anterior exenteration without a perineal phase would probably represent adequate surgical therapy. Because of the patient's young age and performance status, a continent urinary reservoir would be the urinary diversion of choice.

References

1. Lopez MJ, Kraybill WG, Fuchs GJ, et al. Transvaginal parametrial needle biopsy for detection of postirradiation recurrent cancer of the cervix. Cancer 1988; 61:275–278.
2. Averette H, Lichtinger M, Sevin BU, Girtanner RE. Pelvic exenteration: A 15-year experience in a general metropolitan hospital. Am J Obstet Gynecol 1984; 150:179–183.
3. Penalver M, Donato D, Sevin BU, et al. Complications of the ileocolonic continent reservoir (Miami pouch). Gynecol Oncol 1994; 52:360–364.
4. Popovich MJ, Hricak H, Sugimura K, Stern JL. The role of MR imaging in determining surgical eligibility for pelvic exenteration. AJR 1993; 160:525–531.

PHYSICIAN'S RESPONSE

JOANNA M. CAIN

This patient must be presumed to have recurrent squamous cell carcinoma. While not stated in the case, the first step is to document that the mass at the vaginal apex is recurrent cervical carcinoma and not an unexpected new malignancy. Furthermore, from the case presentation, we would have to assume that there were high-risk factors present that led to radiation following radical hysterectomy and lymph node dissection. The details of the previous pathology must be examined to determine if the metastatic workup is adequate. For example, if the cell type was glassy cell and the lymph nodes were positive, a more detailed evaluation of the chest lymphatic structures would be called for before deciding on a course of treatment. If no paraaortic lymph nodes were sampled and this area was not treated, then paraaortic node dissection should be part of the treatment plan. There is no substitute for accurate data and pathology review before further planning proceeds.

Assuming that all the initial evaluation suggests a limited recurrence involving the apex of the vagina and the base of the bladder, the next step required is careful counseling of the patient for a presumed anterior exenteration. At this point, it is unclear whether continent urinary diversion and vaginal sparing (without reconstruction) is a possibility. Therefore, counseling includes much more than simple explanation of survival statistics and the potential risks of such surgery. Counseling must explore the patient's self-image and the changes that could potentially occur in that self-image with stomas—whether a urinary conduit or continent nipple is present. Furthermore, while it is rarely uppermost in a patient's mind at the time recurrent cancer is encountered, the initial opening of issues of sexuality with recurrence and surgical revision of anatomy needs to be opened. In particular, the facts that the vaginal length will be shortened or the sensation altered by a graft along with reassurance that there are ways to address these changes functionally need to be presented. Frequently, this counseling is best done over two sessions and with nurse oncologist involvement and support rather than in one exhausting session. The impact of different counseling styles and methods has never been directly studied, but it is axiomatic that any patient can hear and process only small portions of these data at any one time, particularly when the issue of survival is raised.

The approach to surgical resection needs to be carefully crafted. Clearly the two basic axioms are that surgery should have the potential of affecting overall survival and that conservation of as normal functional anatomy as possible be the result. The first issue in any such surgery is to address the potential areas for silent metastatic disease—for example, paraaortic node dissection or liver evaluation intraoperatively. In the presence of positive findings, management of the central lesion should not go forward if no appropriate therapy exists for the metastatic lesion that is identified. Some lesions, however, might have reasonable therapies available (radiation for paraaortic metastases with no prior radiation), and this critical decision making is done intraoperatively.

From this presentation we assume that the minimal surgery required will be the removal of the urinary bladder and the apex of the vagina. Depending on the length of the vagina following resection, further reconstruction may not be necessary. If further reconstruction is necessary, then myocutaneous flaps (gracilis, rectus, free flaps) can both substantially improve the healing and allow for a potentially functional vagina. The type of urinary conduit chosen is dependent on the status of the bowel. For example, severely radiation-damaged small and large bowel may compromise the variety of continent urinary conduits, so that ileal or small bowel conduit is the only choice. This decision again requires the experience of the surgeon at the time of operation. Extension of the operation beyond this scope should not be done if the margins are surgically free.

Finally, while this patient should be expected to recover well from this surgery, the psychological recovery may be much delayed beyond physiological recovery. Close and continual evaluation for depression and coping problems should be an expected part of the follow-up of this patient.

PHYSICIAN'S RESPONSE

MICHAEL HOPKINS

This patient underwent radical hysterectomy and afterwards received pelvic radiotherapy. I presume, therefore, that she had some high-risk feature, either positive lymph nodes with deep stromal invasion or microscopic positive margins. She now presumably has a central recurrence of disease after maximum treatment, including radical hysterectomy and radiotherapy.

A biopsy of the pelvic mass needs to be done to confirm the clinical impression that this is recurrent squamous cell carcinoma. An evaluation should then be done consisting of a chest x-ray and CT scan to rule out metastatic disease either to the lungs or to the pelvic and periaortic lymph nodes. If a lymphangiogram is available, this can also be done to evaluate for nodal disease. If the metastatic evaluation is negative and the patient agrees, she should be counseled and the recommendation made for a pelvic exenteration. This is the only salvage therapy available that can be performed with a curative intent. Chemotherapy in this situation would be only palliative. The patient needs to be counseled preoperatively concerning the extent of the operation, i.e., removal of bladder, rectum, and vagina. Sexual function and her desire for vaginal reconstruction must be covered prior to surgery. At the time of surgery, if any metastatic disease is encountered, the pelvic exenteration should be aborted.

In a central recurrence, after radiotherapy, usually the bladder and a portion of the rectum need to be removed, as the mass will be adherent onto both bladder and rectum. When the cervix is present, either an anterior or a posterior exenteration is sometimes appropriate, as the uterus and cervix will separate the two structures, allowing for a disease-free margin. When the cervix and uterus are absent, however, the upper vaginal recurrence tends to expand in both directions and involves both the bladder and the rectum. Thus, I would plan for a total pelvic exenteration as my initial treatment and as the best approach to completely control the malignancy. A continent conduit could be constructed and possibly a rectal reconstruction could be done based on the findings at the time of surgery.

In the selected patient population with squamous cell carcinoma, when exenteration is performed only if there is no evidence for metastatic disease, the survival can be as high as 70%. Unfortunately, the survival is decreased with an early recurrence. Recurrence within 1 year of initial treatment portends a poorer prognosis. An ultraaggressive but prudent approach is necessary to try and salvage the life of this patient.

PHYSICIANS' RESPONSE

WATSON G. WATRING
NEAL SEMRAD

In general, patients with stage IB carcinoma of the cervix are treated with radical surgery *or* radical radiation. One must assume that some poor prognostic findings were noted on this patient's final pathology that dictated, essentially, complete retreatment of the area. Despite this extensive treatment, her tumor had regrown to a 4-cm mass within 10 months.

The prognosis for 5-year survival/"cure" with stage IB cervix carcinoma is approximately 80% with either radical surgery or radical radiation. The rationale for surgery is to retain ovarian function without reducing cure rates in smaller lesions. It is clear, regardless of its initial size, that this patient's tumor is behaving in a very aggressive fashion.

There is no effective chemotherapy for recurrent/persistent cervical carcinoma. Minimally effective palliative chemotherapy, such as cisplatin, should be reserved to treat symptomatic patients. Due to its toxic and quality-of-life–reducing side effects, chemotherapy would not be helpful at this time.

This patient needs to be explored for possible exenterative surgery—most likely an anterior or total exenteration. Depending upon her findings at surgery, her treatment would most likely entail an anterior exenteration with Indiana pouch and neovagina construction. With this treatment, an approximately 40% chance for 5-year survival will be obtained (1,2).

If the patient is found to be inoperable at surgery, consideration for chemotherapy and/or hospice referral would be appropriate.

References

1. Robertson, Lopes, Beynon, Monaghan. Pelvic exenteration: A review of the Gateshead experience, 1974–1992. Br J Obstet Gynecol 1994; 101:529–531.
2. Lopez, Standiford, Skibba. Total pelvic exenteration: A 50 year experience at the LS Fischel Cancer Center. Arch Surg 1994; 129:390–395.

54

Locally Advanced Cervical Cancer in a Woman Who Is HIV-Positive

CASE

A 33-year-old woman is found to have a 1.5-cm squamous cell carcinoma of the cervix. The patient is 5 ft, 4 in tall and weighs 160 lb. Past medical history is significant for her being positive for human immunodeficiency virus (HIV). Despite this history, the patient has a good performance status and has not had any opportunistic infections. Evaluation for the presence of metastatic disease is negative.

PHYSICIANS' RESPONSE

BRADLEY J. MONK
MICHAEL L. BERMAN

This patient has a Fédération Internationale de Gynécologie et d'Obstétrique (FIGO) stage IB squamous cell carcinoma of the cervix. Traditionally, these patients have been treated with equal efficacy using either radical hysterectomy and pelvic lymphadenectomy or external-beam irradiation with brachytherapy. The choice between these two options is usually based upon the age and medical status of the patient, body habitus, and tumor size as well as patient and physician biases. Patients should be counseled regarding the risks and benefits of either modality. Surgery is generally associated with some degree of impaired bladder function but less sexual dysfunction. The risk of fistulas is comparable between both choices; however, when they occur following radiotherapy, they tend to be much more difficult to manage successfully than following surgery. Finally, many patients choose surgery over radiotherapy because of the ability to preserve ovarian function and because of the important prognostic information concerning lymphatic spread that can be determined at surgery. In a young, otherwise healthy 33-year-old patient with $1^1/_2$ cm squamous cell lesion, most gynecological oncologists would recommend a radical hysterectomy and pelvic lymphadenectomy with ovarian preservation; however, this patient's body habitus and HIV status can influence this decision.

Although this woman is not morbidly obese, her weight puts her at increased risk of increased blood loss and operative time. Nevertheless, radical hysterectomy in moderately obese women such as this patient is technically feasible and does not compromise outcome. If she were morbidly obese, however, the additional risk of operative and postoperative complications and the technical difficulties that might impair the surgeon's ability to achieve wide lateral clearance of the tumor would warrant a choice of radiotherapy over surgery.

Women with HIV infection represent a small but growing subset of patients with cervical carcinoma. Preliminary data suggest that this human papillomavirus–associated malignancy is more aggressive and carries a worse prognosis in the immunocompromised patient. Among HIV-infected women, the response to treatment and probability of cervical cancer eradication correlates with mean CD4 counts, CD4:CD8 ratios, and the percentage of CD4 cells. Moreover, among those HIV-infected patients with relatively good immune function, surgery can be performed with low risk of infectious complications. Since positive serostatus for HIV alone does not uniformly confer an unfavorable outcome, patients with initially adequate immune status may do well following therapy for cervical cancer. Finally, the impact of antiviral therapy on the survival of patients with cervical carcinoma is currently under study.

Although the CD4 status is not reported in this brief case history, the lack of opportunistic infections suggests that this patient's immune system is relatively intact. Accordingly, treatment recommendations should be similar to those for an HIV-negative patient of similar stage. Nevertheless, her immune status should be studied, and if severe immunocompromise is documented, I would favor primary radiotherapy. Although a radiotherapeutic approach would also limit exposure of HIV-infected body fluid to hospital personnel, clinical judgment in conjunction with the patient's preference should override this consideration during treatment planning.

The risk and benefits of adjuvant radiotherapy following radical hysterectomy among HIV-infected patients with cervical carcinoma have not been studied. Therefore I would not deviate from my standard practice of prescribing 5040 cGy whole pelvic external-beam irradiation if histopathological evaluation of the specimen revealed outer one-third involvement of the cervical stroma, occult parametrial extension, or at least one positive lymph node metastasis.

References

Maiman M, Fruchter RG, Guy L, et al. Human immunodeficiency virus infection and invasive cervical carcinoma. Cancer 1993; 71:402–406.

Monk BJ, Cha DS, Walker JL, et al. Extent of disease as an indication for pelvic radiation following radical hysterectomy and bilateral pelvic lymph node dissection in the treatment of stage I-B and II-A cervical carcinoma. Gynecol Oncol 1994; 54:4–9.

PHYSICIAN'S RESPONSE

ALEXANDER W. KENNEDY

The most critical information in advising this patient about her cervical cancer and the therapeutic options available to her is that her performance status is good and that she has not experienced any opportunistic infections. This information is more important than any arbitrary CD4 cutoff level, although this will probably be above 300 cells per microliter. Given this information, it can be assumed that her life expectancy is substantial and that this is not merely a palliative situation.

The decision to be made, therefore, is between definitive radiotherapy versus radical surgery. While there are certainly institutional biases, most gynecological oncologists would ordinarily advise radical hysterectomy with pelvic lymph node dissection as the preferred management of a small cervical carcinoma in a young patient. I would advise treating this patient as one would despite her positive HIV status and would therefore favor radical surgery to treat her cervical cancer.

Her weight is approximately 15% above ideal, and this does increase her risk of complications. Based upon a review of our own experience (1), patients greater than 80 kg undergoing radical hysterectomy for cervical cancer can be expected to require intraoperative transfusion more often than nonobese patients, and their operative time is approximately 20 min longer. Their risk of postoperative complications as well as their long-term outcome are not substantially different from those of other patients.

Two remaining issues are blood availability for transfusion and protection for the operative personnel. Our blood bank would prefer to deal with allogeneic blood donation in this setting instead of autologous donation of known contaminated blood. Their advice is based upon the risks of handling possibly versus certainly contaminated blood. The operative team must strictly adhere to universal precautions including double gloving and handling of sharp instruments. Her postoperative care and subsequent gynecological follow-up would not be affected by her HIV status. Her long-term survival will probably be determined more by the course of her HIV infection than by that of her cervical cancer. With proper precautions, her therapeutic options should not be limited by her HIV status.

Reference

1. Kennedy AW, Peterson GL, Belinson JL, et al. Recent trends in the surgical management of cervical cancer. Cleve Clin J Med 1995; 62:in press.

PHYSICIAN'S RESPONSE

A. ROBERT KAGAN

The presence of the HIV virus and a cancer of the cervix establishes an *acquired immune deficiency illness* for this patient, with a 5-year survival of 20 to 30%. The absence of opportunistic infections enables me to *assume* a CD4 lymphocyte count above 200. I will assume this is an exophytic (noninfiltrative, nonbarrel) cancer *and* that a CT of the retroperitoneal lymph nodes, complete blood count, and chest roentgenogram are normal. Commonly, a discussion of an operative procedure versus radiation therapy would occur for a 1.5-cm lesion in a 33-year-old patient. However, the added problems to the operating room personnel because the patient is HIV-positive would press me to recommend radiation therapy.

Although initially I expected *increased gut reactions* to irradiation as seen in the oral cavity for Kaposi's sarcoma and/or lymphoma in the patient with acquired immunodeficiency syndrome (AIDS), this expected severe visceral morbidity has *not* occurred in my experience with HIV-positive patients irradiated for cancer of the cervix and/or anal canal.

My irradiation management would be similar to that of a non-AIDS patient, 5000 cGy external-beam irradiation and either 2100 cGy high-dose-rate (preferred) or 2500 cGy low-dose-rate rads to point A. I would not modify my treatment because of the reported increased aggressiveness of cancer in the AIDS patient.

PHYSICIAN'S RESPONSE

WILLIAM J. HOSKINS

This patient has an apparent stage IB squamous cell carcinoma of the cervix. Although most gynecological oncologists would recommend radical hysterectomy and bilateral pelvic lymphadenectomy, the patient can be treated with either radical hysterectomy and pelvic lymphadenectomy or radical radiotherapy with comparable cure rates. This patient is an ideal surgical candidate in that she is young and not obese.

By definition, a woman who is HIV-positive and develops cervical cancer has AIDS. There is clear evidence that cervical cancer, like Kaposi's sarcoma, *Pneumocystis carinii* pneumonia, and pulmonary tuberculosis, indicates a level of immunocompromise that allows the diagnosis of AIDS.

While the diagnosis of AIDS indicates an increased risk of infectious complications following radical surgery, this increase in risk is not sufficient to contraindicate radical pelvic surgery. Although there is some increased risk to health care workers and, in particular, the surgical and anesthesia team because of the patient's HIV infection, this also is not of sufficient magnitude to contraindicate radical hysterectomy and pelvic lymphadenectomy. There is ample evidence that by practicing universal precautions, the risk to health care workers is minimal.

In counseling this patient regarding her options for therapy, it is important that she be informed that the cure rate and major complication rate for the treatment of early invasive cervical cancer is similar using either radical hysterectomy and pelvic lymphadenectomy or radical pelvic irradiation using a combination of whole-pelvis teletherapy and intracavitary brachytherapy. The treatment interval for surgery is shorter and ovarian function can be preserved. It is likely that vaginal function will be more normal following surgical treatment.

There is no known contraindication to pelvic irradiation in patients with AIDS. Although increased radiation reactions in the oral mucosa of AIDS patients have been seen in cases of head and neck cancers, this increased mucosal reaction has not been documented in patients receiving pelvic irradiation.

In summary, this patient has a small, apparently early cervical cancer. There are no contraindications to either surgical therapy with radical hysterectomy and pelvic lymphadenectomy or radical radiotherapy with whole abdominal irradiation in patients with AIDS. Treatment should be carried out according to the wishes of the patient after appropriate counseling. Universal precautions as recommended by the Centers for Disease Control to prevent infection of health care workers should be observed.

References

Hoskins WJ, Ford JH, Lutz MH, Averette HE. Radical hysterectomy and pelvic lymphadenectomy for the management of early invasive carcinoma of the cervix. Gynecol Oncol 1976; 4:278–290.

Perez CA, Camel HM, Walz BJ, et al. Radiation therapy alone in the treatment of carcinoma of the uterine cervix: A 20-year experience. Gynecol Oncol 1986; 23:127–140.

Pluda JM, Brawley OW, Broder S. AIDS and women. In: Hoskins WJ, Perez CA, Young RC, eds. Principles and Practice of Gynecologic Oncology. Philadelphia: Lippincott, 1992:485–506.

PHYSICIAN'S RESPONSE

DAVID MOORE

Based on current Centers for Disease Control definitions, a woman with human immunodeficiency virus infection and invasive cervical carcinoma has acquired immunodeficiency syndrome (AIDS). Although this patient has not manifested any opportunistic infections to date, I would recommend a CD4 count and consultation with an AIDS or infectious disease clinic. A CD4 count $\leq 500/mm^3$ would be an indication for AZT (zidovudine) therapy and portend a poorer prognosis in the treatment of her cervical cancer.

Women with cervical carcinoma who also have HIV tend to do worse than their HIV-negative counterparts, primarily because they tend to present with high-grade, more advanced-stage cancers. Such women with cervical carcinoma usually die from cervical cancer before they die from other AIDS-related complications and should be considered for aggressive antitumor therapy.

The ethical obligation in the care of this patient is best stated by the American College of Obstetricians and Gynecologists: "Seropositivity for HIV should not be a barrier to health care for women. Medical care should be provided to persons in need without regard to the circumstances of infection." This patient has FIGO stage IB1 squamous cell carcinoma of the cervix with a small (1.5-cm) lesion and no evidence of metastatic disease on clinical evaluation. Unless computed tomography has already been performed, I would not recommend it, because the diagnostic yield of CT in early-stage cervical cancer is exceedingly low. Her cancer is amenable to either surgical or radiation therapy. There are no data documenting clear superiority of either treatment from the perspective of overall survival, so I would present both options to the patient and let her choose which treatment she would rather undertake. Should she choose surgery, the number of operating room personnel should be kept to a minimum. I would perform the radical hysterectomy and pelvic lymphadenectomy myself. I work at an academic medical center and teach gynecological surgery to ob/gyn residents, but I feel that it would be unwise to allow an inexperienced surgeon to practice operative technique on a case such as this. According to the series reported by Maiman and colleagues, HIV-seropositive patients with good immune function tolerate elective surgery quite well, seemingly without an increased incidence of postoperative infectious or other complications. Interestingly, three of the four patients Maiman explored for planned radical hysterectomy proved to have more advanced disease and received adjunctive radiation therapy.

References

ACOG Committee on Ethics. Human Immunodeficiency Virus Infection: Physicians' Responsibilities. Committee opinion #130. Washington, DC, American College of Obstetricians and Gynecologists, 1993.

Maiman M, Fruchter RG, Guy L, et al. Human immunodeficiency virus infection and invasive cervical carcinoma. Cancer 1993; 71:402–406.

Telford GL. Contracting AIDS and other blood-borne diseases in the OR. Surg Rounds 1987; 10:30–37.

55

Locally Advanced Cervical Cancer in a Woman with a History of Scleroderma Who Refuses Blood Products

CASE

A 43-year-old moderately obese female is found to have a 3-cm stage IB carcinoma of the cervix. The patient refuses blood products due to her religious beliefs. Physical examination is unremarkable except for the above-noted findings. Radiographic and laboratory evaluation reveals no evidence of metastatic disease. Past medical history is significant for a 10-year history of scleroderma.

PHYSICIANS' RESPONSE

PAMELA J. CARNEY
LINDA F. CARSON

The gynecological literature cites comparable survival rates with both radiotherapy and radical surgery in treating patients with Fédération Internationale de Gynécologie et d'Obstétrique (FIGO) stage IB cervical carcinoma. As such, the decision to select one modality over the other rests on clinical judgment. The physician must take into consideration the patient's overall fitness, any prior history of radiation therapy, concomitant medical illnesses that preclude either surgery or radiation therapy, and, not least, patient preference, including the desire for preserved ovarian and vaginal function.

At presentation, every patient with invasive cervical carcinoma should

426

undergo a thorough clinical, laboratory, and radiographic workup in accordance with FIGO guidelines. Complementary examination techniques, such as computed tomography (CT) or magnetic resonance imaging (MRI), are advisable in this case to search for evidence of extrapelvic spread of disease. Although CT and MRI are not considered in assigning stage in cervical carcinoma, when selectively carried out, these tests can play a valuable role in guiding therapy.

The physician's next task is to weigh the risks and benefits of radiotherapy versus radical surgery and assimilate a therapeutic plan that minimizes morbidity in accordance with each patient's unique circumstance.

This particular woman has a history of scleroderma. Cancer patients with co-existent collagen vascular disease may be at greater risk for complications attendant to radiation therapy than women in the general population. While there are, as yet, no prospective data addressing this question, a number of recent reports in the literature suggest that this may be a valid concern, particularly in those cases where radiation dosages are given with curative intent. These reports vary from complications of severe progressive skin fibrosis to fatal sequelae of bowel perforation in patients receiving standard pelvic radiotherapy doses (1). Alarming reports such as these serve to discourage the use of radiation therapy in a patient with scleroderma when an alternative, equally effective treatment exists.

On the other hand, in contemplating radical surgery, this woman's religious convictions raise valid concerns as well. A patient's refusal to accept a blood transfusion, even in the face of death, presents the physician with a myriad of complex ethical and medicolegal issues. Physicians must accept and respect the patient's autonomy over a sense of duty to do what they feel may be in the best interest of that individual if a situation of life-threatening anemia evolves.

Throughout history, both medical ethicists and our legal system have invariably upheld the patient's right to refuse blood transfusion on the basis of religion. Therefore, in agreeing to provide care for such a person, the physician is obligated to conform with that individual's wishes and thus to avail himself or herself of all possible strategies to avoid life-threatening anemia. The physician must also recognize that even short of transfusion, certain alternative therapies may also be unacceptable within the framework of the patient's beliefs. Preoperative strategies to be considered include the use of erythropoietin or iron therapy as well as nutritional support to bolster hematological reserve. Intraoperatively, crystalloid and colloid should be used judiciously to support intravascular volume. Additionally, the surgeon must pursue meticulous attention to hemostasis. Consideration of the use of red cell salvaging devices, hemodilution, and antifibrinolytic agents such as apoprotein and desmopressin may also be appropriate. Postoperatively, strategies would again include the use of agents to maximize blood production as well as minimizing iatrogenic contributions to anemia by prudent limitation of phlebotomies. Pharmacological agents that might potentially initiate unanticipated hemolytic cascades should also be avoided.

A recent report from investigators at Memorial Sloan Kettering Cancer Center compared perioperative blood transfusion in women undergoing radical hysterectomy in time periods before and after the discovery of transfusion-related HIV infection. This group found that patients undergoing radical hysterectomy, after the knowledge of the risks of HIV transmission, received markedly fewer units of blood than individuals operated on prior to this awareness (0.62 versus 3.5 units). Correspondingly, the women in the more recent period had significantly lower intraoperative blood loss. Additionally, the more current group of participants had a significantly shorter postoperative stay and were discharged with significantly lower mean hemoglobin levels, without any detectable adverse effects on postoperative recovery. This report suggests that simply a heightened concern for risks associated with blood transfusion has played a notable role in decreasing intraoperative blood loss and frequency of blood transfusion in a gynecological oncology population of patients (2).

In summary, the patient described should be counseled objectively as to the potential risks of radiation therapy, including damage to surrounding normal tissues likely affecting vaginal function. In addition, the potential increased risk in women with connective tissue diseases should be discussed. Radical surgical therapy need not be discouraged based on the patient's religious philosophy provided that she accepts a very small risk of surgical mortality due to exsanguination. I would recommend she undergo radical hysterectomy, bilateral salpingo-oophorectomy, and pelvic and periaortic lymphadenectomies.

References

1. Olivotto IA, Fairey RN, Gillies JH, Stein H. Fatal outcome of pelvic radiotherapy for carcinoma of the cervix in a patient with systemic lupus erythematosus. Clin Oncol 1989; 40:83–84.
2. Benjamin I, Barakat RR, Curtin JP, et al. Blood transfusion for radical hysterectomy before and after the discovery of transfusion-related human immunodeficiency virus infection. Obstet Gynecol 1994; 84:974–978.

PHYSICIANS' RESPONSE

SUSAN K. GIBBONS
HENRY KEYS

A 3-cm stage IB cervical cancer can be treated with equal efficacy using either primary radiotherapy or radical hysterectomy. The choice of therapy must be individualized for each patient, with consideration of the patient's eligibility for either treatment modality and her willingness to accept the risk associated with each.

This case brings up two important issues that must be carefully considered in the management of this patient's disease. The first is her religious objection to the transfusion of blood products. Most gynecological surgeons would be uncomfortable undertaking radical surgery without the availability of transfusable blood, especially in a moderately obese female, where limited exposure may make bleeding a bit more difficult to control. The patient may not have the same objections to autotransfusion (assuming that her initial hemoglobin level is adequate), but this may delay surgery. If her presenting hemoglobin level is low, the situation is even more complicated, regardless of the treatment modality used. Hemoglobin levels less than about 10 g/dL have been shown to be associated with compromised outcomes in cervical cancer patients treated with primary radiotherapy, and such patients are usually transfused up to an adequate hemoglobin level prior to the start of pelvic irradiation. Radical surgery with no option of transfusion would obviously be most risky in a patient who is already anemic.

The second issue that must be addressed is the patient's diagnosis of scleroderma. There have been many reports of marked cutaneous and subcutaneous fibrosis following radiotherapy in patients with scleroderma and other connective tissue diseases. Some of the reported patients have had stable connective tissue disease at the time of radiotherapy, with reactivation and severe fibrosis afterward. There are rare reports of visceral encasement due to fibrosis of the bowel or esophagus. Many radiotherapists consider scleroderma to be an absolute contraindication to irradiation if a reasonable alternative treatment exists.

Most importantly, all of the above risks must be discussed thoroughly with the patient, and she must understand the importance of undergoing some sort of curative treatment. If the patient and gynecological surgeon can come to some agreement regarding autotransfusion or avoidance of transfusion, radical hysterectomy would be the preferred treatment alternative. If such an agreement cannot be reached, less conventional alternatives should be considered, such as low-dose irradiation and extrafascial hysterectomy.

References

Abu-Shakra M, Lee P. Exaggerated fibrosis in patients with systemic sclerosis (scleroderma) following radiation therapy. J Rheumatol 1993; 20:1601–1603.

Robertson JM, Clarke DH, Pevzner MM, et al. Breast conservation therapy: Severe breast fibrosis after radiation therapy in patients with collagen vascular disease. Cancer 1991; 68:502–508.

PHYSICIANS' RESPONSE

EDWARD PODCZASKI
RODRIGUE MORTEL

Cervical cancer can be definitively treated with either radiotherapy or radical surgery consisting of radical hysterectomy and bilateral pelvic lymphadenectomy.

These two therapeutic modalities differ as to the nature of treatment, the time course of therapy, and potential complications. Although radical surgery and radiotherapy produce equivalent therapeutic results in early-stage cervical cancer, radical surgery offers a number of therapeutic advantages, especially to the premenopausal patient. Radical surgery in the young patient preserves ovarian function, precludes radiotherapy to the vagina, and avoids potential damage to the lower urinary tract and bowel, which may appear years after the completion of radiotherapy.

The patient described has systemic sclerosis (scleroderma), a generalized disorder of connective tissue characterized by fibrosis and changes in the skin, joints, muscles, and some internal organs, especially the gastrointestinal tract. Proliferative vascular changes can lead to Raynaud's phenomenon and other obliterative lesions of blood vessels. Pelvic radiotherapy to such a patient may be accompanied by a significant risk of acute and delayed morbidity due to gastrointestinal tract injury.

In the clinical situation presented, the 43-year-old woman with an early stage IB cancer of the cervix would appear to be a reasonable surgical candidate. However, the patient is moderately obese, and, more importantly, is a Jehovah's Witness. Although they accept other forms of medical care, most Jehovah's Witnesses refuse to accept blood transfusions. This prohibition usually extends to autologous blood; once physically separated from the body, blood cannot be reinfused. The average blood loss at radical hysterectomy has been quoted as from 800 to 1700 mL. However, the data of Soisson and colleagues provides the most comprehensive picture in terms of overall blood loss. Of 320 patients undergoing radical hysterectomy, 87 (27%) had a blood loss in excess of 2 L. Furthermore, obese patients were more likely to experience a greater blood loss, with 46% having a blood loss in excess of 2 L.

The decision as to mode of therapy is determined by a dialogue between the patient and physician. We feel that this patient would be best treated with radical surgery, given the risks of radiotherapy in this case. However, the refusal to accept transfusion remains a significant problem. If the patient were willing to accept the risks of surgery without transfusion, we would agree to perform such surgery. Although radiotherapy will produce equivalent therapeutic results, such treatment may be accompanied by a greater risk of gastrointestinal and urinary tract injury, given the medical history. If the patient does wish surgery, it is important to enlist the services of an anesthesiologist experienced in the care of Jehovah's Witnesses. Techniques such as hypotensive anesthesia may be clinically useful. Furthermore, many Witnesses accept the use of a cell saver for intraoperative blood salvage, since the blood is in continuous contact with the circulation. Isovolemic hemodilution has also been useful in such clinical situations. One or two units of blood are collected and the patient is fluid-expanded. The blood withdrawn remains connected to the patient by an intravenous line. Following completion of the surgical procedure, the blood is reinfused back into the patient by the same intravenous line.

References

Medsger TA. Systemic sclerosis (scleroderma), localized scleroderma, eosinophilic fasciitis, and calcinosis. In: McCarty JD, ed. *Arthritis and Allied Conditions. A Textbook of Rheumatology,* 11th ed. Philadelphia: Lea & Febiger, 1989.

Soisson AP, Soper JT, Berchuck A. et al. Radical hysterectomy in obese women. Obstet Gynecol 1992; 80:940–943.

PHYSICIAN'S RESPONSE

HUGH BARBER

The patient is reported to have a 3-cm stage IB carcinoma of the cervix. A careful history and physical are essential. Since the patient has an autoimmune disease, laboratory tests for collagen disorder to monitor the progress or stability of scleroderma are important. Certain tests should be obtained preoperatively such as an intravenous pyelogram (IVP), CT scan of the pelvis and abdomen, chest x-ray, electrocardiogram, barium enema, complete blood count and serology, carcinoembryonic antigen (CEA) and small-cell carcinoma antigen (SCCA) tumor markers.

Since the patient is moderately obese and refuses blood products, external and intrauterine plus colpostat radiation is recommended. Prior to the start of radiation therapy, the patient should be examined under anesthesia and have a fractional curettage and an official staging. Histology of the specimen may help in determining prognosis. Keratinizing carcinomas have a better prognosis than small-cell nonkeratinizing carcinomas, which generally have a poor prognosis.

It has been reported that clinical staging (FIGO) is inaccurate judged by staging at surgery. Up to 35% of the cases have been incorrectly staged—most understaged. At least 6% of stage I and IIA lesions are associated with paraaortic node metastases outside the traditional treatment fields and 10 to 20% of stage IB lesions have pelvic lymph node metastases. This information has relevance when one is consulting with the radiation therapist about establishing the radiation therapy fields.

If there is an acute flare-up of the scleroderma, cortisone therapy can be used as needed. There is no contraindication to this.

Following radiation therapy, the patient must be instructed in the use of estrogen vaginal cream so that the walls of the vagina will not agglutinate. Since a premature menopause will follow radiation therapy, a regime of estrogen plus medroxyprogesterone (Provera) is recommended.

It is ideal to follow the patient at 3-month intervals for the first year. A pelvic examination and Pap smear are carried out at each visit. The tumor markers CEA and SCCA should be ordered at 6-month intervals. Since the Pap smear is merely a screening method, any gross lesion must be biopsied. At 1 year, a careful pelvic examination, Pap smear, tumor markers CEA and SCCA, a CT scan of the pelvis and abdomen, an IVP, and a chest x-ray should be performed. An early diagnosis of persistence of disease or recurrence is as vital to obtain a good prognosis as it is in fresh cases. If everything is negative, the patient can be followed at 6-month intervals. There is no time at which it is safe to stop the follow-up regimen.

References

Barber HRK. Manual of Gynecologic Oncology, 2d ed. Philadelphia: Lippincott, 1989.

Averette HE, Jobson VW. Surgical staging: New approaches. In: Coppelson M, ed. *Gynecologic Oncology,* 2d ed. Edinburgh: Churchill Livingstone, 1992.

56

Small-Cell Carcinoma of the Cervix

CASE

A 32-year-old woman presents with mild pelvic discomfort and on pelvic examination is found to have a 3-cm cervical lesion. The tumor appears to be localized to the cervix. Biopsy reveals a small-cell carcinoma of the cervix. There is no evidence of metastatic disease on the remainder of the physical examination or on laboratory or radiographic evaluation.

PHYSICIAN'S RESPONSE

WILLIAM McGUIRE

Small-cell cervical carcinomas, like their counterparts in the lung, are systemic diseases at the time of presentation in the vast majority of cases. Thus, some form of systemic therapy is mandatory as part of the treatment regimen. Due to their rarity, there are no large series regarding management of these tumors. In one series, 3 of 26 patients treated with various modalities and presenting with various stages of disease were alive and disease-free 2 to 8 years following diagnosis, while in another series only 1 of 14 patients is alive at the second posttreatment year.

In this patient, at a minimum, there should be a hysterectomy and staging of regional lymph nodes. A Wertheim hysterectomy may not be necessary, since this is a systemic disease and the more radical hysterectomy does not deal with this problem. Radiation therapy has often been used postoperatively in such patients, but logically and biologically it would seem to be indicated only in those patients with obvious and bulky nodal disease in the pelvis and lower periaortic region.

433

Since most patients with this disease die of systemic manifestations, some form of systemic therapy is appropriate even in patients with disease localized to the cervix after a surgical staging evaluation. This is due to the fact that many patients with stage I disease develop recurrence following both surgery and radiation therapy. There are multiple reports in the literature of small-cell carcinoma of the cervix responding to regimens similar to those used to treat small-cell carcinoma of the lung. The two most commonly used regimens include platinum and etoposide, with platinum given in a dose of 75 to 100 mg/m^2 and etoposide at a dose of 100 mg/m^2 for 3 consecutive days. The alternative is a regimen consisting of cytoxan, doxorubicin (Adriamycin), and vincristine, with cytoxan at a dose of 500 mg/m^2, Adriamycin at 50 mg/m^2, and vincristine at 2 mg.

Thus, for this patient I would recommend an immediate exploratory laparotomy, simple hysterectomy, and sampling of pelvic and possible periaortic nodes. Depending on the results of this staging procedure, the patient could receive radiation therapy to bulky nodal disease that was unappreciated on prestaging evaluation, followed by or preceded by chemotherapy. If there is no evidence of extrauterine disease in the pelvis, the patient should be started immediately on one of the two above cytotoxic regimens, preferably platinum and etoposide, for a total of six cycles. Follow-up should be vigorous during the first 2 years, when most relapses occur. Unfortunately, patients with relapsing disease are typically refractory to additional therapy and expire shortly following relapse.

PHYSICIAN'S RESPONSE

TATE THIGPEN

This patient presents with a limited-stage carcinoma of the cervix, stage IB, which is distinguished by the histology: small-cell carcinoma. Although some have attempted to draw distinctions between pulmonary small-cell carcinomas and those occurring at extrapulmonary sites such as the cervix, (1) the majority of studies point to similarities in clinical course, response to therapy, and markers (2–6). For these reasons, the approach to management of such patients resembles the treatment of small-cell carcinoma of the lung more than the treatment of squamous cell carcinoma of the cervix, the most common histology found in cancer of the cervix.

Although this particular patient has limited small-cell carcinoma of the cervix, initial treatment should consist of chemotherapy. In general, combination chemotherapy is preferred to single agents because multiagent regimens yield better results in pulmonary small-cell carcinoma. The two most commonly employed regimens are CAV (cyclophosphamide 1000 mg/m^2, doxorubicin 50 mg/m^2, and vincristine 1.4 mg/m^2, to a maximum of 2 mg every 3 weeks) and PE (cisplatin 100 mg/m^2 on day 1 plus etoposide 100 mg/m^2 on days 1 to 3 every

3 weeks). The patient should receive four cycles of chemotherapy followed by radiation therapy (both external plus intracavitary) with cisplatin plus etoposide, which are less likely to produce problems during radiation than the doxorubicin-containing regimen. If the patient is a clear responder to chemotherapy and still has residual disease after completion of radiation, an additional four cycles of chemotherapy should be considered.

Certain additional questions should also be considered. Should the patient receive prophylactic cranial radiation if she achieves a complete response? Although no data support the use of prophylactic cranial radiation in small-cell carcinoma of the cervix, this approach has been recommended for patients with limited small-cell carcinoma of the lung who achieve a complete remission. Even in small-cell carcinoma of the lung, the issue remains controversial. Although prophylactic cranial radiation can reduce the incidence of brain metastases from 25 to 5%, its administration to the 75% who do not require it can result in significant sequelae, such as memory impairment. Survival, furthermore, is not improved. Until further evidence supporting the use of prophylactic cranial radiation is presented, this approach should not be a part of the management.

A second question to consider concerns the appropriate approach to management if the patient fails to respond to initial chemotherapy. Because the response to second-line chemotherapy, usually consisting of those drugs not employed in the initial combination, is relatively low, treatment of the local disease should be undertaken, preferably with radiation, although surgical resection is an option. Whether to give second-line chemotherapy as an adjuvant in those in whom the limited disease can be controlled or to await recurrence before giving further systemic therapy is not clear; but four cycles of the alternate combination (CAV) is a reasonable option, which should be employed.

A third question is whether treatment of the local lesion with either surgery or radiation followed by chemotherapy is an acceptable alternative. Anecdotal data support the efficacy of such an approach, (6) but initial chemotherapy is considered to be preferable.

In summary, the patient should receive four cycles of cisplatin plus etoposide followed by radiation therapy. The response rate to chemotherapy should exceed 50%, and the majority of patients will have no evidence of disease at the conclusion of radiation therapy. No further treatment is indicated for those with no evidence of disease. The long-term survival rate for such stage IB patients is not clear but should exceed 25%.

References

1. Chen C, Wu C, Juang G, et al. Serum neuron-specific enolase levels in patients with small cell carcinoma of the uterine cervix. J Formosan Med Assoc 1994; 93:81–83.
2. Lore G, Canzonieri V, Veronesi A, et al. Extrapulmonary small cell carcinoma: a single institution experience and review of the literature. Ann Oncol 1994; 5:909–913.

3. Hoskins P, Wong F, Swenerton K, et al. Small cell carcinoma of the cervix treated with concurrent radiotherapy, cisplatin, and etoposide. Gynecol Oncol 1995; 56:218–225.
4. Abeler V, Holm R, Nesland J, Kjorstad K. Small cell carcinoma of the cervix: A clinicopathologic study of 26 patients. Cancer 1994; 73:672–677.
5. Morris M, Gershenson D, Eifel P, et al. Treatment of small cell carcinoma of the cervix with cisplatin, doxorubicin, and etoposide. Gynecol Oncol 1992; 47:62–65.
6. O'Hanlan K, Goldberg G, Jones J, et al. Adjuvant therapy for neuroendocrine small cell carcinoma of the cervix: Review of the literature. Gynecol Oncol 1991; 43:167–172.

PHYSICIANS' RESPONSE

MICHAEL W. METHOD
BERND-UWE SEVIN

The case presented is consistent with a clinical stage IB1 carcinoma of the cervix. The histopathological subtype, small-cell carcinoma (SCC), is an aggressive tumor with a propensity for rapid recurrence and is associated with a higher mortality rate, stage for stage, than squamous cell carcinoma and adenocarcinoma of the cervix. Even in clinical stage I disease, there is a tendency toward early subclinical hematogenous and lymphatic metastases with frequent recurrences, despite the absence of the usual pathological risk factors. Overall 5-year survival of patients with stage I disease is reported to be as low as 14% (1).

Highly malignant behavior has been found to correlate closely with the histological pattern of the tumor. Diffuse nuclei similar to SCC in other organs correlate with a high frequency of lymph node metastasis and tumor recurrence. Because SCC or neuroendocrine carcinomas of the cervix appear to have the highest incidence of recurrence and the poorest prognosis, it is necessary to distinguish these neoplasms from squamous cell carcinomas. Despite clearly defined morphology in many cases, a group of neuroendocrine tumors with mixed histology appear to have a similarly poor prognosis. These types should have selected immunohistochemical staining performed for both prognostic information and treatment considerations. Flow cytometry should also be considered to define ploidy and S-phase fraction (proliferative DNA index), which has been related to survival time and may have prognostic importance in SCC.

Optimal treatment methods have yet to be established due to the rarity of the tumor, and poor prognosis is noted with standard radical surgical and/or radiation therapy. If any suggestion of distant disease was noted, we recommend primary chemotherapy as described below. From our own experience, small lesions have been treated effectively by radical surgery followed by radiation therapy when the depth of invasion is less than 10 mm. In general, tumors less than 2 cm in size have a survival advantage over those larger than 2 cm. In the absence of physical, laboratory, and radiographic evidence of distant disease, however, a radical hysterectomy with pelvic and paraaortic lymphadenectomy is recommended as initial treatment in this patient unless medical conditions would preclude its safe completion. When surgery is not considered an option, induction chemotherapy followed by standard pelvic radiotherapy is recommended. Alternatively, three courses of neoadjuvant chemotherapy followed by radical hysterectomy with pelvic and paraaortic lymphadenectomy should be considered. Further adjuvant therapy would be based upon the final histopathological findings. In the absence of risk factors—which include deep invasion, positive margins, positive parametria, and/or positive lymph node metastases (LNM)—cytotoxic chemotherapy including DDP (cisplatin) and etoposide (VP-16) should be given for a total of six courses (2). Although the response rates of neuroendocrine tumors to these agents often exceeds 90%, it is unknown whether such treatment will have an impact on survival. One regimen would include DDP at 50 mg/m^2 and doxorubicin (Adriamycin) at 50 mg/m^2 on day 1, with etoposide at 75 mg/m^2 per day on days 1 to 3. Other treatment recommendations replace Adriamycin with cyclophosphamide at 500 mg/m^2, and dose elevations of both DDP and etoposide up to 100 mg/m^2 each.

In patients with positive risk factors (e.g., deep invasion, positive margins, positive parametria, and positive LNM), concurrent pelvic radiotherapy or consolidation pelvic radiotherapy is advised in addition to cisplatin- and etoposide-based chemotherapy (2). The toxicity of such a treatment combination is high, with as many as 70% of patients experiencing severe neutropenia and 40% reporting grade 4 gastrointestinal toxicity. Maximum therapy, however, should be administered to this group early, as prognosis is guarded and any evidence of recurrence ensures a dismal outcome. Finally, it is imperative to provide the patient with an honest summary of her prognosis. Early emphasis should be placed on increasing the patient's and family's support network with referrals to organizations that are prepared to provide added support. Despite aggressive standard therapy, many patients have succumbed to their disease in as little as 8 months after presentation with a clinical stage I lesion.

References

Abeler VM, Holm R, Nesland JM, Kjorstad KE. Small cell carcinoma of the cervix. 1994; 73:672–677.

Hoskins PJ, Wong F, Swenerton KD, et al. Small cell carcinoma of the cervix treated with concurrent radiotherapy, cisplatin, and etoposide. Gynecol Oncol 1995; 56:218–225.

PHYSICIAN'S RESPONSE

RICHARD BARAKAT

This is a 32-year-old patient with a clinical stage IB small-cell carcinoma of the cervix. This patient has an extremely rare cervical carcinoma, which accounts for approximately 1% of all cervical cancers. Unfortunately, these cancers tend to behave in an extremely aggressive manner, with a predilection for early spread to regional lymph nodes and systemic metastasis. An extensive metastatic survey is therefore required prior to undertaking any radical surgical procedure. Since these cancers undergo neuroendocrine differentiation, they may be hormonally active. In rare circumstances, this can cause clinical symptoms such as Cushing's disease due to elevated serum adrenocorticotropic hormone (ACTH) levels. An ACTH level should be obtained if the patient displays any clinical symptoms of Cushing's disease.

Patients with early-stage disease confined to the cervix or upper vagina can be managed with radical hysterectomy and pelvic lymphadenectomy or radical radiation therapy. Of patients undergoing radical hysterectomy for early-stage disease, approximately 50% will be found to have pelvic nodal metastasis. Postoperative pelvic radiotherapy does not appear to be effective, as many patients will fail at distant sites, including bone, brain, liver, and supraclavicular lymph nodes. Five-year survival in patients with early-stage disease is approximately 20%. There is some evidence that patients whose greatest primary tumor diameter is < 2 cm fare better than those whose diameter is greater than 2 cm (1). Patients treated primarily with radical radiotherapy are also prone to extrapelvic failure.

Despite the early-stage of disease at presentation, the dismal outcome experienced by the majority of patients with small-cell cancer of the cervix indicates that traditional modes of therapy are ineffective. There is increasing evidence that patients with small-cell cancer of the cervix may benefit from treatment with combination chemotherapy consisting of cisplatin, doxorubicin, and etoposide. Response rates of 57% have been noted in patients with measurable disease (2). The chemotherapy doses are cisplatin (50 mg/m^2) and doxorubicin (50 mg/m^2) on day 1 and etoposide (75 mg/m^2) on days 1 to 3. This is usually given in an adjuvant manner postoperatively for four cycles in patients such as this, who undergo radical hysterectomy for small lesions. Patients with bulky lesions may benefit from two cycles of neoadjuvant chemotherapy prior to radical hysterectomy or radical radiation therapy. This can be followed by two to four additional cycles of chemotherapy after surgery or radiation. The patient should be followed closely every 3 months for 2 years, every 6 months for 3 additional years, and annually thereafter. Follow-up should include radiological examinations to search for metastatic disease, as distant failures are not uncommon.

References

1. Sheets EE, Berman ML, Hroutas CK, et al. Surgically treated, early-stage neuroendocrine small cell cervical carcinoma. Obstet Gynecol 1988; 71:10–14.
2. Morris M, Gershenson DM, Eifel P, et al. Treatment of small cell carcinoma of the cervix with cisplatin, doxorubicin, and etoposide. Gynecol Oncol 1992; 47:62–65.

PHYSICIAN'S RESPONSE

THOMAS F. ROCERETO

Small-cell carcinoma of the cervix accounts for less than 5% of all cervical cancers. It is a highly aggressive tumor similar to small-cell carcinoma of the lung and behaves quite differently from other types of carcinomas of the cervix. This tumor tends to metastasize earlier than the large-cell squamous carcinomas of the cervix. Its spread frequently is via the hematogenous route to the liver, bone, and brain as well as via the lymphatic route to the pelvic, paraaortic, and supraclavicular lymph nodes.

Grossly these tumors look no different than those of the large-cell variety. Histologically, they consist mostly of small basophilic cells with a characteristic cell and nuclear diameter and area. There is a high mitotic count and no keratinization. Because of the rarity of this type of tumor, the slides should be evaluated by more than one pathologist, with consideration for consultation with a gynecological pathologist.

The pretreatment workup of the patient with the usual carcinoma of the cervix has been limited to the physical examination, routine laboratory studies, chest x-ray, and an intravenous pyelogram. Some institutions substitute a CT scan of the abdomen and pelvis with intravenous contrast for the IVP. Cystoscopy and sigmoidoscopy are performed in patients with greater than stage I disease.

In the patient with the aggressive small-cell carcinoma, the usual pretreatment workup may be inadequate. These patients should undergo a CT scan of the head and chest along with that of the abdomen and pelvis. Bone scan and a bone marrow aspiration and biopsy should be entertained also.

These tumors tend to be more advanced than the clinical stage suggests and recur earlier than the large-cell types. The cure rate for patients with small-cell carcinomas is reported to be between 20 and 80%, with most studies showing less than 50% cure. The median survival in most studies is a year or less.

The traditional treatment modality for a patient with carcinoma of the cervix has been radical hysterectomy with lymph node dissection in early-stage disease and radiotherapy in more advanced stages. This may not be adequate for small-cell carcinomas. It is obvious that this cancer is a systemic disease and should be treated as such. Small-cell carcinoma of the lung has responded to aggressive chemotherapy. Chemotherapeutic regimens that have been used in small-cell carcinoma of the cervix include the combinations of cyclophosphamide, doxorubicin, and vincristine; cisplatin, etoposide, and cyclophosphamide; and cisplatin, doxorubicin, and etoposide. These regimens have been used before and after surgery and/or radiotherapy. Presently there are no large studies using combination chemotherapy with surgery or/and radiation, and, because of the rarity of this type of cancer, it is unlikely that there ever will be adequate studies.

With respect to this case, adequate workup should include CT scans of the head, chest, abdomen, and pelvis as well as a bone scan, along with the routine workup for cervical carcinoma. Assuming that the metastatic workup is negative, radical surgery would be appropriate in a patient of this age with a lesion of this size. The regimen of Morris from the M.D. Anderson Cancer Center should be considered in the treatment of this patient. This regimen includes a radical hysterectomy with a pelvic and paraaortic lymph node dissection followed by six courses of combination chemotherapy. The chemotherapy consists of a 28-day regimen with cisplatin 50 mg/m^2 and doxorubicin 50 mg/m^2 on day 1 and etoposide 75 mg/m^2 per day on days 1 to 3. If lymphatic or other pelvic spread is present at the time of surgery, the chemotherapy should be followed by a course of pelvic radiotherapy.

References

Hoskins WJ, Perez CA, Young RC, eds. Principles and Practice of Gynecologic Oncology. Philadelphia: Lippincott, 1992:612.
Morris M, et al. Treatment of small cell carcinoma of the cervix with cisplatin, doxorubicin and etoposide. Gynecol Oncol 1992; 47:62–65.
van Nagell JR, et al. Small carcinoma of the uterine cervix. Cancer 1988; 62:1586–1593.

PHYSICIAN'S RESPONSE

PETER FLEMING

Small cell carcinoma of the cervix is characterized by a uniform population of small cells with a high nucleus-to-cytoplasm ration, with up to 50% of cases staining positive for neuroendocrine markers, as in small-cell carcinoma of the lung. This histologic type is a variant of the squamous cell carcinoma subtypers, i.e., large-cell nonkeratinizing, large-cell keratinizing, small-cell, and verrucous carcinoma. Small-cell carcinoma is an aggressive tumor demonstrating the capacity to metastasize to regional and distant sites. Van Nagell et al. reported on 2001 patients with invasive cervical cancer treated at the University of Kentucky between 1962 to 1985 (1). Twenty-five cases (1.1%) fulfilled the histological criteria for small-cell cancer. Forty percent of stage IB cases with tumor diameter less than 3 cm were found with pelvic metastases. Forty-two percent of the 12 patients with stage IB experienced recurrent disease, whereas only 4% of the 24 matched keratinizing/large-cell nonkeratinizing cases developed recurrences. DiSaia has reported his personal experience with 14 cases of stages IB and IIA, all treated with radical hysterectomy and postoperative radiation therapy (2). All patients experienced recurrence, 86% within 31 months of treatment.

Hoskins et al. recommend that treatment for this aggressive tumor should be a combined modality incorporating the principles of therapy for small-cell carcinoma of the lung (3). Multiagent chemotherapy, such as cyclophosphamide, doxorubicin, and vincristine, may be administered for two or three cycles prior to standard radiation techniques for carcinoma of the cervix.

References

1. Van Nagell, et al. Small cell carcinoma of the uterine cervix. Cancer 1988; 62:1586–1593.
2. DiSaia P, Creasman. Clinical Gynecologic Oncology, 4th ed. St Louis: Mosby-Year Book, 1993:72.
3. Hoskins WJ, Perez CA, Young RC, eds. Principles and Practice of Gynecologic Oncology. Philadelphia: Lippincott, 1992:612.

57

Cervical Cancer, Adenosquamous (Stage IB, Post–Simple Hysterectomy)

CASE

A 40-year-old banker was experiencing abnormal bleeding for several months. Because of her busy schedule, she told her gynecologist that she was not interested in any complicated testing or conservative procedures, she simply wanted her uterus removed. The physician complied, and even though her Pap smear prior to surgery was normal, the hysterectomy specimen showed an adenosquamous carcinoma of the cervix invading to a depth of 6 mm. There was no obvious vascular space invasion. On finding this, the physician has contacted you, and the patient now presents for advice as to future management. She is now 2 1/2 weeks status post–total abdominal hysterectomy through a Pfannenstiel incision. Her surgery went smoothly without complications and the patient has actually been back at her office for the past 2 days.

PHYSICIAN'S RESPONSE

HUGH M. SHINGLETON

A 40-year-old woman with irregular bleeding for several months who wishes to forgo "complicated" testing presents a diagnostic and therapeutic problem. While it is unlikely that at age 40, the bleeding is due to endometrial carcinoma, a few such cases occur and the diagnosis would be possible with a uterine biopsy or curettage. A common cause of irregular bleeding, especially postcoital bleeding, is cancer of the cervix. The physician treating this patient would have been very wise, in spite of a "negative" Pap smear, to have performed some cervical or endocervical biopsies and even a dilation and curettage at the time of hysterectomy and to have submitted the material for frozen section. Had that been the case, most likely it would have been determined that the woman had a cancer of the cervix and an inappropriate operation could have been avoided. The case also demonstrates another point: physicians should not forgo good clinical judgment and careful preoperative evaluation in order to please an assertive patient such as this.

Given that the total hysterectomy has occurred with a surprise finding of a significant (although small) mixed adenosquamous carcinoma, the patient most certainly requires additional treatment. Without such treatment, the chance of a recurrence and subsequent poor outcome is high. If the entire primary tumor were contained in the hysterectomy specimen (no clinical residual tumor known), 5-year survival would be expected to be in the 70 to 90% range should pelvic irradiation therapy be given promptly (i.e., within 1 to 2 months of the hysterectomy). Poor prognostic signs are known residual tumor at the onset of the postoperative radiation or a prolonged delay (6 months or more) between the hysterectomy and the irradiation therapy. Five-year survival is cut in half by these findings (1).

The matter of whether the tissue type of this particular cervical cancer represents an additional risk factor is somewhat controversial, although adenocarcinomas in general and adenosquamous carcinomas in particular are thought by many to have reduced cure rates. In an American College of Surgeons patterns-of-care study (2), stage 1 adenocarcinomas, adenosquamous carcinomas, and squamous cell carcinomas were found to have similar 5-year survival (83.7%, 76.6%, and 84.1%, $p = NS$, respectively). It was found that adenosquamous tumors seem to fare better with combination therapy (surgery and irradiation) as compared to either surgery or radiation alone (88.1% combined, radiation 77.5%, surgery alone 72.0%).

Reference

1. Shingleton HM, Orr JW. Cancer of the Cervix. Philadelphia: Lippincott, 1995:180–182.
2. Shingleton HM, Bell MC, Fremgen A, et al. Is there really a difference in survival of women with early stage squamous cell carcinoma, adenocarcinoma and adenosquamous cell carcinoma of the cervix? Cancer. In press.

PHYSICIANS' RESPONSE

GUNTER DEPPE
VINAY MALVIYA

My recommendation would be a radical parametrectomy with upper vaginectomy and bilateral pelvic lymphadenectomy. Selective paraaortic lymphadenectomy to be performed in event of positive pelvic lymph nodes at the time of frozen section. The surgical procedure may be carried out either through a midline incision or a Maylard incision, preferably after 4 to 6 weeks (allowing the resolution of local inflammation). Computed tomography of abdomen and pelvis should be done with 5-mm cuts to rule out any paraaortic involvement or hydronephrosis prior to the surgical procedure. Transposition of ovaries should be performed.

Discussion

Recurrence rates following total hysterectomy with a surprise finding of invasive cervical cancer are approximately 60%. Additional therapy is therefore indicated. Survival rates for women treated for cervical cancer by radiation therapy after total hysterectomy range from 71 to 92% when there is no clinical evidence of residual cancer on pelvic examination (1); while patients with gross disease at the start of post hysterectomy treatment had a 5-year survival rate of 39%. The prognostic significance of tumor histology remains unclear, as disparate findings have been reported.

Chapman et al. (1) reported their experience with radical parametrectomy in a series of 18 patients with 72 months of follow-up with invasion deeper than 3 mm and/or lymphovascular space involvement following "simple" hysterectomy. In 15 of 18 patients, no evidence of disease was found in the specimen. One patient of this group received adjuvant postoperative radiation therapy (RT) because of tumor extension to the uterine serosa in the original hysterectomy specimen. Only 1 of 14 of these patients who needed no adjuvant RT had pelvic recurrence 66 months after therapy. Among 18 patients, 2 had microscopic metastatic disease on radical re-operation specimens. One patient had microscopic positive pelvic nodes. Both were treated with adjuvant RT. The patient with positive pelvic nodes died with recurrent disease 24 months later. Also among 18 patients, 1 had obviously positive pelvic nodes and died 8 months later in spite of extended postoperative RT. The actual 5-year survival for 18 patients was 89%. Radiation therapy was therefore avoided in 78% of patients and ovaries were preserved in all 10 patients under the age of 40 who underwent ovarian transposition.

The operative technique of radical upper vaginectomy and parametrectomy can be facilitated by preoperative packing of the vagina to identify the vaginal apex. Sutures are placed on the posterior vaginal wall for countertraction while a bladder flap dissection is performed. The pack is then removed and through-and-through countertraction sutures are placed in the upper vagina; the remainder of the procedure is continued as a radical hysterectomy. The morbidity of the surgical procedure—when comparing OR time, estimated blood loss, and hospital stay—was no different than for a radical hysterectomy.

Radiation therapy, an alternative to the above, leads to loss of ovarian function and a greater frequency of sexual dysfunction than does operative management. Roman et al. presented their experience with 120 patients undergoing "simple" hysterectomy in the presence of invasive cancer of the cervix (2). The 5-year survival rate for 90 patients with no gross disease was 45% (patient population includes those with no clinical evidence of disease but with microscopically positive or negative surgical margins) and 39% for 30 patients with gross disease present before the start of radiation. The site of recurrence in patients with no gross disease was equally divided between the pelvis and distant locations, suggesting that both unappreciated pelvic and distant metastases play a role in recurrence. The treatment complication rate (10% overall with a 6% rate of major complication) is higher than the 3% rate of major complications for patients receiving primary irradiation. The increased morbidity is related to pelvic adhesions and poor geometry for brachytherapy.

References

1. Chapman JA, Mannel RS, DiSaia PJ, et al. Surgical treatment of unexpected invasive cervical cancer found at total hysterectomy. Obstet Gynecol 1992; 80:931–934.
2. Roman LD, Morris M, Mitchell MF, et al. Prognostic factors for patients undergoing simple hysterectomy in the presence of invasive cancer of the cervix. Gynecol Oncol 1993; 50:179–184.

PHYSICIAN'S RESPONSE

F. MONTZ

The most important aspects of this case revolve around educating the referring physician and encouraging him to avoid being "browbeaten" by his patients into practicing medicine that is below the optimal standards. He should not be surprised that the Pap smear was "normal," as the Pap smear is negative in about half of patients with adenosquamous carcinoma of the cervix. Similarly, he should be reminded that exfoliative cytology is of limited value in screening for endocervical and endometrial malignancies. He must remember that an endocervical curettage and an endometrial biopsy would not be considered "complicated testing" and can easily be performed in the office with minimal patient discomfort or time commitment.

There is little information that I would need prior to offering my consultative opinion. However I would want:

1. A thorough rereview of the pathology by a trusted gynecological pathologist, looking specifically at:
    a. Further size characteristics of the invasive component of the lesion
    b. Further definition of the subtype of the adeno component

    c. Determination of vascular space invasion that may not have been obvious on review by the community pathologist

2. A chest x-ray and a CT of the abdomen and pelvis

3. CEA, SCCA, and CA-125 determinations

Assuming that the final pathology review was relatively consistent with the information provided above, I would offer the patient two options:

1. Reexploration with radical parametrectromy/upper vaginectomy, bilateral pelvic lymph node dissection, selected paraaortic lymph node sampling, and a bilateral salpingo-oophorectomy.
2. Whole-pelvis radiation (4500 cGy with a midline block at 4050 cGy) followed by a single application of vaginal brachytherapy using colpostats in an attempt to bring the vaginal epithelial dose to 7500 cGy.

In light of what has been described about this patient and her inferred desire to have her career disrupted as little as possible, I would encourage her to undergo the radiotherapy. During her follow-up, I would recommend:

1. Institution of estrogen replacement therapy 1 week into her radiotherapy course. This should be accompanied by adequate calcium and vitamin D supplementation and physical activity.
2. If she is not coitally active, she should dilate her vagina on a twice-weekly basis using Replens as the lubricant.
3. She should undergo physical examinations every 3 months for a period of 3 years, with exams occurring on an every-6-month basis thereafter for 2 more years.
4. At her visits, she should have a serum CEA, CA-125, and SCCA determinations performed.
5. For the first 3 years, she should have a twice-yearly chest x-ray and a CT scan of the abdomen and the pelvis performed. These examinations should be performed on a yearly basis thereafter for the following 2 years.

References

Benda JA, Platz C, Buchsbaum H, Lifshitz S. Mucin production in defining mixed carcinoma of the uterine cervix: A clinicopathologic study. Int J Gynecol Pathol 1985; 4:314.

Gallup DG, Harper RH, Stock RJ. Poor prognosis in patients with adenosquamous cell carcinoma of the cervix. Obstet Gynecol 1985; 65:416.

Roman LD, Morris M, Eifel P, et al. Reasons for inappropriate simple hysterectomy in the presence of invasive cancer of the cervix. Obstet Gynecol 1992; 79:485.

PHYSICIAN'S RESPONSE

JONATHAN M. NILOFF

This 40-year-old patient, although she has not been formerly staged, presumably has a stage IB adenosquamous carcinoma of the cervix. Inasmuch as she had a Pap smear performed prior to surgery, I assume that her cervix looked grossly normal and therefore that the patient has a small tumor. I will further assume that the pelvic examination was normal. If the patient has not had a careful rectovaginal examination, this should be performed to exclude lateral tumor extension. I do not feel that cystoscopy or proctoscopy will add useful information. This patient's evaluation should be completed with liver function studies, a chest x-ray, and CT scans of the abdomen and pelvis with intravenous contrast. If the CT scan suggests the presence of metastatic adenopathy, I would recommend that this be documented by CT-guided percutaneous biopsy.

The survival among patients with small stage I carcinomas of the cervix managed with radiation therapy after simple hysterectomy is not compromised, compared to those patients managed either with radical hysterectomy and lymph node dissection or primary radiation therapy. I recommend that this patient be managed with radiation therapy. Treatment should be tailored to the findings of the above studies. Important factors include the presence or absence of lateral tumor extension on the pelvic examination, CT evidence of adenopathy, and histological tumor status of the margins of the hysterectomy specimen. If there is metastatic tumor involving high pelvic or paraaortic lymph nodes, then a paraaortic chimney should be added to the radiation field.

This patient should be followed after completing radiation therapy with serial clinical examinations and Pap smears. There is no contraindication to the prescription of estrogen replacement therapy.

PHYSICIAN'S RESPONSE

J. SAXTON

I believe that there are three essential points that guide the decision of management in this patient: (a) histology, (b) depth of invasion, and (c) the lack of index of suspicion on the part of the surgeon that he was dealing with a malignancy, resulting in an inadequate surgical procedure.

In general, most clinicians seem to feel that adenosquamous carcinoma of the cervix has a worse clinical prognosis than a corresponding squamous cell carcinoma. These lesions in general are felt to be more poorly differentiated. They constitute 2 to 5% of the malignant lesions arising in the cervix. The degree of differentiation seems to be based on the adenocarcinoma component of the mixture of adeno and squamous cells. The limited number probably preclude clinical evaluation of these tumors based on the individual grading of the specific adenomatous component.

The FIGO staging system classifies a T_1A_2 lesion with an invasive component of 5 mm or less in depth and 7 mm or less in horizontal spread. No information was given in the case concerning the spread of the lesion, which would seem to carry prognostic significance. Therefore, this lesion technically would be a IB lesion, albeit an early IB. Without definite knowledge of the horizontal spread of the lesion for more specific staging, I would opt for overcompensation with management. I would estimate the risk of nodal involvement to be more in line with an early IB lesion of 15%. The fact that there was no vascular invasion is reassuring. Some authors have reported minimal local regional failure treating small-volume IB lesions with intracavitary radiation only, attesting to a low risk of regional nodal involvement.

Due to the depth of invasion and the risk of nodal involvement, I believe the most accepted procedure in this relatively young patient would have been a radical hysterectomy plus or minus ovarian sparing, with nodal sampling. Because there was no index of suspicion, the nodal inspection may have been suboptimal.

I would recommend a baseline CT scan and postoperative whole-pelvis radiation to a dose of 5000 rads in 5 to 5 1/2 weeks, with or without an intracavitary boost, or chemotherapy. One could make an argument for a cuff boost considering that there was probably no cuff removed.

58

Cervical Cancer, Adenosquamous (Stage IB/Surgical Stage IIIB)

CASE

A 40-year-old woman (gravida III, para III), has a history of postcoital spotting for 6 months. Recently she was admitted to the hospital with heavy bleeding and was found to have an ulcerative lesion of the cervix. The cervical tumor measured approximately $3^1/_2$ cm in size. The parametria and uterosacral ligaments were soft and without nodularity. Cervical biopsy revealed an adenosquamous carcinoma. Preoperative workup included a normal chest x-ray and an intravenous pyelogram (IVP). The patient's preoperative hematocrit was 36% and she had normal blood urea nitrogen (BUN), electrolytes, and liver function studies. She was taken to the operating room for a planned radical hysterectomy and pelvic lymph adenectomy. A paraaortic dissection was done, and on frozen section both right and left paraaortic lymph nodes were determined to be negative. On exploration of the pelvic side wall, the patient had a 3-cm left external iliac lymph node just below the bifurcation of the common iliac. This lymph node was somewhat fixed to the left external iliac vein, although, with careful dissection, it was removed with no obvious gross disease remaining on the vein. At this point, what would be your course of action if there were no other suspicious nodes on the pelvic side wall? In addition, how would you approach this patient if the lymph node were fixed to the vein and could not be resected off the vein?

PHYSICIAN'S RESPONSE

JAMES ROBERTS

This woman presents with a very difficult clinical problem. Data from the University of Michigan (1) have shown that the survival for adenocarcinoma of the cervix with a clinical stage IB carcinoma drops to 28% when even one pelvic lymph node is involved. This survival has been obtained regardless of the treatment: radiation alone, radical hysterectomy with or without radiation, or radical hysterectomy alone. Therefore, innovative therapy is necessary if this woman is to have a prolonged survival.

As a first step, I would continue the resection of her disease and complete the planned radical hysterectomy and pelvic lymphadenectomy. Since the ovaries are rarely involved with this disease, I would retain them in this 40-year-old woman if they appeared normal. I expect to treat this woman with postoperative radiation therapy, so I would transpose her ovaries above the pelvis in the colic gutters. I would also send a 1-cm^3 portion of the tumor for chemosensitivity testing. Following her recovery from surgery, I would begin pelvic and paraaortic radiation therapy. This should commence as soon as possible (within 3 weeks of surgery).

Our data have shown that this approach has resulted in a long-term survival below 30%. We have also found that many of these women will experience recurrent disease outside the radiated field. Thus, this therapy is locally effective, but one must still address the systemic manifestations of this pathology. At this time, the only systemic therapy available is cytotoxic drugs. There are no reports of any agent or combination of agents that are effective in the majority of these women. Therefore, the selection of treatment agent(s) may be best guided by the results of the chemosensitivity testing of the tissue sent at the time of surgery. If it were not possible to obtain this testing, the most active agent against this disease is cisplatin, which should be administered either alone or in combination with another drug.

This approach is quite aggressive and is associated with a moderate amount of morbidity, but it is intended to successfully treat a condition that has a long-term survival rate of less than 30%. The alterative is to approach this woman with *standard therapy*, which would mean radiation alone or surgery and radiation. It must be kept in mind that once this disease recurs, either locally or distantly, it is rarely responsive to any form of therapy.

If one were unable to resect the lymphatic disease, the situation becomes even more complex. One can pursue the same approach outlined for the resectable patient, i.e., remove all the disease possible. This could be approached by using the Cavitron Ultrasonic Surgical Aspirator (CUSA) device to remove the disease from the vein wall or simply by resecting the involved vein. One would then follow up the surgery with the same treatment as in the resectable patient.

Since the approach to this disease is far from established, the treatment plan may be altered by the resources available locally. If intraoperative radiation is available, this modality could be employed after the pelvic lymph nodes were resected. If *high-dose-rate (HDR)* radiation is available, tubes may be placed along the left pelvic side wall to allow for postoperative delivery of HDR. Both of these approaches will address the issue of local control but will still require some form of systemic therapy to treat the threat of widespread disease.

Reference

1. Hopkins MP, Schmidt RW, Roberts JA, Morley GW. The prognosis and treatment of stage I adenocarcinoma of the cervix. Obstet Gynecol 1988; 72:915–921.

PHYSICIANS' RESPONSE

N. NIKRUI
R. SAINZ DE LA CUESTA

For early-stage cervical cancer, either radiation or surgery is the standard treatment of choice. In a young patient, a radical hysterectomy is the preferred treatment because it allows preservation of ovarian and sexual function. When a surgeon encounters a positive pelvic lymph node at the time of surgical exploration, the dilemma to continue or to abort the procedure will arise. In the first case, where there are negative paraaortic nodes and debulkable pelvic disease, it is reasonable to complete the operation and give postoperative adjuvant radiation and chemotherapy. In the case where nodal disease is not debulkable, as in the second scenario, the textbooks' practice would be to abort the surgery and treat the patient with postoperative radiation. However, the 5-year survival and quality of the life of this patient is probably going to be very poor. Therefore we would suggest debulking the tumor by excising the nondissectable node with Cavitron Ultrasonic Surgical Aspirator (CUSA) and complete a limited radical hysterectomy for treatment of the primary lesion. It would be important at the time of surgery to mark the involved node with hemo clips to help the radiation oncologist identify and include the site of disease in the radiation field. We would recommend postoperative radiation therapy using external beam to the pelvis, including the chain above the involved node. The patient should also receive an intraoperative boost to the involved area after termination of external-beam therapy. We also recommend platinum-based combination chemotherapy.

The survival rates of women with stage IB cervical cancer drop 20 to 30%

when there is lymph node involvement. Furthermore, patients with negative nodes who have recurrent disease can be cured by secondary therapy, whereas those patients with involved lymph nodes who relapse are rarely salvageable. Based on these findings, several investigators recommend postoperative pelvic irradiation to patients with resected positive pelvic lymph nodes. Although a decrease in the frequency of pelvic recurrence has been reported, few authors have been able to show a survival advantage for patients receiving radiation therapy compared to those who do not. The literature suggests that patients with one risk factor do well. However, tumor size, depth of tumor invasion, and capillary-lymphatic space invasion may be the only independent risk factors that substantially alter the disease-free interval in patients with early-stage cervical cancer. Women with grossly positive but completely resected pelvic node metastases have been found to have the same relapse-free rate as those with only microscopic disease. Therefore, the decision to give postoperative whole pelvic radiation to the patient who had all nodal disease removed should be based on these pathological findings (1).

Several investigators advocate platinum-based adjuvant chemotherapy for patients with high-risk cervical cancer. Multicentered randomized trials are needed to determine the value of chemotherapy alone compared to chemotherapy plus radiation therapy. The aim of these studies is to decrease pelvic and distal recurrence and possibly make unresectable disease resectable. Therefore our recommendation to use chemotherapy in these two difficult cases would be based on these ongoing studies (2).

References

1. Gregoria Delgado et al: Prospective surgical-pathological study of disease free interval in patients with stage I squamous cell carcinoma of the cervix: A Gynecologic Oncology Group study. Gynecol Oncol 1990; 38:352–357.
2. Jones WB. New Approaches to high risk cervical cancer. Cancer Suppl 1993; 71(4):

PHYSICIAN'S RESPONSE

PETER FLEMING

This patient present with an adenosquamous carcinoma of the cervix, stage IB (surgical stage IIIB) by virtue of the demonstrated 3-cm left external iliac lymph node, somewhat fixed to the adjacent vein. If the node is resected with no gross residual disease on the vein and there are no other suspicious nodes on the pelvic side wall, the patient would be a candidate for postoperative external radiation therapy to the pelvis—i.e., 45 to 50 Gy with standard fractionation techniques. The treatment field would extend cephalad to the L3-L4 interface in order to cover the next adjacent lymph node region (common iliac). The rationale for the latter adjunctive treatment is possible reduction in the incidence of pelvic tumor recurrence and the prolongation of survival. Multiple uncontrolled studies on the effect of postoperative irradiation or no postoperative irradiation on 5-year survival rates (stage IB and IIA) indicate results varying from 43 to 63% and 40 to 59%, respectively (1). Kinney et al. reported a 5-year survival of 72% for a surgery-only group and 64% for a postoperative irradiation group (2). The incidence of pelvic recurrence was 67% in the surgery-only group and 27% in the adjuvant postoperative irradiation group.

In the situation wherein minimal macroscopic disease remains at the resection site, intraoperative iodine-125 seeds in suture may be utilized as a permanent brachytherapy adjuvant. This procedure will deliver approximately 80 to 100 Gy in 60 days elapsed time to a point 0.5 cm perpendicular to the planar midpoint. In the case of large-volume residual tumor, including vessel encasement by tumor, an intraoperative iridium-192 temporary interstitial implant may be considered, delivering a dose of approximately 25 Gy at 40 to 50 cGy/hr.

References

1. Hoskins W, et al. Principles and Practice of Gynecologic Oncology. Philadelphia: Lippincott, 1992:617.
2. Kinney, et al. Value of adjuvant whole pelvis irradiation after Wertheim hysterectomy for early-stage squamous carcinoma of the cervix with pelvic nodal metastases: A matched-control study. Gynecol Oncol 1989; 34:258–262.

PHYSICIAN'S RESPONSE

A. ROBERT KAGAN

The incidence of positive lymph nodes in a patient with a visible lesion confined to the cervix can vary, with an *overall* incidence of 20%. A $3^1/_2$-cm lesion in a 40-year-old gravida III might just cover the entire cervix, which, adding the histology of adenosquamous carcinoma, would make the incidence of positive nodes closer to 40%. A CT of the pelvis would have revealed a 3-cm node unless the patient were very thin. Excluding extenuating circumstances—for example, pelvic inflammatory disease, ulcerative colitis, or diverticulitis—a 3-cm node in a patient with cancer of the cervix is metastatic cancer. When in doubt, a 3-cm lymph node can be aspirated for a cytological diagnosis with a fine needle under CT guidance.

After the *high* external iliac node was *removed*, I would advise abandoning the surgical procedure in favor of irradiation therapy. I foresee that if the planned surgery is carried out, postoperative irradiation will be asked for. In this situation, the radiation will not improve survival but will increase the probability of complications.

The prognosis of this patient is very poor: a 5-year survival of 15%. The cervix drains to nodes in the parametrium, obturator, external iliac, and common iliac regions. The node in this patient is at least a third-echelon node. I would assume that the lymph node chains inferior to the removed lymph node are positive.

If the lymph node were *left* at the common iliac bifurcation, I think that further surgery would be contraindicated. Irradiation management would be similar except for a wide boost to the lymph node, which I hope would be clipped with clips of recognizable size. Survival in my opinion would be close to zero.

59

Cervical Cancer, Squamous Cell, IB, 3- to 5-mm Invasion

CASE

A 29-year-old woman, gravida I, was treated for an abnormal Pap smear with cryotherapy 2 years ago. At her most recent presentation, her Pap smear showed CIN3. This was followed by a colposcopy and loop electrosurgical excision procedure (LEEP), which showed a squamous cell carcinoma of the cervix invading to a depth of 4 mm. The lesion involved about 30% of the circumference of the LEEP specimen, but the margins were clear of invasion as well as dysplasia. The overall length of the LEEP specimen was 1.5 cm if one combines the first-pass specimen (using a 2- by 0.8 cm loop) with the endocervical specimen (using a 1- by 1-cm loop). The patient has come to you for consultation in terms of her future management.

PHYSICIAN'S RESPONSE

MAUREEN JARRELL

The patient described in this case has a stage IB squamous cancer of the cervix by both the classifications of the Society of Gynecologic Oncologists (SGO) and the Fédération Internationale de Gynécologoie et d'Obstétrique (FIGO). The size of the tumor exceeds the 3-mm depth of invasion defined by the SGO and the width of the tumor exceed the 5- by 7-mm maximum tumor size designated by FIGO. Information is lacking regarding tumor differentiation, lymphovascular space involvement, pattern of invasion, and tumor volume, all which have been shown to be prognosticators for this disease. The fact that the margins were clear is reassuring, although sometimes the surgical specimen provided by LEEP is less than optimal for evaluation of margins.

The management of small stage IB squamous cancers (3 to 5 mm) is controversial and has produced a number publications in the last 5 years that contain thought-provoking arguments regarding less radical therapies. All of the authors have urged prospective studies to look at this problem; however, at this time such studies do not exist.

Although there are scattered reports of similar tumors treated by conization or extrafascial hysterectomy (1,2), there are an equal number of reports of positive lymph nodes when radical surgery was performed (3). The incidence is estimated to be 7.4% (4). This patient should not be treated by conization or simple hysterectomy but should be treated by some form of radical hysterectomy and pelvic lymphadenectomy after allowing 6 to 8 weeks for healing from the LEEP.

In order to determine the appropriate hysterectomy, the tumor should be studied further. If possible, despite the two-step excision, the size, horizontal spread, or volume of the tumor should be estimated. If the histology is poorly differentiated or there is lymphovascular space involvement, radical hysterectomy and lymphadenectomy should be performed. If neither of these factors is present and the horizontal spread of the tumor is no greater than a 2-cm sphere (5), modified radical hysterectomy and lymphadenectomy should be performed.

Should the patient refuse hysterectomy despite the recommendation, she should be treated minimally with pelvic lymphadenectomy and close follow-up with Pap smears and ECC every 3 months for 2 years and then every 6 months for a minimum of 5 years.

References

1. Girardi F, Burghardt E, Pickel H. Small FIGO stage IB cervical cancer. Gynecol Oncol 1994; 55:427–432.
2. Yaegashi N, Sato S, Inque Y, et al. Conservative surgical treatment in cervical cancer with 3 to 5 mm stromal invasion in the absence of confluent invasion and lymphvascular involvement. Gynecol Oncol 1994; 54:333–337.
3. van Nagell JR, Greenwell N, Powell DF, et al. Microinvasive carcinoma of the cervix, Am J Obstet Gynecol 1983; 145:981–991.
4. Sevin BU, Nadji M, Averette HE, et al. Microinvasive carcinoma of the cervix. Cancer 1992; 70:2121–2128.
5. Kinney W, Hodge D, Egorshin E, et al. Identification of a low risk subset of patients with stage IB invasive squamous carcinoma of the cervix possibly suited to less radical surgical treatment, Gynecol Oncol 1993; 49:107.

PHYSICIAN'S RESPONSE

M. DWIGHT CHEN
LEO B. TWIGGS

The significance of depth of invasion in cervical cancer has been a source of controversy for the past two decades. In particular, gynecological oncologists have struggled to clearly define those invasive lesions that have minimal potential for metastatic foci and risk of recurrence. This would certainly have both therapeutic as well as prognostic implications, since conservative treatment options may be curative and avoid some of the morbidity associated with either radical surgery or radiotherapy.

There is consensus of opinion that lesions invading less than 1 mm into the cervical stroma can truly be considered "microinvasive" with minimal risk of metastatic disease; therefore, either a simple hysterectomy or a cone biopsy with free margins could be considered definitive therapy. Whether other lesions can also be classified in this category is far less certain. In 1988, the FIGO attempted to define microinvasive disease by subdividing it into two groups: stage IA1, which refers to "preclinical" carcinomas diagnosed only by microscopy, and stage IA2 disease, which comprised those lesions invading up to 5 mm in depth and no wider than 7 mm. Unfortunately, these parameters were established for data comparison only and were not meant to be used as treatment guidelines.

Since 1974, the Committee on Nomenclature of the SGO has adopted an alternate, more restrictive definition of microinvasive carcinoma of the cervix: it is limited to lesions that invade the cervical stroma to a depth of up to 3 mm, with no evidence of lymphovascular space involvement (LVSI). Many gynecological oncologists currently utilize this definition in tailoring treatment options for their patients. The exclusion of LVSI differs from the FIGO definition, and much debate exists as to the significance of LVSI. The other difference between the SGO and FIGO definitions is whether a lesion that invades 3 to 5 mm into the cervical stroma can be conservatively treated (i.e., with a cone biopsy or simple hysterectomy).

Two essential questions must be addressed in this particular case: (1) is a cone biopsy sufficient to remove the entire primary lesion and (2) is this patient at risk for metastatic disease? Greer et al. have published data concerning the adequacy of cone biopsies in FIGO stage IA2 cervical cancers (1). They reported that of 17 patients who had negative margins in a cone biopsy specimen, 4 (24%) had residual invasive disease in the hysterectomy specimen. Thus, a cone biopsy may not be adequate in completely removing the primary lesion.

In answering the second question, the Gynecologic Oncology Group (GOG) recently reported on the multi-institutional experience of cervical cancer with 3 to 5 mm depth of invasion (2). This is one of the few studies in which a large number of patients in this particular category underwent radical hysterectomy and complete surgical staging, including pelvic lymphadenectomy; therefore accurate patterns of spread of disease could be determined. It was found that 4.3% of patients (6/138) with 3- to 5-mm disease had pelvic lymph node metastases. Further analysis of the data did reveal that 0 of 51 patients who had an adequate cone biopsy and no residual disease at hysterectomy demonstrated pelvic lymph node involvement; unfortunately, the gynecological oncologist is unable to use these data preoperatively in planning a surgical procedure precisely because of Greer's findings.

Based on these studies, the patient in this case is at risk for both residual disease and lymph node involvement. Since she is premenopausal and assuming there are no concomitant problems precluding surgery, she should be offered a surgical staging procedure (either via an extraperitoneal laparotomy or by laparoscopy). If there is no gross evidence of extrauterine disease, a modified radical hysterectomy can be performed. Primary radiotherapy could also be offered, but the surgical approach may better preserve both ovarian and coital function. A modified radical hysterectomy will remove some of the parametrial tissue at risk while decreasing postoperative morbidity over a standard type III radical hysterectomy. If fertility is a crucial issue to this patient, she should be referred to an experienced infertility program that specializes in oocyte retrieval and surrogate pregnancies.

References

1. Greer BE, Figge DC, Tamimi HK, et al. Stage IA2 squamous carcinoma of the cervix: Difficult diagnosis and therapeutic dilemma. Am J Obstet Gynecol 1990; 162:1406–1411.
2. Creasman WT, Bundy BN, Zaino RJ, et al. Early invasive carcinoma of the cervix with 3-5 mm of invasion-risk factors and prognosis. Presented at the 25th Annual Meeting of the Society of Gynecologic Oncologists, Orlando, FL, February 1994.

PHYSICIAN'S RESPONSE

JOHN CURTIN

The standard therapy for this unfortunate young woman is radical hysterectomy and bilateral pelvic lymphadenectomy. The reason for this radical treatment is the risk of lymph node metastasis associated with early invasive carcinoma of the cervix when the depth of stromal invasion exceeds 3 mm and/or there is evidence of lymphovascular space invasion (LVSI). In collected series, the incidence of pelvic lymph node metastasis is essentially zero when the depth of invasion is less than 3 mm and there is no LVSI. In contrast, in a series by van Nagell et al. (1), when there is 3 to 5 mm of invasion, the incidence of pelvic nodal metastases ranges from 0 to 14% and the collective average incidence is 8%.

The correct staging of this patient cannot be determined from the current pathology report. While the depth of stromal invasion is clearly stated, the lateral extent of the invasive component is only alluded to by the description of a 30% involvement of the cone specimen. The FIGO guidelines for distinguishing stage IA2 cancers from stage IB cancers is by both the depth of invasion and horizontal extent. It could be assumed from the pathological description that in this case the lateral extent will exceed the upper limit of horizontal extension allowed by FIGO for stage IA2 cancers, which is 7 mm. This distinction is important only for proper classification of the patient and would not change the recommendation for treatment.

Prior to surgery the patient would require only the standard preoperative evaluation; additional medical imaging studies such as an intravenous pyelogram or computed tomography are unnecessary. The patient should be encouraged to donate autologous blood prior to surgery. The surgical procedure will include a radical hysterectomy and bilateral pelvic lymphadenectomy. Removal of the ovaries is not required, thus preserving normal hormonal function. The only accepted alternative to radical surgery is whole pelvic and intracavitary radiation therapy, but this is not considered the preferred method of treatment for a young woman. A recent unproven method of radical trachelectomy (removal of the entire cervix) combined with laparoscopic pelvic lymphadenectomy has been reported in an abstract by Dargent and colleagues. In their series of young women with early invasive cervical cancers, this procedure was performed with the goal of fertility preservation. A cervical cerclage is required before pregnancy. In their initial report, 5 women were able to conceive and deliver term infants; however this approach can only be viewed as an unproven method with an uncertain risk of recurrence.

References

van Nagell JR, Greenwell N, Powell DF, et al. Microinvasive carcinoma of the cervix. Am J Obstet Gynecol 1983; 145:981.
Dargent D, Brun JL, Roy M, Remy I. Pregnancies following radical trachelectomy for invasive cervical carcinoma. Gynecol Oncol 1994; 52:105.

PHYSICIAN'S RESPONSE

MICHAEL GOLDBERG

This is a 29-year-old woman with one child who developed carcinoma of the cervix after failed cryotherapy. Whether or not a biopsy was taken prior to that procedure is not stated. Following a Pap smear, which showed CIN III, the patient underwent a LEEP procedure revealing 4-mm depth of invasion of a squamous cell carcinoma beneath the basement membrane. Although we are told that 30% of the circumference of the LEEP specimen was involved by tumor, the margins of the specimen are clear not only of invasion but of dysplasia. The LEEP specimen was taken in two parts, and it would be of interest to know whether the larger specimen or the endocervical 1- by 1-cm loop both contained dysplastic epithelium. In either case, for the purposes of this discussion, it is assumed that margins free not only of invasion but of dysplasia in a malignancy not known for "skip" characteristics would have the same validity as a formal cervical conization with equally free margins.

The major question in this case is whether or not this patient can be considered to have microinvasive carcinoma of the cervix and therefore be considered for conservative management. Microinvasion defines a subset of squamous cell carcinoma in which the mortality/morbidity of radical therapy is equal to or greater than the mortality/morbidity of the disease itself. Definition of this subset hinges on defining a group with an extremely low incidence of recurrence and lymph node involvement. The SGO defines microinvasive squamous cell carcinoma as a tumor with less than 3 mm of invasion beneath the basement membrane and no lymphovascular space involvement. The 1985 FIGO definition of microinvasion included stage IA2 with invasion of 5 mm or less in depth from the basement of the epithelium and 7 mm or less in horizontal spread. Within the calendar year, it is expected that FIGO will adopt the SGO definition and abandon this latter staging. The main reason for this is a demonstration from pooled data that patients with a depth of invasion of 3.1 to 5 mm have a risk of up to 7.4% for lymph node metastases and 5.4% for invasive cancer recurrence (1). It is critical in this case to evaluate the histological specimen for the presence of lymphovascular space invasion. In the presence of demonstrable lymphovascular space involvement along with 4-mm invasion, this patient must be considered as having truly invasive carcinoma of the cervix, and radical hysterectomy with pelvic and paraaortic lymphadenectomy would be indicated. If, on the other hand, there is demonstrated absence of confluent tongues and lymphovascular space invasion, there is more latitude for "conservative" management. In the latter situation, the decision hinges on whether this patient is *committed* to future fertility and whether or not she wishes to accept the *risk* involved in conservative management. The patient must be advised of the risks involved in accordance with the statistics previously mentioned. She must understand that the presence of lymph node involvement means that the disease may progress without our ability to monitor it via Pap smears or scans, such that distant spread may be the first sign of persistent/recurrent disease. If the patient, after proper counseling, understands that risk and wishes to accept it and is doing so for the express purpose of preserving fertility (and provided that she understands the need for close follow-up), in my opinion no further immediate treatment would be indicated. Under any other circumstances, I believe the patient should undergo radical hysterectomy with lymph node dissection, offering her definitive safety of the proper cancer operation. At age 29, barring other factors (i.e., familial ovarian carcinoma), ovarian preservation would be advised.

References

1. Sevin BU, et al. Microinvasive carcinoma of the cervix. Cancer 1992; 70:

PHYSICIAN'S RESPONSE

HOWARD W. JONES, III

I strongly urge a personal review of the cone specimen slides in all patients with superficially invasive cervical cancer. When the gynecologist sits down with the pathologist and looks at the microscopic sections, it is much easier to appreciate the extent of invasive tumor and to get a better understanding of the risk of nodal metastases. The new cervical cancer staging classification adopted by FIGO in 1994 defines stage IA2 as tumors invading 3.1 to 5.0 mm below the basement membrane with a lateral extent of < 7 mm. The lateral extent of this lesion is not described in the available report and no mention is made of the presence or absence of lymphovascular involvement. Although the issue is controversial, most gynecologists in the United States feel that lymphovascular space involvement indicates a higher risk of pelvic lymph node metastases. Therefore most of these patients and patients such as this one, who has invasive cancer > 3 mm deep, have been treated by radical hysterectomy and pelvic lymphadenectomy in this country.

From the description available, it sounds as if this patient has a small but nevertheless truly invasive cervical cancer. Her margins are reported to be negative, but the validity of this report depends on the number of sections, and so on. In a large series of cone biopsies, Peterson-Brown et al. (1) reported that 12.5% of women who had repeat cone or hysterectomy after a cone with a "negative" margin had residual intraepithelial disease in the cervix. In addition, Copeland et al. (2) reported a 5.7% incidence of pelvic lymph node metastases in a literature review of 157 patients with 3- to 5-mm invasion.

The therapeutic options for this patient include (a) careful follow-up with no further therapy at this time, (b) simple hysterectomy, or (c) modified radical hysterectomy and pelvic lymphadenectomy. I feel that the greatest risk to her life is the 4–5% incidence of pelvic nodal metastases, and I would therefore recommend a modified radical hysterectomy and pelvic lymphadenectomy, which has a low risk of significant morbidity in a young, healthy patient.

References

1. Paterson-Brown S, Chappatte OA, Clark SK, et al. The significance of cone biopsy resection margins. Gynecol Oncol 1992; 46:182–185.
2. Morris M, Mitchell MF, Silva EG, et al. Cervical conization as definitive therapy for early invasive squamous carcinoma of the cervix.

60

Cervical Cancer, Adenocarcinoma "Microinvasive"

CASE

A 27-year-old woman, gravida O, had a Pap smear that showed atypical endocervical cells. A cone biopsy was done by her local physician, and it showed adenocarcinoma in situ. The patient was referred for consultation. The slides were reviewed and a repeat Pap smear 12 weeks after the cone biopsy showed reactive endocervical cells not felt to be compatible with adenocarcinoma in situ. The patient was then seen for her next Pap smear 7 months following the cone biopsy, which revealed atypical endocervical cells, and this was followed by a loop electrosurgical excision procedure (LEEP). The LEEP showed adenocarcinoma in situ with one small area (five glands) interpreted as early invasion. The margins were clear. An endocervical curettage at the time of the LEEP was negative.

PHYSICIAN'S RESPONSE

VICKI SELTZER

Prior to discussing the patient's options with her, I would carefully review all her Pap smears and histological specimens. I would want to assess the dimensions of the LEEP and evaluate its adequacy. I would want to confirm the diagnosis of early invasive adenocarcinoma and distinguish this from adenocarcinoma in situ. I would want to assess the grade of the lesion.

I believe that the proper approach for this problem is a hysterectomy. If the patient wished to preserve her reproductive capacity, I would discuss extensively

463

the risks of this approach with her. If she strongly wishes to preserve her reproductive capacity, this could be done, but I believe that the attendant risk is significant and I would definitely discourage it.

Andersen reported on 36 consecutive cases of adenocarcinoma in situ of the cervix, including 8 cases of early stromal invasion found on cone biopsy. All early invasive adenocarcinomas had uninvolved margins of the cone biopsy, but residual disease was found in 4 of 6 cases in hysterectomy specimens.

If this young woman strongly wishes to have a child, I would encourage her to consider options such as utilizing assisted reproductive technologies.

If the patient's uterus were left in place, I would be concerned about both persistence of disease and also the difficulties of diagnosing recurrent disease. In Andersen's series of 32 patients with adenocarcinoma in situ who had previous Pap smears, 16 had benign cytology within the last 3 years and 5 had benign cytology within the last 12 months. All 3 cases of adenocarcinoma in situ with coexisting early invasion without squamous lesions had been preceded by 1 to 6 negative smears.

In Andersen's series, preoperative colposcopy was performed in 32 patients and was considered "normal" in 10. In these "normal" cases, punch biopsies and ECCs were important in detecting an abnormality. Therefore, if the patient is not willing to have a hysterectomy, I would do pelvic exams with Pap smears, colposcopies, and biopsies, including ECC, initially at 3-month intervals. However, I believe that the likelihood of persistent or recurrent disease is high if initial treatment is by cone biopsy and I would discourage this approach.

Reference

Andersen ES, Arffmann E. Adenocarcinoma in situ of the uterine cervix: A clinico-pathologic study of 36 cases. Gynecol Oncol 1989; 35:1–7.

PHYSICIAN'S RESPONSE

R. GERALD PRETORIUS

If the patient did not desire fertility, I would have advised hysterectomy at the time of the initial consultation. If fertility is not an issue, hysterectomy is indicated when adenocarcinoma in situ of the cervix is found on conization, because the margins of the cone are not good predictors of whether there is disease remaining in the cervix and because neither Papanicolaou smear, endo-cervical curettage, nor colposcopy accurately detects recurrence.

If the patient desired fertility and her conization removed the transformation zone but not the majority of the endocervical glandular epithelium, my initial management (regardless of whether the margins on the first cone were positive or negative) would be to perform a second conization in which the cone specimen was roughly cylindrical, about 2.5 cm deep, and about 1 cm wide at its base. This technique, described by Bertrand et al. (1), assures that the majority of the endocervical glandular tissue has been sampled. If, on repeat conization, no invasive cancer was found and the margins were clear, I would, with some misgivings, follow the patient with Papanicolaou smears and endocervical curettage every 4 months.

If the patient's initial conization did not remove the majority of the endocervical glandular tissue and, 7 months later, she underwent LEEP excision with clear margins showing invasive adenocarcinoma in a total of five glands, I would advise that she undergo a second conization to exclude a larger invasive adenocarcinoma (the technique would be Bertrand's). If the second conization revealed no invasive cervical cancer, then I would advise simple hysterectomy 6 weeks following the second conization. If the second conization revealed invasive cancer with a volume greater than 250 mm^3, vascular space invasion, or depth of invasion greater than 3 mm or if the margins of the second cone were positive for invasive cancer, I would advise modified radical hysterectomy with pelvic node dissection.

The decision to perform simple hysterectomy despite the finding of a small invasive adenocarcinoma of the cervix is made with some trepidation. Though microinvasive adenocarcinoma of the cervix has been defined by Burghardt (2) as an invasive cancer less than 7 mm wide and less than 5 mm deep, there are too few cases reported to determine whether this definition is restrictive enough to allow less than radical treatment. Given the lack of data, I treat small adenocarcinomas of the cervix as I treat small squamous cancers (the rules stated above are my rules for small squamous cancers). Though I have conserved fertility by treating some small squamous cancers with conization alone, I would be reluctant to treat any invasive adenocarcinoma of the cervix with less than hysterectomy because of the difficulty in detecting recurrence.

References

1. Bertrand M, Lickrish GM, Colgan TJ. The anatomic distribution of cervical adenocarcinoma in situ: Implications for treatment. Am J Obstet Gynecol 1987; 157:21–25.
2. Burghardt E. Pathology of early invasive squamous and glandular carcinoma of the cervix (FIGO Stage Ia). In Coppleson M, ed. Gynecologic Oncology, 2d ed. Edinburgh: Churchill Livingstone, 1992:609–630.

PHYSICIAN'S RESPONSE

THOMAS MONTAG

This 27-year-old nulligravid woman has recurrent adenocarcinoma in situ (ACIS) of the cervix with a small focus of microinvasion. The LEEP margins were clear and the endocervical curettage was negative. It would be interesting to know if the initial cone biopsy margins were clear.

Simple hysterectomy is the treatment of choice for women who do not wish to preserve fertility. Pelvic lymph node sampling should be considered, since recurrence involving the pelvic side wall, suggesting lymphatic spread, has been reported.

For patients who have not completed childbearing, the effectiveness and safety of cone biopsy alone as therapy for ACIS is undetermined. In a recent review (1), patients with ACIS diagnosed by cone biopsy with positive margins were noted to be at high risk for residual ACIS or early invasive adenocarcinoma. Of 34 women, 21 (62%) with ACIS and positive cone margins had persistent ACIS in the subsequent hysterectomy specimen. In contrast, 4 of 50 women (8%) with uninvolved cone margins had residual ACIS. The authors report 18 women with ACIS and uninvolved margins treated only with conization (1). All 18 patients were relapse-free after a median follow-up of 3 years (range 1.5 to 5 years).

Additional study is necessary to establish the safety of cone biopsy as treatment for ACIS. A recent report (2) is concerning, although the number of patients is small. Of 9 patients with ACIS and negative margins on cone biopsy, 4 (44%) had residual ACIS in the hysterectomy specimen (2). These authors conclude that the status of margins on cone biopsies containing ACIS does not predict the presence of residual disease in the hysterectomy specimen.

Nevertheless, my recommendation for this patient, if she wishes to preserve her fertility, is close follow-up, with pelvic examination and Pap smears every 3 months for 2 years. After that, the intervals can probably be extended to every 4 to 6 months. The patient must be apprised of the risks of recurrence as well as the fact that the safety of this conservative approach has not been established. She must agree to close follow-up.

References

1. Hopkins MP, Roberts JA, Schmidt RW. Cervical adenocarcinoma in situ. Obstet Gynecol 1988; 71:842.
2. Im DD, Duska LR, Rosenshein NB. Adequacy of cone biopsy margins in adenocarcinoma in situ of the cervix as a predictor of residual disease. Presented as a poster at the Society of Gynecologic Oncologists Annual Meeting, San Francisco, February 18–22, 1995.

PHYSICIAN'S RESPONSE

MAUREEN KILLACKEY

The diagnosis of endocervical adenocarcinoma in situ in a young nulliparous woman present both pathological and clinical problems. All cytology, conization,

LEEP, and curettage slides should be carefully reviewed by an experienced gynecological pathologist and the clinician who has examined this patient colposcopically. I am most concerned about the area of gland involvement interpreted as early invasion and would request several expert pathological opinions. Assuming that the focus of early invasion, negative margins, and endocervical curettage are confirmed, the patient's desire for fertility must be determined.

Whatever the patient's wishes, I would recommend a repeat conization to evaluate other additional areas and depth of invasion. If pregnancy is not an issue and the second cone does not show further invasion, an extrafascial or vaginal hysterectomy would be recommended. If the patient wishes to maintain her childbearing potential and the second cone is negative, my discussion would consist of the following:

1. There are few data about the safety of conservative management of patients with cervical adenocarcinoma in situ or early cancer. Specifically, follow-up with Pap smears, endocervical curettage, and colposcopy may be inadequate.

2. The negative status of the second cervical conization margins does not predict the presence of residual disease in the uterus.

3. The patient's human immunodeficiency virus (HIV) status should be determined; if it is positive, conservative follow-up may not be appropriate.

4. The patient and her partner should be carefully evaluated for lower-genital-tract human papillomavirus (HPV) and all lesions eradicated.

5. Within reason, I would advise the patient not to delay attempts to achieve pregnancy.

References

Poynor EA, et al. Management and follow-up of patients with adenocarcinoma in situ of the uterine cervix. Abstract #4, Society of Gynecologic Oncologists, 1994 meeting.

Im DD, et al. Adequacy of cone biopsy margins in adenocarcinoma in situ of the cervix as a predictor of residual disease. Abstract #87, Society of Gynecologic Oncologists, 1995 meeting.

PHYSICIAN'S RESPONSE

KENNETH D. WEBSTER

Adenocarcinoma in situ of the uterine cervix (AIS) was first described in 1953. The number of patients diagnosed with AIS at the Cleveland Clinic Foundation has increased in recent years. From 1980 to 1989, a total of 18 patients were treated for this condition. In the last 5 years, 34 patients have been diagnosed with AIS. Management of AIS has been controversial.

A recent review of 52 patients with AIS was completed at our institution. In all but one patient, AIS was detected from an abnormal Pap smear. Hysterectomy was the primary treatment in 7 patients and none had recurrent disease (mean follow-up, 102 months). Of 45 patients treated with conization, 18 had positive endocervical margins; 24 had negative margins, and 3 had conization specimens with margins not specified. The 3 cases with unspecified margins showed no recurrence (mean follow-up, 93 months). Of the 24 cases with negative margins, 2 were treated with hysterectomy and showed no residuum and 2 had recurrence of AIS after 15 and 27 months.

Of 18 patients with positive margins, 6 underwent hysterectomy and 2 of those had residual disease; 4 had a second conization (2 residual AIS) and 8 had close follow-up (1 recurrence). After the second conization, 2 of the 4 patients had recurrence of AIS and were treated with a third conization. One of these had an invasive carcinoma.

In this 27-year-old patient, a conservative approach (i.e., no additional therapy) can be permitted only if she wants a pregnancy in the very near future. The histology must show no invasion beyond 3 mm and no vascular space involvement. If the patient is not reliable for follow-up, is not desirous of near future fertility, or the above histological requirements are not satisfied, she should have a hysterectomy.

Reference

Wildrich T, Kennedy A, Belinson J, et al. Adenocarcinoma in-situ of the uterine cervix: Management and follow-up of 52 patients. Abstract submitted to American College of Obstetricians and Gynecologists, Annual Meeting 1995.

61

Cervical Cancer, Squamous Cell, Stage IIA

CASE

The patient, a 58-year-old woman, gravida IV, para IV, is 5 ft, 6 in tall and weighs 180 lb. She had been experiencing a bloody mucous discharge for approximately $2^1/_2$ months when she came to the gynecologist's office. At the time of her visit, her physician, suspecting she had an invasive cancer of the cervix, performed a cervical biopsy and referred the patient to a gynecological oncologist. On examination, the patient was found to have an exophytic squamous cell carcinoma of the cervix measuring 4 cm in diameter on the cervix and extending approximately $1^1/_2$ cm centrally posteriorly and on the anterior vaginal fornix. The parametria were clear. There was no evidence of pelvic side-wall nodularity. The patient was in good physical condition, taking no medications. Chest x-ray was normal. An abdominal pelvic computed tomography (CT) scan was normal. Complete blood count (CBC), serology (SMA12), electrolytes, blood urea nitrogen (BUN), and creatinine were all within normal limits.

PHYSICIANS' RESPONSE

A. MENZIN
S. RUBIN

This patient appears to have a large but early cervical cancer. Though radiological evaluation has failed to identify regional or distant metastases, the clinical staging has not yet been completed. Prior to therapy, proctoscopy and cystoscopy would

469

be valuable to assess for spread of tumor to contiguous structures. Management options for a patient with stage IIA disease (as described for this patient) are notably different than for those for a patient with stage IV cancer (e.g., bladder involvement).

If one assumes that the findings after the completion of clinical staging favor a stage IIA designation, several therapeutic modalities are available to this woman. The 5-year survival rate for patients with stage IIA squamous cell carcinoma of the cervix varies between 70 to 85%. In both retrospective and prospective trials, rates of survival and pelvic tumor control are statistically equivalent between radiotherapy alone and radical surgery. One should note that women with stage IIA cervical cancer may comprise a spectrum in which the cancer may extend well into the middle third of the vagina. Only those patients whose lesions extended minimally onto the fornix are reasonable candidates for surgical resection.

The recommendation for primary therapy is based on a number of factors. The patient's physical condition may militate against an operative approach if medical issues are severe. Though technically feasible, radical dissection in the obese patient is a challenge and may expose the individual to greater risk of operative complications than the nonobese patient would face. Certain character- istics, particularly size and location, of the primary lesion can be critical. Radical resection needed to remove lesions with extensive vaginal involvement may pose undue risk as compared to radiotherapy. Some authors have recommended primary treatment with radiation for large or barrel-shaped cervical tumors, often followed by an adjuvant extrafascial hysterectomy. Evidence to support this approach is, however, lacking. The use of radical hysterectomy after primary radiotherapy adds little to outcome and substantially to morbidity.

The nature of the morbidity associated with the treatment of cervical can- cer must impact significantly on a patient's choice of therapeutic modality. Radical surgery clearly has a greater incidence of short-term complications, including pneumonia, atelectasis, venous thrombosis and pulmonary embolism, fistulas of bladder, ureters, or rectum to the vagina, and nearly ubiquitous atony of the bladder due to extensive transection of autonomic nerve pathways in the retroperitoneum. With current modalities using high-energy sources and effective brachytherapy techniques, radiation can be delivered with minimal short-term sequelae. Though the disfiguring cutaneous injuries are gone, long- term complications may not become apparent until 2 or more years after treat- ment, particularly in the case of bowel fistulas, intestinal dysfunction, and chronic urinary symptoms.

Other critical issues relate to the preservation of ovarian and sexual function. Operative management allows for the possibility of ovarian preservation, but recent evidence does note that ovarian function may be decreased following hysterectomy (as indicated by age at the onset of menopausal symptoms). Several authors have reported experience with ovarian transposition to decrease the rate of ovarian failure after adjuvant radiation therapy, but this practice has its own set of potential problems. In this 56-year-old woman, ovarian preservation should not weigh in the therapeutic decision. However, the physician should consider the patient's current sexual activity and her plans for the future. Though vaginal resection associated with radical surgery does shorten the functional length of the canal, the vaginal epithelium retains its pliability and transudative lubrication in the postoperative patient. The vagina in the radiated patient is considerably less pliable as well as dry and foreshortened. These changes often make resumption of sexual function difficult in the 70 to 85% of women cured by primary therapy.

Our recommendation is for examination under anesthesia, cystoscopy, and proctoscopy followed by exploratory laparotomy if stage IIA is confirmed. At exploration, we recommend a frozen-section evaluation of paraaortic lymph nodes and, if negative, a radical hysterectomy with bilateral salpingo-oophorectomy and bilateral pelvic lymph node dissection. Consideration can be given to adjuvant chemotherapy and/or radiotherapy following surgery if prognostic factors warrant.

PHYSICIANS' RESPONSE

SUSAN K. GIBBONS
HENRY KEYS

Although this tumor does not strictly meet the usual definition of a "bulky" or "barrel-shaped" cervix cancer (because it is exophytic), its 4 cm diameter warrants discussion of tumor size and its effect upon prognosis. Stage for stage, large-diameter cervical lesions are associated with increased incidence of lymph node positivity, increased rates of local and distant recurrence, and decreased patient survival. This discrepancy is seen in patients treated with standard (conventional) radiotherapy, as well as those treated with radical hysterectomy.

A number of treatment strategies have been devised to improve the prognosis of patients with large cervical tumors. In general, radical hysterectomy is not recommended because patients will so often require postoperative irradiation for positive margins, parametrial involvement, or positive lymph nodes, and this combination of therapies carries an increased risk of complication. When primary radiotherapy is used, the treatment volume may be the pelvis only, or it can be extended to include the para-aortic lymph nodes. In either case, the proportion of the total central dose that is delivered by external beam irradiation is increased, in order to allow shrinkage of the tumor prior to intracavitary implant. If tumor shrinkage is inadequate to allow an optimal intracavitary implant, an interstitial implant can be used instead. The total central radiotherapy dose (external beam plus intracavitary or interstitial implant) is increased, to address the larger tumor burden implicit in a bulky lesion.

Alternatively, a variety of combined modality approaches are under investigation. These include neoadjuvant chemotherapy (followed by radical hysterectomy or radiotherapy), radiotherapy with concurrent chemotherapy for radiosensitization, and primary radiotherapy followed by TAH/BSO.

In the case of the patient presented, a cystoscopy should be performed to complete her clinical staging. Assuming this study is negative, her disease would be classified as stage IIA. I would recommend primary radiotherapy, for several reasons. Despite its exophytic growth pattern, the large size of her tumor puts her at increased risk of local recurrence after radical hysterectomy. Also, exophytic tumors generally respond very well to irradiation, so she should have good tumor shrinkage prior to intracavitary treatment. Finally, one of the most significant long-term side effects of pelvic radiotherapy, ovarian ablation, would not be of consequence in this postmenopausal patient. Concurrent chemotherapy may radiosensitize the tumor, and it may decrease the risk of distant failure; however, this approach must still be considered investigational at this time.

If she is eligible for a randomized clinical trial comparing two or more reasonable treatment options, randomization may be the best recommendation of all. As always, the risks and expected benefits associated with all available treatment options should be thoroughly discussed with the patient.

References

1. Fuller AF, Elliott N, Kosloff C, Hoskins WJ, Lewis JL. Determinants of increased risk for recurrence in patients undergoing radical hysterectomy for stage IB and IIA carcinoma of the cervix. Gyn Oncol 1989:33:34–39.
2. Lowrey GC, Mendenhall WM, Million RR. Stage IB or IIA-B carcinoma of the intact uterine cervix treated with irradiation: A multivariate analysis. Int J Rad Oncol Biol Phys 1992:24:205–210.

PHYSICIAN'S RESPONSE

GEORGE W. MORLEY

On reviewing this case history, one wonders whether or not this patient has had previous Pap smears and, if so, what the results were. If this patient had had annual Pap smears in the past, I suspect that the existing lesion would have been detected at a much earlier date and thus her chance of survival would have been improved. In addition, the past medical and social history would be of interest; however, it would serve no useful purpose in the outline of a therapeutic program for the existing condition.

As far as prognosis is concerned, there are a couple of points in her favor in that this is an exophytic lesion and it is of the squamous cell variety; however, the histological grade is not reported. The diameter of the cervix measures 4 cm, thus placing this lesion at the dividing point in regard to treatment. A number of people would treat this patient with total pelvic irradiation if it were 4 cm or greater, whereas a more aggressive, surgically oriented gynecological oncologist would consider a radical hysterectomy and pelvic and paraaortic lymph node dissection. However, if it were thought to be a barrel-shaped type of lesion, then x-ray therapy would be the treatment of choice in most instances. There are still others who would treat this patient with combined therapy by reducing the radiation therapy and then following this with an extrafascial hysterectomy and regional lymph node dissection. The treatment of choice in this situation is still somewhat controversial.

Given that this disease has already extended approximately 1 to $1^1/_2$ cm into the anterior vaginal fornix, the question then arises whether this is a stage IIA or IIB invasive carcinoma of the cervix with involvement of only the vaginal mucosa versus a lesion with parametrial involvement. The pretreatment assessment of these patients should include the standard workup followed by cystoscopy, CT scanning, and/or intravenous pyelography (IVP) and lymphangiography. Some feel that CT scanning is a reasonably well established part of the pre-treatment evaluation for carcinoma of the cervix and thus an IVP and lymphangiogram is not necessary; however, others think that CT scanning may produce false-positive results. In well-trained hands, the lymphangiogram increases the accuracy of determining the exact extent of the disease, especially if this is followed with a fine needle aspiration in the presence of suspicious or positive lymph nodes. If the cystoscopy revealed bullous edema only, then one should seriously consider staging this lesion as stage IIB carcinoma of the cervix. I am not a particular proponent of an extraperitoneal nodal evaluation, but if done, this has fewer complications than does the transperitoneal approach. The use of magnetic resonance imaging (MRI) in the future will certainly lessen the need for surgical staging.

In regard to treatment, one should divide the therapy into two parts; i.e., stage IIA and stage IIB carcinoma of the cervix. A number of people in this country and elsewhere treat stage IB and IIA similarly, with either a radical hysterectomy and pelvic lymphadenectomy or with full-course pelvic radiation therapy. This latter treatment would consist of 4500 to 5000 rads delivered to the whole pelvis through both external-beam radiation and intravitary cesium, utilizing the Fletcher-Suit technique. Others think that radical surgery should be reserved for stage IB, and that stage IIA and higher stages should be treated with full-course irradiation. These individuals feel that the limits of involvement are better defined by separating the diseased cervix proper from disease beyond the cervix.

As one discusses radical surgery further, if one chooses to use the Rutledge classification of extended hysterectomies, then this would be considered a class III radical procedure. A class II radical hysterectomy is often referred to as a modified radical hysterectomy and should be reserved for a much lesser lesion of the cervix.

Surgery and radiation therapy are certainly complementary, and optimal results can be obtained with either form of treatment. Surgery does have the advantage of requiring a shorter treatment period, and in the earlier lesions it does remove the primary lesion and limits the injury to the surrounding tissue. Ureteral complications either as a fistula or stricture are complications related to radical hysterectomy, but the incidence has been markedly reduced through improvements in technique and less traumatic handling of the ureters during this dissection. Bladder dysfunction to some degree is a common post-operative complaint; however, this is usually of short duration.

Many gynecological oncologists recommend postoperative whole pelvic irradiation for those patients with parametrial invasion, nodal metastases, or positive surgical margins. This is thought to decrease the local recurrence rate; however, often extrapelvic disease has already occurred. Once this has been detected, systemic chemotherapy must be considered as additional adjunctive therapy.

Girardi and associates (1) reported a close correlation between involvement of the parametrial lymph nodes and the lateral pelvic lymph nodes. Of the patients with negative parametrial nodes, only 26% had positive pelvic lymph nodes; however, 81% of patients with positive parametrial lymph nodes also had metastasis to the pelvic nodes. This is a very important finding that endorses the need to include the entire en bloc dissection in the diagnostic and therapeutic approach to this disease.

Finally, from a review of the literature over the past several years, the 5-year survival rate for those patients treated with radiation therapy were stage IB, 88%; stage IIA, 75%; and stage IIB, approximately 60%. For those patients treated with radical surgery and in separating the results into those with positive pelvic lymph nodes versus negative pelvic lymph nodes, the 5-year survival rates were stage IB and positive nodes, 45%; with negative nodes, 91%. The overall survival was 83%. Similarly, for stage II, the 5-year survival rates were positive nodes, 42%; negative nodes, 77%. The overall survival was not reported (2).

Again, earlier diagnosis plus earlier onset of therapy equals better prognosis.

References

1. Girardi F, Lichtenegger W, Tamussino K, Haas J. The importance of parametrial lymph nodes in the treatment of cervical cancer. Gynecol Oncol 1989; 34:206.
2. Knapp RC, Berkowitz RS, eds. Gynecologic Oncology. New York: Macmillan, 1986.

PHYSICIAN'S RESPONSE

MARK D. ADELSON

Patients do present in this older age group with primary cancer of the cervix, but it is becoming more common for such patients to present in their twenties and thirties. Has this patient had routine gynecological follow-up, including a yearly Pap smear? Were these Pap smears correctly read? Were atypical squamous cells of undetermined significance (ASCUS) or a squamous intra-epithelial lesion (SIL) present? Cervical cancer should be almost entirely preventable with regular Pap smears, and investigation of abnormal Pap smears by colposcopy (including ASCUS). If the metastatic workup is negative, she has a stage IIA cancer, with a 25% incidence of lymph node metastasis. A CT scan negative for metastatic disease does not eliminate the possibility of lymphatic spread, for it is not sensitive for disease under 2 cm. In order to avoid an unnecessary laparotomy in patients with larger-volume disease, for whom the chance of lymph node metastasis is higher, their lymph nodes could be removed laparoscopically. It is possible to perform this laparoscopic staging just prior to planned laparotomy for radical hysterectomy. It is also possible to perform a laparoscopic radical hysterectomy in addition to the nodal staging (1). At laparotomy, I perform a modified radical hysterectomy since there is no clear evidence that a formal radical produces a better cure rate than lesser resection. The nerve sparing technique using the CUSA (2) allows me to remove the anterior portion of the cardinal ligament (pars vasculosa), sparing the dorsal portion, which carries the nerve supply to the rectum and bladder. The significant morbidity accompanying radical hysterectomy is bladder weakness/voiding dys-function, which can be minimized by performing a modified radical hysterectomy or using the nerve-sparing technique. The nerve-sparing approach allows resec-tion of the entire ventral cardinal ligament up to the pelvic wall (including the sentinel node(s).

An informed consent discussion needs to be carried out with this patient, clearly stating the material risks and benefits of radiation versus surgery. In the absence of nodal metastasis, the 5-year survival should be equivalent for both modalities (85%). If one should find pelvic nodal metastasis after radical hyster-ectomy, radiation therapy would be advised. In the presence of nodal metastases, radiation therapy may result in a better survival rate than radical hysterectomy alone. It is unclear whether radiation therapy after radical hysterectomy improves survival, but the standard of care is adjunctive radiation in this setting. We may be able to perform a nerve-sparing approach laparoscopically, and this is being considered for future investigation. If there is no gross evidence of metastasis, I complete the lymphadenectomy, including periaortic sampling, and proceed to radical hysterectomy. In the presence of nodal metastasis, lymphovascular space involvement, close surgical margins, or parametrial involvement, adjunctive radiation therapy would be advised.

References

1. Querleu D. Case report: Laparoscopically assisted radical vaginal hysterectomy. Gynecol Oncol 1993; 51:248–254.
2. Yabuki Y, Asamoto A, Hashiba T, et al. Dissection of the cardinal ligament in radical hysterectomy for cervical cancer with emphasis on the lateral ligament. Am J Obstet Gynecol 1991; 164:7–14.

PHYSICIAN'S RESPONSE

JOHN CURRIE

In deciding on treatment options for stage IIA carcinoma of the cervix, the clinician must take several factors into consideration. Ideally, surgical therapy is probably better treatment for a relatively young patient; a 58-year-old woman in good general health would fit in this category. Although preservation of ovarian function is not an applicable issue at this age, avoidance of sexual function problems associated with radiation therapy is a pertinent issue. Thus, if the patient, given the alternative between surgical and radiation therapy, chose the former, type III radical hysterectomy (Clark-Wertheim) would be an ideal treatment. Of course, the surgeon should take care to ensure that a true radical dissection was performed; a healthy vaginal margin is essential. Such a radical extirpation is beyond the training capabilities of many surgeons, and expertise in performing a true radical hysterectomy is mandated in this case.

An acceptable alternate treatment is radical radiation therapy, administered by a radiation oncologist with expertise in treating gynecological neoplasms. The case as presented could be treated with standard ports and dosages.

If clinical trials are available, this patient could also be considered for such. Pertinent studies are under way; for instance, surgical therapy in this patient would allow entry into a trial comparing postoperative radiation therapy versus such therapy accompanied by systemic chemotherapy. The patient, because of the stage and size of the lesion, has certain risk factors for recurrence; entry into clinical trials would offer the best options for contemporary treatment.

Treatment of this patient present challenges to the gynecological oncologist. Regardless of mode, appropriate therapy should result in a very good survival rate.

62

Cervical Dysplasia; Persistent CIN1

CASE

A 37-year-old woman, who for the past 2 years has been having Pap smears done every 4 months because of CIN1. Two years ago she had a colposcopy done that showed CIN1. This was followed by biopsies and cryotherapy. An endocervical curettage at that time was normal. Eight months after the cryotherapy, CIN1 again returned on her Pap smear, and this has remained the case since. Colposcopy reveals some evidence of cervical CIN1 as well as a couple of areas in the right fornix suggestive of flat condyloma. The patient expresses concern to you that she is worried she may develop cancer and she is now seeking your advice.

PHYSICIAN'S RESPONSE

ALEXANDER W. KENNEDY

Patients with Pap smears indicating atypical squamous cells of undetermined significance (ASCUS) or low-grade squamous intraepithelial lesion (LG-SIL) are being encountered with increasing frequency. This is partially, at least, due to changes in the reporting terminology incorporated into the Bethesda system. In our clinical practice, we manage patients with ASCUS or LG-SIL in an identical fashion. These patients are seen promptly, and foremost in their management must be an intensive educational effort to allay their fears of having cancer and to understand the significance of their current findings. Patients need to understand at the outset that the goal of Pap-smear screening is not to have a "normal" Pap smear but rather to prevent cervical cancer.

In order to provide prompt and efficient care at the lowest possible cost, we have trained a nurse colposcopist to manage these patients with minor abnormalities on Pap smears. The patient is provided with extensive educational counseling and literature to understand the significance of her findings and to explain the complexities of human papillomavirus (HPV). We stress the need for careful follow-up and educate patients that the low-grade lesions are usually not associated with the viral subtypes related to carcinoma in situ and invasive cancer. We counsel them that the goal of the initial triaging is to exclude more serious underlying lesions and then to work out a follow-up schedule.

We do not perform cryotherapy for low-grade lesions and have elected, in reliable patients, to follow them without treatment once more severe lesions have been excluded. With the colposcopic findings presented, we would remove the abnormal-appearing area on the cervix as well as within the vagina if this can be done easily. We would then recommend that the patient return for repeat screening colposcopy by our nurse, along with a Pap smear, in 6 months. Unless more significant findings than CIN1 are encountered, the patient is advised to be followed by serial Pap smears; repeat colposcopy or other intervention is not advised unless a more significant finding such as high-grade SIL is suggested. We emphasize to patients that the risk of low-grade lesions progressing to cancer with an intact immune system is small, and interventions that may lead to impairment of fertility or cause cervical/vaginal scarring are avoided. We have been satisfied with this management protocol and patients have been very accepting of this scheme once proper educational efforts have been conducted.

PHYSICIANS' RESPONSE

THOMAS V. SEDLACEK
MAX A. CLARK

This patient presents with a very typical history reflecting the difficulties in clinical management of a patient with low-grade squamous intraepithelial lesions. The initial diagnosis based on colposcopically directed biopsy was presumably confined to the portion of the cervix, since the endocervical curettage was normal. Cryotherapy was an appropriate management technique for a 35-year-old woman. Subsequent Pap smears have continued to show CIN1, and evidence of flat condylomata in the vaginal fornices at the most recent colposcopic examination is consistent with a regional distribution of HPV.

We recognize that inter- and intraobserver variation in interpreting both cytology and histology is high in the low-grade spectrum of intraepithelial neoplasia. We would expect roughly only a 30% correlation between observers. Thus, this patient may, in fact, have no disease, may have subclinical HPV infection with a latent HPV infection, or may have a premalignant condition bound to progress to cancer unless it is treated aggressively.

Recent work strongly indicates that HPV infection is a regional infection. When the cervix is involved, there is a high likelihood of involvement of both the vagina and the vulva. Attempts at eradiating subclinical HPV have proven to be fruitless. More recent attempts at managing subclinical HPV have emphasized improving the immune system, treatments with interferon, or treatment with topical 5-fluorouracil. There are significant disadvantages to each of these treatment programs. Interferon is expensive, it causes flulike symptoms, and its efficacy in treating subclinical disease has not been established. Topical 5-fluorouracil has demonstrated efficacy in treating clinical warts but is of unproven efficacy in treating subclinical disease. In addition, recurrence rates are high, in the range of 30 to 50%, and some patients suffer unacceptable vaginal ulceration and develop adenosis of the vagina, which is quite troublesome.

Precursor lesions, which are destined to develop into cancer, are characterized by chromosomal aneuploidy and atypical mitotic figures; they are usually HPV types 16 or 18. While the positive predictive value of HPV typing has not been established, if this patient were found to have HPV 6 or 11 inhabiting her vagina or vulva, she and the physician could be reassured that the likelihood of progression is nil. Similarly, if her biopsy results show no evidence of atypical mitotic figures, this would indicate a low likelihood of progression.

Immune-modulating chemicals or medicines such as steroids and low-dose chemotherapy can compromise the patient's immune system and impair the delayed hypersensitivity system's handling of the HPV. Therefore these drugs should be avoided. In a similar fashion, cigarette smoking, recreational drug use, and high alcohol intake have been correlated with an increased risk of high-grade CIN. Infection with the human immunodeficiency virus is similarly associated with an increased risk of developing CIN.

Recommendations

1. Repeat colposcopy with complete evaluation of cervix, vagina and vulva.
2. Strongly suggest that patient stop smoking, using recreational drugs, or overutilizing alcohol.
3. Monitor the patient with endocervical and ectocervical Pap smears every 6 months and a colposcopy every year for the next 2 years. Treatment is indicated only for CIN 2 or 3; if, after this period of surveillance, no lesion worse than CIN1 is noted, further colposcopy should be restricted to cytology showing high-grade SIL.

References

Sedlacek TV, Peipart, Post JF. Genital human papillomavirus infections. Grad Obstet Gynecol 1991; 2:

Riva JM, Sedlacek, et al. Extended carbon dioxide laser vaporization in the treatment of subclinical papillomavirus infections of the lower genital tract Obstet Gynecol 1989; 73:25.

PHYSICIAN'S RESPONSE

HOWARD D. HOMESLEY

Risk factors that may be pertinent to this patient should be reviewed. Risk factors for cervical dysplasia appear to be smoking, oral contraceptive use, and multiple sexual partners. The association of nutritional factors with cervical dysplasia has been examined through a case-control study. The insufficient intake of vitamin A, riboflavin, ascorbate, and folate is associated with an increased risk of cervical dysplasia (1).

Although it may not be the case in this particular patient, human immunodeficiency virus (HIV) infections in women now account for 40% of all HIV infections worldwide, and the majority of the infections are due to heterosexual transmission. In the United States, 12% of acquired immunodeficiency syndrome (AIDS) cases occur in women in certain high-prevalence areas. Both squamous cell neoplasia of the cervix and HIV infection are in part sexually transmitted, associated with oncogenic types of human papillomavirus, which is an implicated carcinogen associated with several cancers. Therefore, an association between cervical cancer and AIDS can be anticipated on the basis of common sexual behavioral risk factors.

Although this may not be the case in this particular patient, more and more often HIV testing should be considered in patients presenting with cervical dysplasia.

The management of patients with mild dysplasia on cervical smears remains uncertain. Laser vaporization can be used for treatment of patients with a satisfactory colposcopic examination. Where the cervical intraepithelial neoplasia extends into the cervical os, laser excisional cone may be necessary. The success rates with vaporization and/or excisional cone are high because this can be done under direct visualization. The flat condylomata would be amenable to vaporization.

The use of loop electrosurgical excision of the cervix as an office procedure is feasible with few complications, minimal discomfort, and provision of a pathology specimen. This could be performed in this patient with procurement of a separate endocervical specimen to assure clear endocervical margins.

With the advent of loop excisional cones, cold-knife conization is rarely indicated and would be unnecessary except perhaps where there would be a need to distinguish between microinvasive and invasive cancer.

The least invasive and most inexpensive recommendation is to reassure this patient of proven reliability for follow-up that she has a 90 to 95% chance for spontaneous regression of the lesion. The condylomata, if necessary, could be managed with weekly intravaginal 5-fluorouracil for 2 to 3 months.

Transvaginal hysterectomy would be a consideration only in a patient with gynecological indications for hysterectomy.

Reference

Liu T, Soong SJ, Wilson NP, et al. A case control study of nutritional factors and cervical dysplasia. Cancer Epidemiol Biomarkers Prevention 1993; 2:525–530.

63

Ovarian Cancer, Epithelial (Early Disease, Unstaged)

CASE

The patient, a 46-year-old woman who is a Jehovah's Witness, is 5 ft, 1 in tall and weighs 350 lb. She has undergone an emergency laparotomy for acute abdominal pain. At the time of surgery, her right adnexa was torsed. A right salpingo-oophorectomy was done to solve the acute situation. Fortunately, her incision healed up nicely postoperatively and she was discharged home on her fourth postoperative day. At that time the diagnosis returned as a grade 2 papillary serous carcinoma of the right ovary. Her postoperative course was smooth. Postoperative computed tomography (CT) could not be done due to the patient's size. A preoperative CA-125 was 81. Postoperatively, the patient's hemoglobin was 13.5; her liver function test as well as renal function tests and electrolytes were all normal. The patient has had no previous operations. She is on no medications and has no previously diagnosed illnesses.

PHYSICIANS' RESPONSE

JUDY CHENG
WILLIAM MANN

Ovarian cancer is the leading cause of death in gynecological malignancies and the fifth leading cause of death from cancer in women. Serous papillary cystadenocarcinoma is the most common histological type, accounting for 35% of malignant epithelial tumors, and is bilateral 40 to 60% of the time. Extraovarian

482

spread is common, and only 15 to 25% of patients present at stage I. The mean disease-free interval, including all stages, is 11.7 months, with a 5-year survival of 37%, median survival of 31 months, and recurrence rate of 66.5%. Patients with advanced disease have a dismal prognosis, with a 5-year survival of < 20%, while patients with stage I disease have a 5-year survival of approximately 85%.

The Gynecologic Oncology Group has defined low-risk patients as those with stage IA or IB disease with grade 1 or 2 histological differentiation. Grade 3, stage IC or Stage II are considered high risk for early ovarian carcinoma. DNA diploidy, patient age < 50 years, residual disease < 1 cm, minimum CA-12 < 35, and CA-125 half-life of < 12 days are considered favorable prognostic signs.

The patient is a Jehovah's Witness with no other medical problems and a good hemoglobin level. Besides her obesity and religious beliefs, probably precluding transfusion, she is a good surgical candidate. She should be offered a meticulous and comprehensive surgical staging laparotomy including total abdominal hysterectomy, left salpingo-oophorectomy, peritoneal washing, omentectomy, biopsies of adhesions and suspicious lesions, and bilateral pelvic and paraaortic lymphadenectomy. If she is fortunate enough to have stage IA or IB disease, no additional adjunctive therapy is needed. She would expect to have a 5-year disease-free survival of 91% and overall survival of 94%. However, if advanced disease is found, adjunctive chemotherapy is indicated. We currently favor platinum and paclitaxel (Taxol) as our first-line therapy. Treatment usually consists of six cycles and CA-125 levels are followed, although we recognize negative levels may be associated with minimal disease. In this particular patient, while we do not feel surgical staging to be contraindicated by obesity and in fact find that this procedure can be accomplished with minimal blood loss, nonetheless the patient must be offered the alternative of either no adjunctive therapy and simply following her, clinically and with CA-125 levels, or alternately treating her with chemotherapy and not completing her surgical staging prior to therapy. Of these two options, while we still feel repeat exploration would be our preference, our second recommendation if this were declined would be to institute a set number of courses of platinum and paclitaxel. We would be particularly concerned if a CA-125 were noted to be elevated 4 to 6 weeks postoperatively or at any other time in the future. In this setting, of a CA-125 beginning to rise, we would recommend reexploration to the patient. At that time, we would complete her surgery and any cytoreductive surgery needed and then institute paclitaxel/platinum regimen.

If the patient declined adjuvant chemotherapy and also reexploration, we would then follow her with clinical examinations and CA-125 measurements. We have not found CT scans or magnetic resonance imaging to be of value in this setting, as these tests are rarely positive unless clinical symptoms and findings exist, and they are quite expensive.

References

Rosman M, Hayden CL, Thiel RP, et al. Prognostic indicators for poor risk epithelial ovarian carcinoma. Cancer 1994; 74:1323–1328.

Soper JT. Management of early staged epithelial ovarian cancer. Clin Obstet Gynecol 1994; 37:423–438.

PHYSICIANS' RESPONSE

LARRY J. COPELAND
JAMES L. NICKLIN

The dilemma of making recommendations for an ovarian carcinoma that has not been appropriately staged, unfortunately, is not an uncommon one. A frozen section of the right ovary at the time of the first laparotomy would have prevented this problem. We assume that the patient's chest x-ray shows no effusions. The preoperative CA-125 is not much help, since this slight elevation could have been secondary to the inflammatory response associated with the torsion or, in a patient of this weight, there may be a chronic high baseline from fatty infiltration of the liver. While CT imaging would require moving the patient to another facility (college of veterinary medicine), the information gained would be unlikely to offset the patient's distress and humiliation with this process. Another consideration would be to perform an OncoScint scan. If positive, this could justify surgical exploration to complete primary debulking. We also assume that there is not a significant family history of ovarian carcinoma.

The patient should be presented with the following management options:

1. Undergo a repeat laparotomy with completion of the surgery (hysterectomy, left salpingo-oophorectomy, omentectomy) and comprehensive staging. Additional treatment will then be influenced by the staging results. *If the staging is negative,* making this tumor stage IA, grade 2, the usual recommendation would be that she be followed with a close posttreatment surveillance program. Early detection of a recurrence in a patient who weighs 350 lb is probably a fallacious concept since one is limited to a severely compromised physical examination and a CA-125. On this basis, some would present an argument to treat the patient even if the staging procedure were negative. *If the staging is positive* (any residual metastatic disease), it would be appropriate to proceed with chemotherapy— paclitaxel and platinum (see doses below). Considering that she is a Jehovah Witness, we would probably recommend cisplatin instead of carboplatin.

2. Proceed with chemotherapy—cisplatin 75 mg/m^2 and paclitaxel 135 mg/m^2 over 24 hour at 3-week intervals for three or six cycles. The patient's morbid obesity would necessitate dose adjustments—initiating treatment based on a body surface area of 2 with subsequent adjustments would seem appropriate.

Without staging information, we would recommend that she receive six cycles. While we would probably not recommend a second-look procedure, the absence of an accurate primary staging procedure could motivate some to be more enthusiastic about considering a second-look laparotomy.

3. Proceed with no therapeutic intervention and follow the patient with a surveillance program of complete physical examination and CA-125 every 6 to 8 weeks for 6 months, then every 2 to 3 months for 2 years, and then every 3 to 6 months. Weight reduction counseling would be appropriate. One could also consider performing an OncoScint scan at between 6 and 9 months.

The patient should be informed as completely and objectively as possible about the pros and cons of each of the above treatment options:

1. Pros: (a) If metastatic tumor is present, there is probably therapeutic advantage to having it removed. (b) This is the most accurate way to confirm if metastatic tumor is present. (c) The decision to either administer additional treatment or withhold treatment would be more universally agreed upon if the staging were completed. (d) Removal of the contralateral ovary would be desirable due to the high frequency of bilaterality of these tumors. (e) The morbidity and expense of chemotherapy could be avoided if the staging is negative.

Cons: (a) While the patient tolerated her first surgery well, the potential for complications is magnified by the patient's obesity. (b) Some may argue that the patient requires chemotherapy regardless as to the staging findings. (c) Surgery delays intervention with chemotherapy.

2. Pros: (a) This avoids surgical morbidity. (b) There is no delay in instituting chemotherapy.

Cons: (a) This may mean unnecessary treatment if the tumor is stage IA. (b) The contralateral ovary is at increased risk for a similar primary in the future.

3. Pros: (a) This is the least expensive (at least initially). (b) There is least risk from treatment morbidity.

Cons: (a) If occult metastatic disease is present, the delay in therapeutic intervention could result in less effective treatment and a compromise in survival, possibly including a lost opportunity for cure.

Hopefully, the patient would be able to make an informed decision from the above options. If she requested additional guidance, we would inform her that we would encourage a close family member or personal friend toward option 1. However, given that the patient is aware of the various risks and limitations, any of the options should be considered within the realm of acceptable care.

PHYSICIANS' RESPONSE

JOHN CARLSON
CHARLES DUNTON

The patient has an unstaged, invasive serous carcinoma of the ovary, grade 2. The surgery was performed on an emergency basis and the malignancy unsuspected at the time of surgery. Because of the patient's body habitus, imaging studies cannot be performed. However, even if she could be imaged by a modified magnetic resonance imaging or CT scanner (such as the unit available in a veterinary school), such a scan would have limited clinical value. It is very unlikely that small-volume (< 1 cm) metastases could be visualized and, if bulky metastases were identified, the patient would justifiably warrant reexploration for cytoreductive surgery.

We have three options for this patient's care:

1. Observation only
2. Empiric chemotherapy
3. Reexploration for definitive surgery including total abominal hysterectomy/left salpingo-oophorectomy (TAH/LSO) and staging assessment

I personally recommend option 3. Despite her age and unwillingness to receive blood products, she is otherwise healthy and should be able to tolerate a planned procedure given the usual safeguards and prophylactic measures to minimize the risk of infection and thromboembolic complications.

The patient is 46 years old, and I would include a contralateral oophorectomy as an essential component of the surgery, considering the 30 to 50% risk of bilaterality with a serous cancer, and I would include a hysterectomy as prophylaxis, considering her obesity risk factor for eventually acquiring uterine cancer. Although surgical staging and retroperitoneal lymphadenectomy might be technically challenging, the literature indicates nearly a 30% risk of metastatic disease in this setting and the surgicopathological staging data are essential for proper determination of prognosis and the need for chemotherapy. Staging may eliminate the need for chemotherapy should this prove to be a stage 1A, grade 2 tumor, although this is a controversial area.

The option to observe this patient only without further intervention is, in my opinion, unconscionable, considering her age, general medical status, and probable good prognosis even if small-volume metastases are encountered.

Similarly, I would hesitate to treat this patient empirically with chemotherapy in lieu of surgical reexploration. Since optimal cytoreduction improves the clinical response to chemotherapy and since her actual disease status is unknown, I would reserve this option only for medically inoperable patients or those refusing reexploration.

PHYSICIAN'S RESPONSE

EDDIE REED

This case presents several practical problems and offers limited "objective" data on which one can base one's decisions. These problems include the patient's substantial obesity, the fact that she is a Jehovah's Witness (and presumably does not accept blood products), and that her operation was done for emergency reasons with the incidental finding of malignancy. Fortunately for the patient, an early-stage tumor was found (stage I, grade 2). Unfortunately, it appears that a complete "cancer operation" was not performed, and there is no mention of the presence of ascites or the possible rupture of the tumor mass.

In this situation, after the patient's recovery from emergency surgery, the CA-125 might be quite helpful. If the CA-125 is persistently elevated and/or rising over several weeks to months, this is strong evidence of persistent/residual disease. Under this circumstance, the possibility of reexploration should be seriously discussed with the patient and her family. Since the patient is obese, the level of difficulty of performing a complete staging operation is increased and may be associated with an increased risk of operative complications. This is a substantial consideration in a patient who is a Jehovah's Witness, since one's ability to intervene may be limited by the wishes of the patient and/or her family. If the CA-125 is persistently elevated and/or rising and if a "cancer operation" is contraindicated by the patient's wishes, one has to discuss with the patient the possibility of chemotherapy at some point. This consultant would wait for clear abnormalities on physical examination and/or radiographic studies (CT scan, for example) before initiating a chemotherapy regimen. Even then, biopsy confirmation of metastatic disease would be desirable. Some studies suggest that the interval between an elevated CA-125 and apparent ovarian cancer can be many months in some patients.

If the CA-125 normalized after the patient's emergency surgery, this consultant would recommend following the patient with monthly visits for at least 1 year, with regular visits of decreasing frequency thereafter. Patients who normalize their CA-125 after initial debulking surgery pose an interesting problem. In this patient, who was incompletely staged, normalization of the CA-125 could represent "debulking" with persistent low-volume residual disease, or it could represent true eradication of a stage I lesion. Since the question of surgery is not straightforward in this type of patient, this consultant would discuss the pros and cons of watchful waiting with the patient and her family. Whereas an aggressive approach would be seriously considered if the patient requested it, my recommendation would be to "watch and wait."

The study of early-stage disease by the Gynecologic Oncology Group (GOG) clearly shows that for patients with stage 1, grade 2 disease, no additional therapy is needed after adequate surgery. Although this patient was incompletely staged, my recommendation to watch and wait would be based on the surgical considerations discussed above, along with the fact that stage 1 disease has such an excellent prognosis.

References

Young RC, Walton LA, Ellenberg SS, et al. Adjuvant therapy in stage I and stage II epithelial ovarian cancer: Results of two prospective randomized trials. N Engl J Med 1990; 322:1021–1027.

Podczaski E, Whitney C, Manetta A, et al. Use of CA125 to monitor patients with ovarian epithelial carcinomas. Gynecol Oncol 1989; 33:193.

Index of Cases

About the Editors

MAURIE MARKMAN is the Director of the Cleveland Clinic Cancer Center and Chairman of the Department of Hematology/Oncology at the Cleveland Clinic Foundation, Ohio, as well as Professor of Medicine at the Ohio State University School of Medicine, Columbus. A contributor to over 25 medical journals and the editor of several books, he is a member of the American Association for Cancer Research, the American Federation for Clinical Research, the American Society of Hematology, and the American Society of Internal Medicine, among many others. Dr. Markman received the M.D. degree (1974) from the New York University School of Medicine, New York, and the M.S. degree (1989) in health policy and management from the New York University Graduate School of Public Administration, New York.

JEROME L. BELINSON is Vice-Chairman, Division of Surgery, and Chairman, Department of Gynecology and Obstetrics, at the Cleveland Clinic Foundation, Ohio, as well as Professor at the Ohio State University, Columbus. The author or coauthor of numerous textbook chapters and journal articles, he is a member of the American College of Obstetrics and Gynecologists, the Society of Gynecologic Oncologists, the American Society of Clinical Oncologists, and the New England Cancer Society. Dr. Belinson received the B.A. degree (1965) from Drury College, Springfield, Missouri, and the M.D. degree (1968) from the University of Missouri Medical School, Columbia.